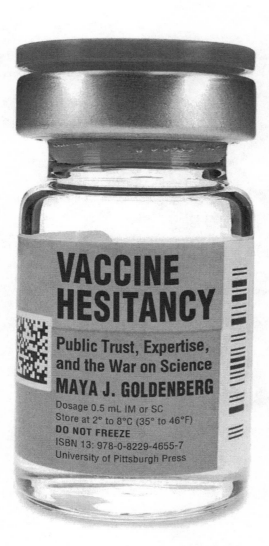

# VACCINE HESITANCY

Public Trust, Expertise, and the War on Science

**MAYA J. GOLDENBERG**

Dosage 0.5 mL IM or SC
Store at 2° to 8°C (35° to 46°F)
**DO NOT FREEZE**
ISBN 13: 978-0-8229-4655-7
University of Pittsburgh Press

# SCIENCE VALUES AND THE PUBLIC

Heather E. Douglas
Editor

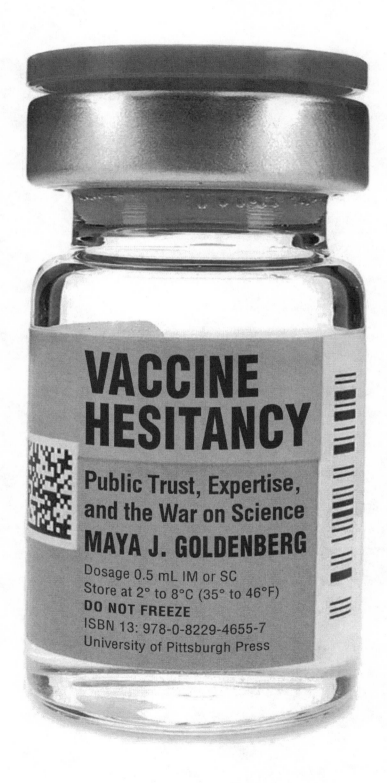

**Published by the University of Pittsburgh Press, Pittsburgh, Pa., 15260**
Copyright © 2021, University of Pittsburgh Press
This paperback edition 2021
Manufactured in the United States of America
Printed on acid-free paper
10 9 8 7 6 5 4 3 2 1

Cataloging-in-Publication data is available from the Library of Congress

ISBN 13: 978-0-8229-6690-6
ISBN 10: 0-8229-6690-5

Cover design by Alex Wolfe

*For my parents*

# CONTENTS

# PREFACE

This book is the culmination of five years of research, writing, and revising. As I prepared to submit the final version of the manuscript to my publisher, the COVID-19 pandemic swept the globe, creating new realities, challenges, and tests for public health, medicine, science, and government. In the chaos and fear that have ensued, there have been wonderful glimpses of the best of humanity, but also devastating failures and a tragic loss of life. I have grappled with the extent to which the major theses of this book needed reconsideration given the new realities. After much reflection I have concluded that the relevance of what is investigated in this work is more important than ever. The COVID-19 pandemic is a clear global test case in public trust between health and government bodies and members of society.

Being in the midst of a crisis places limits on the ability to understand and evaluate its immediate and longer-term implications. This is a shared challenge for individuals and small and large institutions alike. We move forward with the best that we have and hope that it stands up through the storm. Rather than wait for clear skies as this crisis subsides, I have chosen to release this book with the hope that it can be used as a clarifying source for guiding next steps for public health, medicine, and science—especially in the drive for a safe and effective vaccine. Vaccine hesitancy and refusal will undoubtedly feature in yet unknown ways. There will surely be more to say as the pandemic progresses, but this book should be read within the context of understandable unknowns at this time.

# ACKNOWLEDGMENTS

I remember reading the explosive investigative report exposing Andrew Wakefield for fabricating data in his infamous 1998 study linking vaccines to autism. The three-part report (Deer 2011a; 2011b; 2011c) had just come out, and like many readers at the time, I expected vaccine hesitancy to end right there. Yet vaccine hesitancy endured, and the frequency of measles outbreaks attributed to pediatric vaccine refusal by parents climbed in the years that followed. I wondered what evidence was going to convince people to drop this concern. As a philosopher of medicine working on how knowledge claims are constructed and justified in health care, I was in a good position to find out.

My first finding was that I was asking the wrong question, as I initially assumed that vaccine hesitators were missing some key scientific evidence that kept them from embracing the strong scientific consensus on vaccine safety and efficacy. But my research, which engaged science communications, sociology of expertise, public health sciences, behavioral sciences, social sciences, health equity scholarship, history and philosophy of science, health and science journalism, and qualitative research involving vaccine hesitant parents, enriched my understanding of the complexity of vaccine hesitancy. I developed an alternative thesis that I defend in this book; namely, that vaccine hesitancy is a problem of poor public trust. The solution lies in strengthening public trust in scientific institutions.

I want to acknowledge the wide and disciplinarily diverse research community into vaccine hesitancy that informed my philosophical investigation and analysis. These researchers span numerous disciplines and continents and brought many different findings, theories, and challenging perspectives to my attention.

I want to thank Mark Solovey for encouraging me to take the first step in writing this book: contacting a few academic publishers to gauge their interest in a philosophy of science monograph on vaccine hesitancy. When four out of five publishers expressed interest in seeing a book prospectus, I felt encouraged to pursue this long research project, ultimately with guidance and patience from Abby Collier at University of Pittsburgh Press. Thanks to the University of Guelph and my colleagues in the Department of Philosophy and the Bachelor of Arts and Science Program for their support. I have many people to thank for reading drafts of the prospectus and book chapters, and for engaging me in interesting conversations. They include: Tara Abramson, Katie Attwell, Robyn Bluhm, Kirstin Borgerson, Matt Brown, Jim Brown, Shannon Buckley, Amy Butchard, Gideon Chemel, Ben Chin-Yee, Sharyn Clough, Lorraine Code, Michael Cournoyea, Sharon Crasnow, Colleen Derkatch, Michelle Driedger, Heather Douglas, Kevin Elliott, Carla Fehr, Jon Fuller, Patrick Garon-Sayeh, Jennifer Gibson, Daniel Goldberg, Devon Grayson, Kristen Intemann, Clara Juando-Prats, Sauvanne Julien, Nadine Laraya, Mark Largent, Heather MacDougall, Christopher McCron, Tara Mendola, Samantha Meyer, Mark Navin, Jamie Nelson, Kieran O'Doherty, Daniel O'Quinn, Janet Parsons, Jennifer Reich, Alison Thompson, Ross Upshur, and Pam Wakewich. There are surely more that I am neglecting to mention (with apology).

It is difficult to do this kind of intense work without the love and patience of my family. Special thanks to Gideon, Talia, and Lev. Also, my parents, Aviva and Andrew, my grandmother Edith, and my sister, Keren.

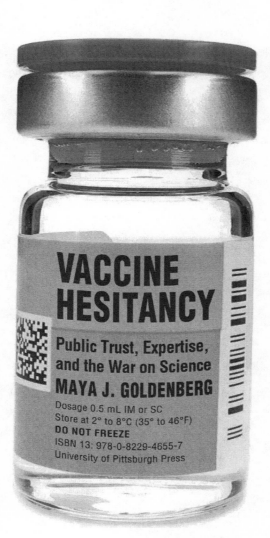

# INTRODUCTION

## VACCINE HESITANCY IN THE INDUSTRIALIZED NORTH

I n January 2019 the World Health Organization (WHO) listed "vaccine hesitancy" as a top ten global health threat, sharing the distinction with known killers like air pollution, climate change, and population displacement due to conflict and war (World Health Organization 2019).[1] The WHO's "Ten Threats to Global Health in 2019" was an eclectic list, ranging from drug-resistant pathogens to noncommunicable diseases related to obesity and physical inactivity and to the health impacts of climate and humanitarian crises. Consistent with a population health approach to health promotion (Evans et al. 1994; Valles 2018),[2] the list incorporated both "upstream" and "downstream" causes of poor health. Some, like Ebola and dengue, are proximal causes of morbidity and mortality, while others, like fragile and vulnerable settings and air pollution, are "upstream causes," or socially mediated determinants of health. Vaccine hesitancy stands out on this list of factors for negative health outcomes for being an attitude, as opposed to a pathogen or context. Indeed, despite a strong scientific consensus in favor of vaccines, vaccine hesitancy persists and impairs public health strategies for infectious disease control.

Vaccine hesitancy refers to an attitude of ambivalence regarding vaccines. It is distinct from vaccine refusal, which is a behavior. Vaccine hesitancy runs along a spectrum from mild to severe uncertainty about whether vaccines are safe, effective, and necessary. While attitudes and behaviors are linked, vaccine hesitancy does not fully determine vaccine acceptance or refusal. When deciding on childhood vaccines, some hesitant parents will vaccinate according to the recommended schedule, some will refuse all vaccines, and others will pursue modified schedules. These alternative schedules might be selective, where children receive some vaccines but not others; temporally delayed, where children begin immunizations when they are older and the schedule is administered over a longer period of time; or some combination of both. Some parents seek to unbundle combination vaccines like the MMR (measles, mumps, rubella) or the MMRV (measles, mumps, rubella, varicella) in favor of separate vaccines for each disease administered over multiple healthcare visits rather than in one appointment.

Vaccine hesitancy is a relatively new research priority for public health. Previously, research had instead focused on rates of vaccine acceptance and refusal (Dubé et al. 2013; Yaqub et al. 2014). The WHO Strategic Advisory Group of Experts (SAGE) on Immunization recognized this growing research need as early as 2001. Their meeting reports detailed difficulties across the globe for eradication programs due to vaccine hesitancy.[3] The 2011 SAGE meeting report warned that hesitancy surrounding vaccines and immunization services, as well as vaccine refusal, threatened to undermine decades of progress and the objectives of the WHO's Decade of Vaccines Global Vaccine Action Plan (2011–2020). The group requested the establishment of a working group on vaccine hesitancy, and in 2012, the Strategic Advisory Group of Experts Working Group on Vaccine Hesitancy was formed. The new group was convened to address the gap between public perception of vaccines and the scientific consensus (Schuster, Eskola, and Duclos 2015).

This research shift also reflected a growing agreement among public health researchers that vaccine *hesitancy* was a more informative analytic concept than vaccine *refusal*. In the industrialized[4] North,[5] where vaccines are widely available due to relatively stable health systems infrastructures, the great variation between vaccine hesitancy and refusal is important. American survey data measure 20 to 40 percent of American parents with small children harboring some uncertainty about vaccines, with the wide variance explained by how tightly one limits the range of ambivalent attitudes (Opel et al. 2011; Largent 2012).[6] In Canada, a 2017 survey revealed roughly 25 percent of parents with young children are vaccine hesitant (Greenberg, Dubé, and Driedger 2017). Hesitancy numbers are much higher than rates of refusal of childhood vaccines, which sit steady at 2 to 3 percent in both countries. In France, pediatric vaccination rates are lower than optimal, but far less dramatic than the country's rates of vaccine hesitancy. One in three people in France think that vaccines are unsafe, and France measures the highest rates of vaccine hesitancy in the world (Wellcome Global Monitor 2019).

Not only does "hesitancy" capture a larger subset of the population than "refusal," but focusing only on vaccine uptake and refusal rates and neglecting the underlying attitudes is likely to lead us to underestimate the challenge of maintaining vaccination programs in the future. It is in the interests of public health to know what makes some hesitators vaccinate their children despite their misgivings, while others do not. Further, it is in the interest of public health to understand what efforts can be made to tip the scale in favor of vaccine acceptance. While committed vaccine refusers may not budge on the issue, many vaccine hesitators may be reached in order to turn the dial from skepticism to confidence in vaccines (Leask 2011). Conversely, failing to communicate effectively with this group can harden vaccine-skeptical views, turning vaccine hesitators into vaccine refusers (Leask et al. 2012).

One of the first tasks of the SAGE Working Group on Vaccine Hesitancy was to define the concept. A 2014 report offered the following definition: "Vaccine hesitancy refers to delay in acceptance or refusal of vaccination despite availability of vaccination services. Vaccine hesitancy is complex and context specific, varying across time, place, and vaccines. It is influenced by factors such as complacency, convenience, and confidence." The group's report articulated the scope and determinants of vaccine hesitancy (for a summary, see MacDonald et al. 2015), both of which pointed to the context specificity of vaccine hesitancy. The determinants are captured in the report's "Three C's": complacency, convenience, and confidence. Complacency (i.e., willingness to go along with the recommended schedule) is determined by individuals' perception of the risk and value of vaccines. Convenience refers to the accessibility of the vaccines (cost, availability, etc.), while confidence refers to "trust in the effectiveness and safety of vaccines, the system that delivers them, including the reliability and competence of the health services and health professionals and the motivations of policy-makers who decide on the needed vaccines" (MacDonald et al. 2015).

Those factors explain what the data show—that vaccine hesitancy varies among different populations. There are geographical, ideological, historical, and philosophical differences that create pockets of highly vaccine-confident individuals and clusters of vaccine-hesitant and vaccine-refusing people. These communities may live near each other, thus creating tension within schools, neighborhoods, towns, and cities.

The SAGE Working Group's definition of vaccine hesitancy also captures the numerous levels of concern surrounding vaccines. Research shows that public concerns are not confined to vaccine safety but include vaccine policies, recommendations, and costs. All these factors make public decision making related to vaccine acceptance complex: it is not driven by scientific evidence alone, but rather depends on a mix of scientific, psychological, sociocultural, and political reasons (Larson et al. 2011).

While it is tempting to think that vaccine hesitancy and refusal are products of misinformation on social media and the sway of celebrity "anti-vaxxers," vaccine hesitancy is as old as vaccines themselves. The first vaccine, Edward Jenner's[7] cowpox inoculation[8] against smallpox, invented in 1796, met religious objection on the grounds that the vaccine introduced into human bodies "substances originating from God's lowlier creatures," namely cows (Edward Jenner Society 2019; see Morgan and Poland 2011). Such were the localized anxieties of Jenner's time. Today, vaccine skeptics like Andrew Wakefield, Barbara Loe Fischer, Meryl Dorey, and (until recently) Jenny McCarthy are the products, not the causes, of contemporary vaccine anxieties.

Anti-vaccine influencers are vilified by health experts and journalists, yet their crafted vaccine-skeptical messages often give voice to fears that were already simmering. American historian Elena Conis ties vaccine skepticism to a fast-growing vaccine schedule and a cultural backdrop, originating in the socially transformative late 1960s, that questioned establishment practices and put many societal norms under scrutiny (Conis 2015a). The environmental movement of the 1960s brought concerns about toxic chemical exposure to public attention, as well as antipathy toward big industry. The patients' rights and women's health movements entrenched a new norm of patient autonomy and challenged the paternalism and unquestioned authority of medicine and other expert institutions (Conis 2015a; 2015b). It is against this cultural backdrop, Conis argues, that contemporary challenges to vaccines and vaccination practices began to grow. Another American historian, Mark Largent, situates modern American vaccine anxiety in changes to the vaccine schedule in the early 1990s, when the list of mandatory vaccines began to grow and some fringe critics vocalized concerns (Largent 2012, 36). Both Conis and Largent agree that it is "modern American cultural and ideological notions, not the centuries-old religious opposition to vaccination, [that] form the basis of today's anti-vaccination movement in the United States" (Largent 2012, 36).

Comparative research into vaccination programs converge on one common denominator: vaccination programs are highly politicized. In 2019 several US states considered the removal of nonmedical exemptions for school-entry immunization requirements, while other states relaxed restrictions. In Europe, anti-vaccine views have been folded into populist political movements. The success or failure of vaccine programs are determined by multiple levers of vaccine confidence: in the product, the provider, and the policy (Larson et al. 2015), as well as the broader government and/or nongovernmental organizational infrastructure supporting vaccination programs.

## VACCINE HESITANCY AND SOCIAL PRIVILEGE

A unique feature of vaccine hesitancy in the industrialized North is that the most vocal vaccine hesitators and refusers are affluent and educated, that is, they are people who are largely supported by the systems of power and privilege in place. This is an unusual trend in public health and health promotion, wherein higher wealth and education typically predicts more active pursuit of good health (i.e., eating healthy food, exercising, time for leisure).[9] In America, much attention has been drawn to the staggeringly low rates of vaccination among wealthy coastal Californians (Yang et al. 2016; McNutt et al. 2016; Bonnerfield 2015),[10] whose resistance to vaccines has been described by leading vaccine advocate Dr. Paul Offit as "an ignorance ironically cloaked in education, wealth, and privilege" (Offit 2014).[11] The connection between affluence and vaccine resistance and refusal is visible in other parts of the United States and in other high income countries like Canada (Parmar 2019), Australia (Soekov 2018; Calligeros 2015) and New Zealand (Meier 2017; Duff 2019).

The comparative global data on vaccine hesitancy (Wellcome Global Monitor 2019) finds the highest rates of vaccine hesitancy in the most economically developed nations and the lowest levels in countries on the other end of the development spectrum. Bangladesh and Rwanda have the highest reported levels of vaccine confidence in the world, followed closely by Ethiopia and India (Wellcome Global Monitor 2019). The chief executive of Gavi, the Vaccine Alliance,[12] Seth Berkley, has commented on this division: "In developing countries, where deadly diseases like diphtheria, measles or whooping cough are more common, I've seen mothers queue for hours to make sure their child is vaccinated . . . It is in wealthier countries, where we no longer see the terrible impact these preventable diseases can have, that people are more reticent. This reticence is a luxury we can ill afford" (in Bosely 2019). The presumed connection between negative vaccine sentiments and privilege is reinforced by broad global compar-isons. However, along with oversimplifying the picture of vaccine hesitancy in the industrialized North, comments like Berkley's also misrepresent the state of vaccine confidence in the Global South. While some populations in low- and low-middle-income countries clamor for access to childhood vaccines amid poor access to healthcare, other lower-income countries struggle with pernicious cul-tural associations of vaccine programs with state-sanctioned genocide or foreign imperialism (Leach and Fairhead 2007). Rumors circulate in Nigeria that polio vaccines offered to Muslim children are infected with HIV and cause infertility (Nwaubani 2016); in Gambia, that they strengthen childhood soldiers and make them more violent (Leach and Fairhead 2008; 2007, chapters 5 and 6). Pakistani health workers have been killed in response to rumors that they were promoting poisonous polio vaccines (Shahzad and Ahmad 2019).

The enduring picture of vaccine hesitancy in the industrialized North as a problem of privilege is incomplete due to gaps in the research. Most research into vaccine hesitancy in high income countries has been conducted on white participants, where the link between higher household income and increased vaccine hesitancy holds strong (Smith et al. 2004). Only recently has a widely used measurement tool for vaccine hesitancy, the Parent Attitudes about Child-hood Vaccines (PACV), been tested and validated for use on inner-city racialized American populations (Orr and Beck 2017).[13] Without the availability of reliable research tools, there has been limited opportunity for important cross-cultural comparison in vaccine hesitancy. Studies into vaccine hesitancy tend to mention the lack of racial and ethnic diversity within their study populations as a limita-tion of the study. Yet a strong effort to reverse this limitation by actively recruit-ing and retaining people of color as participants in vaccine hesitancy studies has not transpired. Instead, convenience sampling[14] and survey research that permits self-selection bias[15] are still widely used for recruitment. All the while, the scant research that is available on vaccine hesitancy among racialized Americans sug-gests that underexploration in this area is a major oversight that contributes to a limited understanding of vaccine hesitancy within more affluent countries.

A study involving six small focus groups on Black American mothers' atti-tudes about vaccination (Shiu et al. 2005) revealed high levels of apprehension. The fifty-three Atlanta-based participants were concerned about adverse events following immunization, expressed distrust of medical professionals, and want-ed more information about vaccine ingredients, vaccination, and the rationale for state-level vaccination requirements for school and daycare entry. The study had no comparison group and therefore lacked generalizability. A follow-up survey study (Shiu et al. 2006) pursued comparison of vaccine safety attitudes by race and ethnicity in order to offer more generalizable findings that could be statistically analyzed. The study designed questions based on the initial focus group findings and administered the questions to a nationally representative sample.[16] The survey results showed that Black and Hispanic participants with low income and less education had more negative attitudes toward vaccines and toward their child's healthcare providers than white participants (Shiu et al. 2006). When asked to rate their level of vaccine concern from 1 to 5, with 5 indicating "very concerned," 40 percent of Black parents and 32 percent of Hispanic parents ranked their concern as 5 compared with 15 percent of white parents. Lower levels of education and household income were also significantly associated with high-level concern (Shiu et al. 2006, 246). Compared to white parents, Black parents were more likely to want more knowledge about vaccine ingredients to ensure they are safe, to not trust their child's healthcare provider, to disagree that their child's healthcare provider was easy to talk to, and to agree that school or daycare immunization rules influenced their decision to immunize (Shiu et al. 2006, 247). Gellin et al. (2000) had similar findings in a nationally representative phone survey involving sixteen hundred participants. Both Shiu et al. (2006) and Gellin et al. (2000) found Hispanic parents to be more likely to want to know more about vaccine ingredients than white parents (Shiu et al. 2006, 247; Gellin et al. 2000, 1100).

Prislin et al. (1998) found that Black Americans had greater doubts about the protective value of vaccines, resulting in decreased vaccine acceptance, when compared with Hispanic and white Americans. Freed et al. (2010) conducted a national telephone survey and found Hispanic parents to be more concerned about the serious adverse effects of vaccines, and yet at the same time more likely to follow their doctors' vaccine recommendations, than comparison groups. They were also less likely to have ever refused a vaccine. This last finding highlights that disempowerment, rather than vaccine confidence, can underlie vaccine uptake within marginalized communities. Lacking social privilege and economic capital compels some groups to vaccinate despite harboring vaccine concerns. In this sense, it is the privileged in the industrialized North that are most afforded the right to be vocal about their hesitations, a legacy of historical and ongoing oppression.

Nonetheless, the narrative of vaccine hesitancy as a folly of "affluenza,"[17] the unhealthy and unwelcome psychological and social effect of affluence, still endures in vaccine discourse and research. For example, Wagner et al. (2019) noted that "more affluent individuals in high-income countries appear to be more vaccine hesitant and may have lower vaccine uptake" and cited research by Dempsey et al. (2011), Luthy et al. (2009), and Hedge et al. (2019). Yet the cited authors fail to justify the claim.

Dempsey et al. (2011) studied parental preference for alternative vaccine schedules and found that while being white and having a higher income increased the likelihood of pursuing an alternative schedule, so did not having a regular healthcare provider (which is not typical of affluent Americans). Furthermore, the researchers noted that survey respondents might have employed different understandings of "alternative schedule," which would skew the results. While the researchers were referring to delayed and selective vaccine schedules favored by parents who think the national vaccine schedule is dangerous, respondents could have self-identified as following a delayed/alternative vaccine schedule because they were behind on immunizations due to poor access to healthcare (an attribute of low socioeconomic status). In the end, the connections between alternative vaccination and vaccine hesitancy, and vaccine hesitancy and affluence, are not fully formed. The second cited study, by Luthy et al. (2009), investigated vaccine hesitancy in Utah, using a study population that mostly self-identified as white (70.4 percent of the seventy-one participants who identified their race). The research team offered no subgroup analysis of racial differences in vaccine attitudes, perhaps because the validity of any comparison would be questionable. The final paper cited by Wagner et al. (2019) in alleged support of the thesis that vaccine hesitancy in high income countries is a problem of affluence and privilege offered a comparative look at race and socioeconomic status as determinants of pediatric vaccine compliance; however, the authors, Hedge et al. (2019), were unjustified in their interpretation of the data to suggest affluence was the primary predictor of vaccine hesitancy. Hedge et al. (2019) mapped immunization information from the Michigan Care Improvement Registry to the state's census data to determine neighborhood variations in vaccine uptake. The researchers found the lowest levels of childhood vaccination rates in the wealthy white Detroit suburbs, followed closely by low vaccination rates in mostly Black inner-city Detroit neighbourhoods. They reasoned that low levels of childhood vaccination in the affluent suburbs were a consequence of vaccine hesitancy. Vaccine hesitancy research supports this interpretation. The explanation for low vaccination rates in communities with low socioeconomic status were assumed by the researchers to be a consequence of poor access to healthcare.

While poor access to healthcare is associated with undervaccination (Smith et al. 2004; Bhat-Shelbert et al. 2012), there was no justification for assuming that poor access captured the entirety of underserved populations' relationships to vaccines; the question of whether vaccine hesitancy played a role here was not asked. In summary, vaccine hesitancy is understudied in marginalized groups. The research narrative of vaccine hesitancy as a problem of affluence follows from a limited scope of investigation, and, though popular, does not distinguish between being vaccine hesitant and being *vocally* vaccine hesitant because of social privilege. Further study and deeper investigation must be undertaken to capture the complexity of vaccine hesitancy in diverse populations.

## THE WAR ON SCIENCE FRAMEWORK

The term *war on science* is commonly used in (mostly American) English-language journalism.[18] *National Geographic's* March 2015 magazine cover[19] featured the title "The War on Science" followed by the smaller script:

Climate Change Does Not Exist
Evolution Never Happened
The Moon Landing Was Fake
Vaccinations Can Lead to Autism
Genetically Modified Food is Evil

The bold text and sparse imagery is foreboding. The pages of the magazine give no further explanation about the supposed war, and how the listed public controversies tie into a war on science. The feature article makes no mention of such a war in its analysis of "Why Do Many Reasonable People Doubt Science?" (Achenbach 2015). Instead, the meaning of the stark cover page was taken to be understood; *National Geographic* readers were assumed to already know that science is under attack.[20] Writing in the *Scientific American Blog* two years later, environmental scientist and public speaker Jonathan Foley captures the anxious sentiment: "Make no mistake: There is a War on Science in America . . . This attack on science, and on knowledge itself, goes beyond anything we have seen in America before. And it is not only dangerous to science, it is dangerous to our nation and the world" (Foley 2017)

Defenders of science find moral high ground in a tandem defense of science and democratic values, arguing that the universal findings of science are expressions of humanity's curiosity without deference to private interests, be they religious, corporate, or other. Questioning the scientific consensus is thereby understood as threatening cherished democratic ideals. Thus, the stakes of this "war" are understandably high. As a whole, the *war on science* refers to conflict between science and society, as well as to the worry that science may not win.[21] Many English-language editorials and nonfiction books now instruct readers on who is waging this war, why it matters, and what we can do about it (Otto 2016; Rosenberg and Rest 2018; Foley and Arena 2018; Editorial Board 2017; Parker 2017). The metaphor itself, however, is never examined. How well does it frame the tensions between science and society? How does it shape response to the problem?

Wars and battle metaphors frame the issue as us versus them, good versus evil. Such framing minimizes the need to understand the perspective of the other, or to find compromise. Vaccine hesitators and refusers are uncharitably represented in popular media, and sometimes in academic sources, as scientifically illiterate (chapter 1), irrational (chapter 2), and willfully antiscience and anti-expertise (chapter 3). All the while, the actual concerns of vaccine hesitators are dismissed or ignored, leaving little room for workable solutions. Under the war framework, outreach is misdirected; at the same time, ineffective communications often harden vaccine skeptical sentiments and increase public resentment.

Wars erupt when political negotiation and compromise have been exhausted or are anticipated to end in deadlock. Communications researchers explain that framing an issue as a battle suggests that people need to choose sides and vanquish their opponents to succeed, thereby making it harder to find a reasonable path forward (Nisbet and Scheufele 2009). The war on science metaphor should therefore be applied cautiously, for both descriptive and prescriptive reasons. In this book, I argue that characterizing vaccine hesitancy and refusal as a war on science is both descriptively inaccurate and normatively unhelpful.

Appeals to the good science of vaccines, the public health importance of high vaccination rates, and the prudence of strictly enforced vaccination laws feature daily in many news feeds. At the same time, representations of the people who challenge the public benefits of vaccination are typically limited to caricature.[22] This happens despite available social science research into vaccine hesitators. Vaccine hesitant parents are the subjects of qualitative studies—surveys, interviews, ethnographies—all of which lend small bits of understanding regarding why parents hesitate regarding vaccines and what could be done to reduce those misgivings. An alternative story emerges from the research to show vaccine hesitators are not, for the most part, hateful, ignorant about science in general, chemophobic,[23] or selfish. They want to do what is best for their children and struggle to operationalize that aim because, by my reading, they have low trust in scientific and medical experts, the very people tasked with guiding parents to make healthy choices for their children. This interpretation of the situation as a crisis of trust arises from sociological analysis of parent testimonials and is philosophically supported by a robust science studies literature on science and trust, specifically the role of trust in knowledge production and legitimation (see chapter 5).[24]

The contrivance of an unreachable enemy "anti-vaxxer"[25] structures limited possibilities for resolution of the supposed war. Public health and government bodies have historically oscillated between persuasion and regulation for addressing vaccine hesitancy and refusal (Colgrove 2006). The war metaphor affects these efforts by creating an image of vaccine hesitators and refusers as persistent and obstinate; if this image is true, then persuasion is impractical and ineffective for addressing the dangerous situation. The high stakes war language makes stringent regulation, such as punitively enforced vaccine requirements with narrow exemption criteria, both justified and necessary. This "hardline approach" to vaccine compliance is increasingly supported by vaccine advocates working in public health and government (noted by Rainford and Greenberg 2015) and science journalism (noted by Goldenberg and McCron 2017).

In this alleged "war on science," the enemy is fought by besieged vaccine proponents. Healthcare workers, public health practitioners, and science researchers combat torrents of online misinformation and are often targeted and harassed for these efforts (Karlamanglasta 2019; Georgiou 2019). The war on science metaphor can appeal to battle-weary vaccine advocates who hold that the science is settled and wonder why some members of the public are not convinced. The "death of expertise" might be particularly appealing to physicians and nurses, who find themselves debating vaccine safety and efficacy with patients who read something on the internet. After all, it certainly *feels* as though science and scientific expertise are under attack.

But public refusal to follow vaccine recommendations in fact comprises many things beyond a supposed "war on science": a political act that refuses community solidarity and rebuffs shared responsibility for public health, a suspicion of scientific and medical institutions that have participated in historical social injustices,[26] a rejection of government intrusion on personal affairs, a reinstitution of family autonomy, a demand for less medical intervention and less corporate medicine (especially for children), and to some, a sign of good parenting. Vaccination is as much a civic act as it is a personal health decision (Kaufman 2010). The welfare of the many depends on the actions of individuals. Population-level protection (herd immunity[27]) is achieved when most otherwise healthy individuals are vaccinated. Because the risks associated with most vaccines are borne by the youngest members of the population (as recipients of childhood vaccinations), the public reaction of unease to any perceived problem with a vaccine is justified. Further, because vaccination requires government-led coordination, funding, and enforcement to achieve the collective goal of public health, public perception of vaccines is imbricated with the larger ethical tension between individual choice and collective need. The debate also highlights a specific political flashpoint in contemporary liberal democratic society, namely, the question of when the autonomy of the family can and should be pierced by the state.

While the arguments over vaccines are often centered on the science—with vaccine advocates pointing to the strong consensus on vaccines and vaccine skeptics collating their own research in order to generate a narrative of suppressed science demonstrating vaccines to be unsafe, ineffective, or unnecessary—the science largely serves as a placeholder for the values at stake. Similarly, research into environmental science policy controversies shows that it is not the science of science-based policy decisions that is dividing the publics,[28] but the values at stake in contentious policy decisions (Sarewitz 2004; Carolan 2008). At issue is what follows practically from accepting the science as true. This finding is applicable to childhood vaccine controversy as well. Both sides of the dispute make scientistic efforts to rise above political debate (chapter 4) when they furiously point to the science to justify their claims. The evidence, however, serves as proxies for the values that are on the line, such as individual liberties vs. common goods, medical progress vs. "natural" living, what duties we have toward others and toward future generations, among other values debates. None of these issues are easily settled and, importantly, none will be settled by the science of vaccines.

It is only through the lens of the alleged war on science that vaccine hesitancy appears to be an intractable problem. This book offers a rethinking of vaccine hesitancy. I argue for an alternate framework to better capture the phenomenon. This framework, a crisis of trust, recasts vaccine hesitancy as a sign of poor public trust of medical and scientific institutions rather than a war on scientific knowledge and expertise. Such a recasting permits new formulations for understanding and addressing this divisive public health issue.

## REFRAMING VACCINE HESITANCY AS A CRISIS OF TRUST

Frameworks structure how we view a problem and respond to it. The framing of vaccine hesitancy and refusal as a "war on science" and rejection of expertise is of little service to the effort to increase vaccine confidence and protect public health. It reduces the controversy to the status of vaccine science. But vaccine debates are about much more than vaccines, instead capturing a cluster of temporally, geographically, and historically specific concerns. In liberal democratic societies, those concerns include how technology shapes our lives; who decides and/or regulates technological intrusions on our lives; knowledge and power; science for the people vs. science for corporate interests; government overreach; individual liberty and family autonomy; globalization, multiculturalism, pluralism; community cohesion; health disparities; income inequality; and other issues.

These are concerns about justice and values rather than scientific knowledge, yet both the status of vaccine science and the integrity of science as a knowledge-producing enterprise figure prominently in the airing of these anxieties. The supposed war on science is happening amid a trend of public disaffection and distrust within OECD countries (Dalton 2004; Pharr and Putnam 2000; Roger 2010), as growing numbers of people are losing the conviction that democratic systems are governed equitably, with institutions and experts working for the benefit of everyone rather than privileging the interests of the few.[29] The "age of distrust" has been characterized by *New York Times* editor Roger Cohen as the feeling by "ordinary folk" in advanced industrialized nations that "the system is rigged, that elites are not in it for the people, but rather the money" (2016). This feeling, according to Cohen, has invited this historical moment's surge in nativist, authoritarian, and closed-border politics, in tandem with a cultural shift away from liberalism. These trends, by his account, challenge "some of the very foundations of the postwar world and the spread of liberal democracy—free trade, free markets, more open borders, fact-based debate, ever greater integration."

Scientific production of universal knowledge is a key feature of liberalism's governing apparatus insofar as science produces the common ground (facts) for political engagement. Scientific facts are supposed to be nonpartisan and thereby acceptable to all sides of political debate (see chapter 4). Yet some perceive science as an agent of state power rather than a means for generating universal knowledge.[30] For example, the 2018 Wellcome Global Monitor found that about one in five individuals feel excluded from the benefits of science (Qaisar 2019; Wellcome Global Monitor 2019), and 3M's 2019 annual State of Science Index found one-third of its fourteen thousand respondents, from around the world, were skeptical about science (3M State of Science Index 2019).

But where Cohen sees collapse of liberal institutions and others see a war on science and the death of expertise, I see a crisis of trust in scientific institutions and governing agencies. True, crisis can be the prelude to a catastrophic event, like a war on science or the end of expertise. It can also invite a different kind of social change. Against the apocalyptic decrees that arise from the war and death metaphors characterizing much of the discourse of vaccine hesitancy and public resistance to science more generally, the language of crisis encourages a rethinking of strategies and a redeployment of resources in order to avoid catastrophe. Crisis marks an unstable time, an important critical juncture that requires careful and thoughtful action. This book is thereby not only a diagnosis of the problem of vaccine hesitancy but also a framework for action by expert members of the broad institutional apparatus that governs health science research, health professional practice, and the regulation of health products.

## OVERVIEW OF THIS BOOK

This book is divided into two parts, each of which presents a framework for understanding and addressing vaccine hesitancy and refusal. Part 1 (chapters 1–4) examines the dominant framework—the war on science and rejection of expertise—showing how the war metaphor shapes most of the academic and public discourse on vaccine hesitancy and refusal, and how vaccine hesitancy is thereby constructed as an unfixable problem necessitating hard line legislative action. The war on science metaphor is evident in the past decade of English-language health sciences research, as well as popular science and politics. In many ways, the description fits, as public controversies over childhood vaccines unfold as battles over scientific evidence. There is, on one side, a significant body of literature supporting the scientific consensus, against which opponents pick out selective and often disreputable counterevidence. Experts and public commentators then think to "win" by parsing out the evidence, for example, by emphasizing the robust consensus and debunking myths about vaccines (i.e., Public Health 2019; Mammoser 2019; Gatenby 2019; Doc Bastard 2019). When those efforts do not persuade the skeptics (and the data shows that it does not), the response has not been to question its terms of engagement but rather to bemoan the tenacity of anti-vaccine views.

The *war on science* is an umbrella term capturing three overlapping popular narratives on vaccine hesitancy: scientific illiteracy among the publics (chapter 1); cognitive biases among the publics (chapter 2); and anti-expertise and science denialism among members of the publics (chapter 3). The focus of all three narratives is, notably, on the enemy publics ("them"), with little attention to the valiant "us" in the war on science. I draw from philosophy of science, social epistemology, and science communications scholarship to generate a more contextual understanding of how scientific claims are incorporated into public understanding and decision-making (chapter 4). I highlight the importance of trust in public uptake of scientific claims, as well as the success of scientific institutions in fulfilling their mandates (chapter 5). Part 2 offers an alternative and enabling framework, a *crisis of trust*, to understand vaccine hesitancy (chapters 5–6, conclusion).

Vaccine hesitancy, I argue, is the result of unsuccessful science-public relations. The success of those relationships, like all relationships, hinges on trust. I aim to show that trust is not secondary to good science in support of vaccination; it is, rather, central to the very controversy over vaccines. Vaccine hesitators and refusers see a failure of scientific integrity around consensus claims in general, and/or vaccines in particular. They frequently report feeling disrespected and silenced by their physicians upon voicing their concerns. They then may turn to unconventional sources. Faced with uncertainty regarding important health decisions, they are reconsidering their reliance on experts and expertise (chapter 6).

Vaccine hesitancy is recharacterized here not as the product of a war on science, but as a sign of poor public trust in scientific institutions. The argument that there exists a public trust deficit redraws the lines of responsibility away from the wayward or misguided publics, toward a reexamination of integrity and relationships in science and medicine. This finding is meant to encourage the broad community of health providers to be part of the solution. I note that those most committed to the war on science framework—scientific experts, public health practitioners, and healthcare providers—often undermine their own unique positions to remedy the conflict when they subscribe to the frustrated view that expertise is dead (chapter 3). Rather than being a casualty of war (chapter 3), expertise is instead recalibrated by the publics in this environment of low public trust in expert institutions (chapter 6). A re-centering of the expert as part of a (healthy) science-publics relationship forms my guiding proposal to work to restore public trust in scientific institutions.

Vaccine hesitancy and refusal is studied intensely by scholars from a wide variety of disciplines, ranging from public health and epidemiology to behavioral psychology, folklore and rhetoric, science communications, history, bioethics, and critical theory. I have benefited from reading widely and incorporating diverse empirical and theoretical insights from this multidisciplinary body of research. I turn a critical lens on English-language health science and communications research, as well as news media, to characterize the two frameworks for understanding vaccine hesitancy considered here. I evaluate them with consideration of research into science and values, the science-publics interface, science and democratic governance, and health equity.

Vaccine hesitancy and/or refusal has received some attention from a small group of humanities scholars (mainly historians). I situate myself most closely in terms of methods with the cultural, conceptual, and textual research of historian of science Mark Largent, who offers a personalized history of American vaccine hesitancy in *Vaccines* (2012); fellow philosopher Mark Navin, who investigates epistemic and ethical dimensions of vaccine denialism and vaccine refusal in *Values and Vaccine Refusal* (2015); and feminist cultural theorist Bernice Hausman. The latter's 2019 monograph *Anti/Vax* was published right as I was finishing the full draft of this book manuscript and so I did not fully benefit from her scholarship in the development of my own thinking. Like Hausman, I used my theoretical orientation (in the philosophy of science, in my case) to offer a reframing of the vaccine debate in what I see as more productive terms. What we, this small group of humanities scholars working on vaccines, have in common is the predilection to see vaccine hesitancy and refusal as signs of something bigger than what is captured in the language of the debate.[31] We all point to broader social structures in which vaccine controversy takes place. I tackle the framing of science and policy in democracy more explicitly than others have previously, making it a central focus of the analysis. I also see the crisis of trust in science and public health as inextricably tied to historical and contemporary structures of inequality and injustice that permeate our institutions and act to solidify power and privilege at the expense of underserved and marginalized groups (chapter 5). Vaccine hesitancy is not primarily a "knowledge deficit" in action (see chapter 1), but a complex set of social, historical, and personal anxieties resulting in the expression of poor public trust in science and the health professions (chapters 5–6, conclusion).

# PART I

A WAR ON SCIENCE

# 1

## THE "IGNORANT PUBLIC"

Recent headlines about measles outbreaks across the country, despite the availability of an effective vaccine, make it hard to escape the feeling that widespread rejection of science is on the rise.

— Kari Fischer

I ntense public resistance to scientific claims on diverse health and environmental issues has invited speculation by concerned officials regarding both the source of the problem and the solution. An influential account came from the London Royal Society's 1985 report, "Public Understanding of Science" (also known as the "Bodmer Report" because the committee was chaired by Dr. W. F. Bodmer).[1] The Bodmer report (1985) is commonly cited as the first to propose the theory that public ignorance of science prevents citizens from making mature, rational decisions in support of scientifically backed policies, although a similar sentiment was expressed earlier by the US National Commission on Excellence in Education (1983). The Bodmer report led to the formation of the Committee on the Public Understanding of Science (COPUS), which used grants and other incentives to initiate change in the attitudes of scientists toward outreach activities (Committee on Public Understanding of Science 1987). Internationally, governments have assembled portfolios on "science and society" (National Science Foundation 1995; House of Lords 2000; Canadian Biotechnology Secretariat 2006; European Commission 2008) intended to address this crisis of public misunderstanding and mistrust. Most have committed to cultivating two-way public engagement with science to foster better expert-lay relations in the often-contentious science-policy nexus.

Vaccine hesitancy and refusal in the industrialized North has been widely interpreted as a reflection of the public's alleged misunderstanding of science. A narrative routinely repeated in the biomedical, public health, and popular science literature focuses on the problem of an ignorant and fearful public, susceptible to misinformation by antiscience interests. The problem of the ignorant public is alleged to explain why, despite concerted health promotion and outreach efforts, vaccine hesitancy continues to persist more than twenty years after the publication of the notorious *Lancet* study that galvanized current anti-vaccine sentiment.[2] According to this narrative, despite both the scientific community's unequivocal rejection of the purported link between the MMR vaccine and autism and the finding that the science that first alleged the link was fraudulent, public fear of childhood vaccines persists and cases of measles, mumps, and pertussis (whooping cough) are on the rise in previously safe geographical locations. Fanning the flames of public mistrust of the scientific consensus, the narrative continues, is a well-organized anti-vaccine movement, comprising self-serving researchers and celebrity spokespeople, mobilized parent groups desperate to assign blame for their children's autism, and a sensationalist media. This toxic combination results in our current, persistent, and growing problem of vaccine hesitancy. Years of intense public health and health promotion efforts to assuage public fears by correcting public misperceptions have been ineffective in countering these forces and elevating rates of vaccine compliance to reinforce herd immunity.

Yet this account also bears the markings of its narrators, the biomedical experts and policy makers who have unilaterally framed the vaccine hesitancy problem and thereby dictated its solution. The problem has been framed as a conflict of science versus ignorance, the former unproblematic and the latter entirely flawed. Here the beginnings of the war on science emerge, bolstered by an already solidified policy perspective focused on the publics, and more specifically the publics' poor comprehension of science, as the root of the problem. The enemy in this so-called war is formed by the political mobilization of the so-called ignorant publics, while the allies organize around the anxiety of science not achieving uptake and the insult of expertise not being respected.

In this chapter, I demonstrate that while the public may indeed be prone to misunderstanding science and failing to appreciate relative risk, these characteristics do not explain vaccine hesitancy. The phenomenon described as "public rejection of science" is better understood as a rejection of the values underlying the scientific consensus. But the science and policy agencies tasked with remedying the problem of vaccine hesitancy do not recognize this alternative set of priorities, instead presuming public ignorance of science. Yet, characterizing one's opponents as ignorant is self-serving, as it permits scientific agencies to dismiss their concerns and input in framing both the problem and the solution. It also insulates scientific institutions from a much-needed reflexive scrutiny of their practices (Wynne 2006). These moves are ultimately self-defeating, as public trust is damaged while health outreach programs miss their target. It is only under the auspices of public ignorance that the vaccine hesitancy problem seems intractable.

## THE WAKEFIELD STUDY AND VACCINE CONTROVERSY

Most chronologies of contemporary vaccine controversy commence with the publication of the notorious 1998 study by British gastroenterologist Andrew Wakefield and colleagues, "Ileal-Lymphoid-Nodular Hyperplasia, Non-Specific Colitis, and Pervasive Developmental Disorder in Children," in the *Lancet* (1998).[3] Published in a top medical journal, this paper offered scientific evidence in support of an association between the MMR vaccine and the onset of autism in children. Years later, the data were found to be fabricated (Deer 2011a), but even prior to this revelation, the evidence presented was weak (Chen and Stefano 1998).

The research team presented an early report of a small case series where they claimed to have identified, using colonoscopy studies in twelve children with autism or related disorders, a new form of inflammatory bowel disease that they called "autistic enterocolitis." They noted that in eight of the twelve cases, the parents attributed the onset of symptoms of autism to the MMR vaccine, which the children had received, on average, six days before their parents first observed behavioral changes. The team postulated a causal sequence in which MMR causes persistent measles infection in the gut (virology had not yet confirmed the finding of measles in the bowels of these children), which produces an enterocolitis that leads to the translocation of typically impermeable peptides into the bloodstream and, subsequently, into the brain, where they affect neurological development and could result in autism symptomology. Early reports offered only speculative causal accounts, and the authors suggested that further epidemiological and virological studies should be done to confirm their hypothesis. If they were correct, epidemiological analysis should show a rising incidence of autism after the introduction of MMR to the United Kingdom's national vaccine schedule in 1988. Virological studies, they said, were "under way" to establish measles infection in the bowel specimens of those children in the study affected by autistic enterocolitis.

The paper's scientific limitations should be clear. As a small case series, it could only build hypotheses (the causal claims) for further testing. This limit is not problematic—it merely invites further study. However, establishing a temporal association via parental recall and testimony *is* problematic, as the source is highly unreliable. The study also suffered from selection bias, as the sample was overrepresented by the children of parents who believed MMR caused their children's autism.

In a commentary that appeared alongside the study, Chen and DeStefano (1998) further indicted the study's methodology. Wakefield et al. were criticized for pursuing nonspecific pathological findings, for offering no clear case definition, and for failing to provide evidentiary warrant for their hypothesis being worth pursuing (as they lacked confirmatory virological evidence). As for the alleged temporal association, the commentators asked: is the finding *"causal or coincidence"*? Among one-third of children with autism, developmental regression is typically reported by parents shortly after the child's first birthday. Because the MMR vaccine is typically administered around that time,[4] the temporal association could be mere coincidence.

The Wakefield et al. study was controversial not only because of its methodology and highly speculative findings but also because of concerns about public fallout once the media picked up the story, so much so that the *Lancet* editors deliberated on the appropriateness of publishing the report (Horton 2004).[5] News outlets had a history of publishing provocative medical research findings and failing to follow up when early theories were discredited or revised (Clarke 2008; Offit and Coffin 2003). The harms to public health that result from media-spun vaccine scares had already been witnessed in the pertussis vaccine controversy of the 1970s and 1980s (Blume 2006).[6]

Complicating matters, Wakefield surprised his colleagues by holding a press conference, timed closely to the study's publication release, in which he suggested that single vaccines—one each for measles, mumps, and rubella—should be offered over a twelve-month period in place of the MMR triple-shot until a potential link between that vaccine, enterocolitis, and autism could be further studied (Offit 2008a). The *Lancet* study offered neither evidential support for the safety or efficacy of the single vaccine, nor any warrant for the proposed twelve-month temporal duration (Fitzpatrick 2004c).

In the months that followed, the study was systematically discredited by the medical establishment. A British Medical Research Council hearing concluded that there was no association between MMR and autism (Department of Health 1998). Following a shocking investigation into Wakefield's financial conflicts of interest (Deer 2004), all but one of his coauthors criticized the study's conclusions as being overly suggestive (Murch et al. 2004). Meanwhile, Wakefield was found to have violated ethics protocol in the study and was consequently stripped of his medical license (General Medical Council 2010). The *Lancet* followed by retracting the study (Editors of the Lancet 2010). Subsequently, *London Times* investigative reporter Brian Deer revealed that Wakefield had fabricated his data, publishing an exposé titled "Secrets of the MMR Scare," a three-part series commissioned by the *British Medical Journal* (Deer 2011a; 2011b; 2011c). At each point of damning revelation of impropriety and serious scientific misconduct, public officials anticipated a resurgence of pro-vaccine sentiment. Yet, this attitudinal shift never materialized. To illustrate, a May 2013 *USA Today* headline read, "Measles Surge in UK Years after Flawed Research" (Cheng 2013).

## RESPONSE TO A LOOMING PUBLIC HEALTH CRISIS

In the United States, vaccine specialist Dr. Paul Offit is the most public face of the scientific consensus position that there is no association between vaccines and autism, and he is celebrated for his outreach efforts to correct misperceptions of vaccine safety (George 2011). In his abundant writing on the subject, which include numerous editorials in biomedical journals (2007b; 2008c) and news sources (2007a; 2008b; 2011b), parenting books (Offit and Bell 1999; Offit and Moser 2011), practical guides for physicians (Offit et al. 2002; Offit and Hackett 2003; Offit and Jew 2003; Gerber and Offit 2009), and popular science books (Offit 2008a; 2011a), he has framed the defensive strategy now emulated by other vaccine advocates.

The vaccine defense strategy involves both negative and positive components. While the negative arm is a vigorous attack of the anti-vaccine message, the positive strategy is the corrective application of a strong body of scientific evidence showing no causal association between autism and vaccines. On the negative side, vaccine advocates highlight the weaknesses of the anti-vaccine message, beginning with the faulty and fraudulent science performed by Wakefield and colleagues (Offit 2008a; Fitzpatrick 2004a). Second, vaccine advocates point to the untrustworthiness of the anti-vaccine pundits, beginning with Wakefield, who had received payment for the *Lancet* study from a barrister representing parents suing vaccine companies for causing their children's autism (Fitzpatrick 2004b, 2004c; Offit 2008a). Other untrustworthy pundits, in this reading, include celebrity spokespeople—especially the once central Jenny McCarthy (Mnookin 2011, 249–61; Offit 2011a, 149–54)[7]—who hypocritically, according to Offit, "indulge their own vanity by using injectable cosmetic botulinum toxin while reviling the same pharmaceutical industry for profiting from vaccines" (Brumback 2011, 1329), as well as disreputable entrepreneurs profiting financially from the growing industry of "alternative" autism research and treatment that is founded on public mistrust of mainstream science (Fitzpatrick 2009, 57–65; Offit 2008a; Hannaford 2013). Third, Offit and others blame the media (Offit 2008a, 176–95; Mnookin 2011, 160–69; Fitzpatrick 2004a, 139–44) and the US vaccine courts for distorting public perception of vaccine safety (Offit 2008a, 156–75; 2008b; 2008c). Fourth and finally, criticism is directed at parent groups who have mobilized support and research advocacy for families of vaccine-damaged children, offered information resources to the worried publics, and garnered media attention and political support for their emotional and unscientific claims. The National Vaccine Information Center (NVIC) in the United States and the British group JABS (Justice Awareness and Basic Support) are strongly reproached for playing an instrumental role in misinforming the publics, misdirecting health resources, engendering spurious controversy, and facilitating declining vaccination rates (Offit 2011a; Fitzpatrick 2004c, 2004d).

With the integrity of the anti-vaccine message undermined, the publics can now presumably be swayed by a generous offering of reliable science. Defenders of vaccines exalt the global health gains produced by mass immunization campaigns and offer a strong body of evidence in support of MMR's safety record. In one such publication, written to assist physicians in addressing the concerns of their vaccine-hesitant patients, Offit and coauthor James Gerber explain that even though Wakefield's MMR-autism thesis was not supported by biological or clinical findings, "several epidemiologic studies were *performed to address parental fears* created by the publication by Wakefield et al." (Gerber and Offit 2009, 456, emphasis added). These studies, the authors seem to suggest, offer no scientifically relevant information but instead serve an important public outreach and educational function. Gerber and Offit enlist them to deftly dismantle three popular hypotheses regarding the dangers of vaccines:

(1)   The MMR-autism thesis;

(2)   Thimerosal-autism thesis—the theory that a mercury-based preservative used in vaccines with inactivated viruses causes autism;

(3)   The vaccines "overwhelm the system" thesis—the theory that too many vaccines are introduced too soon into infants' delicate systems, thereby causing harm, including autism.[8]

Taking on both the MMR-autism thesis and the alternative thesis that autism is caused by the mercury-based preservative thimerosal found in vaccines with inactivated viruses (such as polio and pertussis), the authors review twenty epidemiological studies that uniformly fail to make an autism-vaccine association. They highlight the reliability of the findings and the significance of these studies' convergent conclusion. They note that "these studies have been performed in several countries by many different investigators who have employed a multitude of epidemiologic and statistical methods [ecological, case-controlled, retrospective cohort, prospective studies]" (Gerber and Offit 2009, 460). Furthermore, these studies rely on national vaccine records, which provide reliable historical data for excellent descriptive and observational studies. These records permit examination of national rates of autism before and after the introduction of the MMR combination vaccine into national schedules, as well as before and after thimerosal was reduced to trace amounts in vaccines (in response to public pressure, pro-vaccine advocates insist, and not because of sound safety concerns). These large-scale programs allow for a high level of statistical power, and the data are often comparable for meta-analysis due to similar vaccine constituents and schedules across national borders. Electronic medical records also facilitate accurate analysis of outcome data.

The evidence against the last theory—that vaccines can overwhelm the system—is more difficult to convey in accessible terms, as it comes from mathematical modelling of an infant body's theoretical capacity to respond to immunological challenges. Offit relies on basic immunology and reassurances instead. In an interview with a parenting magazine, he declared: "Children have an enormous capacity to respond safely to challenges to the immune system from vaccines . . . A baby's body is bombarded with immunologic challenges—from bacteria in food to the dust they breathe. Compared to what they typically encounter and manage during the day, vaccines are literally a drop in the ocean" (Howard 2005). Writing to healthcare audiences, he elaborates that "the average child is infected with four to six viruses per year . . . The immune response elicited from the vast antigen exposure of unattenuated viral replication supersedes that of even multiple, simultaneous vaccines" (Gerber and Offit 2009, 459).

Offit's claims can be sourced to the work of immunologists Cohn and Langman (1990), who calculated an average young child's immunological capacity and found it to far exceed the roughly two dozen vaccine antigens that they receive as part of routine childhood vaccination. Knowing that antibodies, the component of the immune system most capable of protecting against infection, are made by B cells, and that B cells make antibodies against only one epitope (an immunological unit), the calculation can be made by estimating the number of B cells in the bloodstream against the average number of epitopes contained in a vaccine, and the rapidity with which sufficient antibodies could be made against any offending epitopes (Offit 2011a, 174).[9] From this, Offit concluded that "babies could theoretically respond to about a hundred thousand vaccines at one time" (174).[10] Furthermore, those vaccines induce an excellent immune response to future pathogens.

With arguments mounted against all three "shifting hypotheses,"[11] Gerber and Offit confidently conclude: "These [epidemiological] studies, in concert with the biological implausibility that vaccines overwhelm a child's immune system, have effectively dismissed the notion that vaccines cause autism. Further studies on the cause or causes of autism should focus on more-promising leads" (2009, 460). The conclusion we can draw from this exercise is that the positive or corrective strategy operates with the working assumption that vaccine hesitancy occurs because the publics misunderstand the science.[12] With Offit and others reporting the consensus view as confidently as they do, perception of the publics' ignorance is only reinforced. The thinking is that, with many epidemiological studies failing to find a link between vaccines and autism[13] and clinical and virological studies unable to reproduce the Wakefield research team's findings, the scientific evidence refuting Wakefield et al.'s (1998) findings is solid and the scientific consensus clear and unambiguous. The only reasonable account of why vaccine hesitancy persists, it would seem, is an ignorant public unable to understand what the evidence means.

A 2002 editorial on vaccine hesitancy coauthored by members of the Department of Vaccines and Biologics at the World Health Organization explicitly endorses this disparaging view of the publics (Clements and Ratzan 2002). The authors describe the British publics as "misled and confused" by anti-vaccine misinformation, writing, "Because of the huge amount of media coverage of the safety of MMR, the public, not unreasonably, have come to the conclusion that there is no smoke without fire; there must be some truth in all this alarmism" (Clements and Ratzan 2002, 22).[14] The authors continue: "Once the peoples' mind is made up, it may be very difficult to change it. Members of the general public are less likely to be able to detect flaws or inconsistencies of argument, analyse the risk benefit ratios, or identify omissions in evidence presented to them. The public may focus more on the presence or absence of risk rather than the relative risk of a situation" (22). Commentators frequently endorse this view,

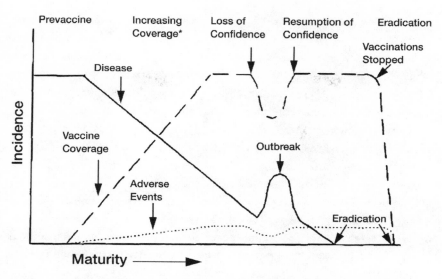

FIGURE 1.1. Natural History of an Immunization Program (Chen et al. 1994).

characterizing the declining vaccination rates as a problem of vaccines being "a victim of their own success" (Lewis 2004; Offit in Howard 2005;[15] Taverne 2005; Janko 2012). This refrain is visually captured in a graph created by Robert Chen, head of Vaccine Safety at the Center for Disease Control and Prevention (CDC), which presents public reaction to vaccines as a recurring historical progression (see fig. 1.1). At first, people are afraid of the serious infectious diseases that they have witnessed in their lifetimes ( "Prevaccine" in fig. 1.1) and parents readily accept immunization ( "Increasing Coverage" in fig. 1.1). This is what happened in the United States in the 1940s with diphtheria, pertussis, and tetanus (DPT), the 1950s with polio, and the 1960s when the MMR vaccine was introduced. In the next phase, as vaccines reduce disease prevalence dramatically, vaccines become "a victim of their own success." A new focus on side effects (whether real or imagined) occurs, and immunization rates plateau ("Loss of Confidence" in fig. 1.1). In the final stage, vaccine fear continues to rise, while immunization rates fall. Rates of preventable disease then increase, as we see now in many outbreaks of measles, mumps, and pertussis. Eventually, we return to something the like first phase ("Resumption of Confidence" in fig. 1.1) (Chen et al. 1994).

The graphic conveys passive publics, motivated by fear rather than sound judgment and lacking in the critical thinking abilities needed to appreciate the long-term benefits of vaccines. These publics also lack the skills to question the motives and opinions of dissenters and to resist the emotional sway of fear mongering.

Of course, those same epistemic vices structure vaccine compliance as well. This has implications for how public health outreach efforts are organized. Health officials widely recognize the importance of public support in achieving public health goals, and so the importance of engaging the publics and garnering their trust lies in more than just academic aspiration or political promise. Even Clements and Ratzan finish their disparaging assessment of the "misled and confused" public with a quick nod to the current vogue of science and the publics: "Because of these and other potential problems in communicating with the public, professionals somehow need to draw them into a participatory process in any risk communication efforts" (2002, 22). But it is unlikely that these health researchers are looking for genuine participation from ignorant and irrational people. Instead, the pro-vaccine message works to create the conditions for mass public compliance—by shutting down dissenting views and amplifying the pro-vaccine message. Yet, both tactics have failed to shift attitudes and behaviors regarding vaccines.[16] First, Wakefield's credibility in the eyes of vaccine resisters seems to be bolstered by efforts to discredit him. Instead, he is seen as a maverick, speaking truth to power, while the scientific establishment looks suspect in a seemingly organized effort to suppress "inconvenient truths" (Habakus and Holland 2012, 5; see also Holland 2012).[17] This view is reinforced by a generalized disdain for the cozy relationships between academic medicine and Big Pharma. Paul Offit's ties to the vaccine industry are particularly disliked (Atkinson 2008; Koch 2009), earning him the nickname Paul "for-profit" Offit (Mercola 2009). Second, the amplified pro-vaccine message does not reach its intended audience because it does not address the concerns of the vaccine-hesitant public, a point which we will now explore.

## A CHALLENGE TO PUBLIC MISUNDERSTANDING OF SCIENCE

Health officials were initially surprised by public backlash against vaccine recommendations and reassurances of their safety. A strong scientific consensus is supposed to be the antidote to such occurrences; it functions to "certify facts for the lay public" (Ranalli 2012) and thereby placate public fears or misgivings by offering expert-driven definitive answers that the publics can trust. The publics' questioning or challenging of the consensus view suggests that the consensus is not serving this purpose. There are several reasons why the publics might not accept the consensus view. One is that they cannot understand the scientific content of the consensus. A second possibility is that the publics fail to appreciate its epistemic stature (i.e., the reliability and knowledgeability).[18] The third and least-considered explanation is that some of the previously secure relations of trust between science and the publics that gave consensus claim their epistemic weight no longer hold. To date, government bodies have mostly accepted the first explanation.

The scientific and policy establishments' casting of the publics as ignorant seeks to absolve these institutions of the responsibility to listen to the concerns of anxious parents. Here, I challenge the characterization of the publics as ignorant or resistant to science and do so without minimizing the general publics' predictable lack of knowledge of the complex science of virology, immunology, epidemiology, and other sciences relevant to vaccine safety. Public dissent does not originate in antiscience ideology or a misunderstanding of the science. Instead many parents approach the question of vaccine safety from a different perspective, namely, concern for their children; this approach makes the presence of rare but serious adverse events a safety priority rather than, as health officials may see it, a reasonable risk.

This individualized approach to risk has been observed in social scientific research into parental attitudes toward vaccination (Evans et al. 2001; Poltorak et al. 2005; Leach and Fairhead 2007; Yaqub et al. 2014). Leach and Fairhead, for instance, noted this phenomenon in surveys and interviews with British mothers and a few fathers participating in community-based postnatal groups in the early 2000s (Leach and Fairhead 2007). This was a time of heavy media coverage in Britain of the MMR-autism debate, precipitated by the circulating rumor that then-prime minister Tony Blair had chosen not to vaccinate his infant son. The personalized approach adopted by most of the study participants contrasted the characterization of vaccine safety by health research, policy, and promotion agencies as a public health question, answerable at the population level. These parents expressed vaccine fear that would not be relieved by reassurances that MMR was safe for the general public. They wanted to know: "Is MMR safe for *my* child?"[19]

The interviewees and survey respondents, who came from both a range of socioeconomic backgrounds and subscribed to a range of political views, were asked about their perceptions of vaccine safety, where they turned for advice and support, and finally, how they intended to act on the options of either vaccinating, not vaccinating, or paying out-of-pocket for an alternative (spread out, reduced, or unbundled) vaccine schedule at a private clinic. Parents, with their copious reflections based on experience and observation of their own children, were widely found to hold a distinctively personalized view of their children's health, immunity, and whether their child should have the MMR vaccination. Against the vision of passive publics wholly susceptible to overblown media reports of vaccines' questionable safety record, these parents typically did not endorse either the mainstream reassurances or the dissenting view, not because they were still undecided, but because they were not interested in generalities. Many parents readily allowed that "MMR might be safe but not for my child" (Leach and Fairhead 2007, 57).

Leach and Fairhead found that this commonly held view toward MMR (or vaccines in general) was often undergirded by detailed reflection by parents on their child's particular strength or vulnerability, immune system characteristics, and family health history (Leach and Fairhead 2007, 57; see also Poltorak et al. 2005). The danger or lack of danger presented by the MMR vaccine was not evaluated in general terms but in relation to parents' assessments of their child's health pathway since birth and their genetic heritage. Some survey responses included: "My first daughter had milk intolerance and was very ill for the first two years of her life. We didn't vaccinate her with MMR because she was quite weak" (Leach and Fairhead 2007, 58). "I was more frightened of the potential side effects of measles should I decide not to get Luke vaccinated. Had he been a poorly sickly baby with allergies I might have considered single jabs" (58). Some parents included a family history in their decision-making, such as relatives with autism, arthritis, allergies, and autoimmune problems (58). Others incorporated consideration of broad characteristics such as the child's birth timing, maturity, sleep patterns, and behavior (Yaqub et al. 2014). Some even worried about the possibility of unknown and undetected "weaknesses" in a child, which can be understood to signify fear of even a slim chance of serious adverse events (Leach and Fairhead 2007, 58–59).

These accounts do not align with current scientific understanding of immune response. But this effort by parents to figure out their own children's risk of adverse events should not be read as ignorance of science or as an antiscience view. Instead parents appear to be incorporating established knowledge that immune responses do vary into their decision as to whether to vaccinate their children and trying to fill the knowledge gap regarding preceding or causal events. This personalized approach is also not clearly demonstrative of fear or selfish disregard for public health (albeit the latter is threatened by this behavior). Instead it highlights a parent's priority—the well-being of the children under their care.

Additionally, this approach toward vaccination accords with other health-promoting influences on parents' thinking. In what sociologist Deborah Lupton (1995) characterized as the "new public health" that emerged in the 1970s, public health discourse adopted the language of choice, empowerment, personal responsibility, and participation. The positive connotations attached to those terms came to shape the "new" public health citizen, patient, and parent into experts on—and advocates for—their own and their children's health and well-being (Petersen and Lupton 1996). It should therefore be no surprise that qualitative research into parental attitudes toward vaccination has found that many respondents prioritize choice regarding their child's vaccine schedule, for example in having the option to select single versus combined shots (Brown et al. 2010, 4244). Parents also regarded themselves as personally responsible for making those choices. Brown et al. reported that "parents felt that personal research was *expected of them*" (Brown et al. 2010, 4244; my emphasis).

It is within this framework that current expert parenting advice in both European and American contexts promotes "active, child-centred, and personalized approaches for improved child health and developmental outcomes" (Leach and Fairhead 2007, 51). The individual particularities of each child are frequently highlighted in the many parenting books available on sleep-training infants, negotiating toddler tantrums, helping your child succeed in school, and so on. Similarly, when it comes to healthcare, with the exception of the "vaccine question," parents are strongly encouraged by their pediatricians and other frontline health workers to actively engage in their children's healthcare and to be experts on their own child. This allied approach is seen to be better for children's health and better for overburdened healthcare systems that frequently download health work onto the individual or caregiver in the name of "personal responsibility." In asking for active parents and compliant vaccinators, the public health establishment seems to want to have it both ways.

## MISSING THE MARK IN HEALTH PROMOTION AND COMMUNICATIONS

The presumption of ignorance can preempt genuine effort to understand the publics' concerns. With this alternative account of the nature of vaccine anxiety among the general public in place, we can now appreciate the missed opportunities by public health agencies to properly reach their audience.

Leach and Fairhead's subjects wanted to make informed decisions regarding vaccinating their children and sought support for doing so. They typically consulted social networks of parents, including parent-lobby groups, for non-judgmental discussion and access to the information they needed. The children's pediatricians were generally not consulted in this process of inquiry, not because parents feared reproach but because they felt that the physicians had to support the "official" line (Leach and Fairhead 2007, 64; see also Evans et al. 2001 and Yaqub et al. 2014).

Government agencies confronting vaccine hesitancy have followed a didactic model, establishing information campaigns meant to educate parents regarding sound science, the social good, and the balance of risk (Leach and Fairhead 2007, 79). For instance, in a Health Canada promotional leaflet titled "Misconceptions about Vaccine Safety," parents read:

> Misconception: Vaccines are not safe.
> The Facts: Vaccines are among the safest medical products available. Prior to approval they are extensively tested and they continue to undergo rigorous ongoing evaluations of their safety when on the market. Serious side effects such as severe allergic reactions are very rare. On the other hand, the diseases that vaccines fight present serious threats. Diseases like polio, diphtheria, measles and pertussis (whooping cough) can lead to paralysis, pneumonia, choking, brain damage, heart problems, and even death. The dangers of vaccine-preventable diseases are many times greater than the risk of a serious adverse reaction to the vaccine (Health Canada 2011).

Here the sound science and assessment of risk were expressed relative to population-level analysis; they therefore do not address the concerns of parents assessing the risk in relation to their own children. While the claim that severe adverse events are very rare is meant to be reassuring, it sidelines the very issue that the parents interviewed by Leach and Fairhead are worried about.

It should not have surprised anyone that the mandatory education sessions introduced in Ontario in 2017 for parents seeking nonmedical exemptions for school-entry vaccine requirements would have a "zero percent conversion rate" among the thousands of parents who had attained "Vaccine Education Certificates" as of March 2019. The program has been described as "a colossal waste of time and money" by some health policy experts and may have caused damage and hardened anti-vaccine views among parents who "found it insulting to have the government force them to be 're-educated'" (Kirkey 2019).

Parent advocacy groups like JABS (Justice Awareness and Basic Support), on the other hand, engage parents on their own terms. These groups were founded on the belief that parents know their children best and thereby have insight into their health not afforded to physicians and medical scientists (Hobson-West 2007). Other vaccine skeptical groups highlight the importance and value of informed consent, for example, iCAN (Informed Consent Action Network[20]) and The Informed Parent.[21] Members of these groups share tales of having their concerns regarding vaccination dismissed by health professionals; similarly, those claiming their children were harmed by vaccine bewailed being routinely ignored (Evans et al. 2001; Leach 2005, 8; Kirby 2006, 9–31). While some accept that a serious adverse event after vaccination is extremely rare, they think that research into the factors precipitating those rare events should be a priority. Indeed, JABS and other British parent lobby groups have outlined their own set of research priorities, with emphasis on studying rare but serious adverse events that they associate with vaccines, and their public communications have called upon the British government to direct resources into pursuing these lines of investigation (see, for example, Fletcher n.d.). This is not antiscience; it is a demand for participation in setting the research agenda. For these parents, mainstream insistence that, to quote the Health Canada (2011) brochure, "it is often very difficult to determine if a 'reaction' was directly linked to a vaccine or was an unrelated 'event' which would normally occur in a population," is grounds for further research rather than secondary to the overall social benefit that vaccination programs provide.

Starting in the early 1990s, when British parent networks perceived the scientific establishment to be ignoring their concerns, they organized popular epidemiological research into this question. JABS was an early user of web-based surveys, where parents' responses were collected and volunteer researchers analyzed any suggested patterns (Leach and Fairhead 2007, 85). Several theories have grown from this exercise in "citizen science" (Irwin 1995). The identification of common symptoms has led some parent-researchers to conclude that their alleged vaccine-injured children do not have "autism" as per ICD-10 criteria[22] but a novel syndrome linking bowel disorder and autistic symptoms (Trowther 2002). Wakefield and his research team later named this syndrome "autistic enterocolitis," and although this disease category remains controversial, even vaccine advocates like Michael Fitzpatrick think it warrants further investigation (Fitzpatrick 2004b). It should not be surprising that citizen scientists find dissonance with the mainstream insistence that MMR does not cause autism. This is not the hypothesis that many parent advocates are exploring.

Parent researchers are also exploring the possibility of "co-factors" that make an admittedly small number of children vulnerable to vaccine harm. This line of inquiry focuses on the family histories of afflicted children. The JABS survey claims to have highlighted a number of allergies common to the families of these children—asthma, eczema, hay fever—or a history of febrile convulsions or epilepsy. They wonder if a small subset of children with certain allergies can have allergic responses when presented with several vaccines at once (Leach 2005, 13; Leach and Fairhead 2007, 85). This theory speaks to the individualized framing of the vaccine safety question observed in the qualitative research on vaccine attitudes among parents. While the safety of vaccines is sufficiently established for public health purposes, parents want to know if vaccines are safe for *their* kids. Parent researchers argue that population-level studies are "too broad-brush" to pick up patterns associated with rare adverse events from MMR (Leach 2005, 17). Instead the science supporting parents' concerns is grounded in clinical case histories and medical and biological processes in individual children.

Parent researchers also insist that the high number of parents reporting autistic symptoms appearing *after* receiving the MMR vaccine regardless of the child's age sufficiently undermines the official claim that autism's onset can be coincidental rather than causal (Trowther 2003). This theory is difficult to defend, however, as it is beset by the problems of sampling and reporting bias.

The point here is not to argue for the epistemic adequacy or inadequacy of these hypotheses. Regardless of their scientific merit, these proposals—which were organized systematically in a 2003 report by parent-researcher David Trowther—provide important insight for health agencies into both what the publics want and how they measure institutional response to these demands. For instance, theories regarding how combination vaccines may interact with the genetic illness histories of particular bodies, the details of which are highly speculative but allowable within the expected limits of popular epidemiology, are instructive insofar as they highlight concerned parents' desire to know *which* children will respond badly to vaccines. So is the charge that epidemiological studies are not sensitive enough to pick up patterns associated with rare adverse events. Trowther's report was widely circulated among parent lobby groups and is still available on-line.[23] Yet I am not aware of any acknowledgement or response to this report by any public health bodies.

To be sure, I am not suggesting that the publics should definitively redirect the public health research agenda, but I will maintain (uncontroversially, I think) that the publics have a stake in establishing its priorities. I have aimed to show that many members of the publics configure the vaccine safety question differently, focusing on the particularities of individuals rather than overall response rates at the population level. While there are difficulties with some of the parent-driven theories, what we have here is, at minimum, the issues upon which health communicators ought to be engaging public stakeholders, rather than the current practice of defining both the problem and the solution for the supposedly ignorant publics. It should be of little surprise that public outreach efforts are not changing public perception. To interpret vaccine hesitancy as a misperception of the probabilities of harm is to ignore the normative dimensions of risk assessment. Trivializing public concern as confused "risk perception" also damages public trust, the very ingredient needed for effective health promotion efforts (Wynne 1996).

This is not an apologia for lay perspectives but a reminder that these voices are part of the expert-lay communicative relationship that fosters the trust so necessary for a well-functioning democratic society increasingly reliant on scientific experts and advisors for negotiating complex social and policy issues. Rather than characterizing lay publics as deficient, an approach whereby "outreach" is appropriately limited to scientific education, scientific and governmental bodies should elicit public participation in framing the issues that the publics care about. This is the best way that public health agencies can meet their mandate of enabling and promoting pro-health behavior among their constituents.

While not a panacea, early two-way communication with the anxious publics could have better directed public health outreach efforts. Public health agencies could have learned that the publics did not only need education into the astounding global health gains that vaccines have afforded us. Resources could have been directed away from repetitive epidemiological studies into the autism-vaccine link. In a dialogical expert-lay exchange, questions can be refined, redundancies and dangerous theories can be collaboratively rejected, and a coherent research agenda that is acceptable to both expert and lay perspectives can be formed. Dialogical communicative practices also encourage trust by the publics (Grasswick 2010, 394), many of whom find the confident, absolutist declarations of vaccine safety to be disingenuous. Public health is a community effort, requiring buy-in from many stakeholders, including the general public. Good relationships must be built and maintained in order to succeed.

The link between communication and trust building has some intuitive appeal and is already presumed in policy makers' *dernier cri* of championing two-way communications to gain the publics' trust. But some attention should be given to *why* communicative practices between scientific bodies and the publics encourage the publics' trust. Heidi Grasswick (2010) lays some of the groundwork for this conceptual link in her analysis of the important public function of scientific whistleblowers. The reason that (credible) whistleblowers gain public attention is because there exists a lay expectation that scientific communities share significant knowledge with the general public, or at least with those who stand to be greatly impacted (whether helped or harmed) by this information. The whistleblower exposes the failure of scientific institutions in fulfilling this expectation to participate in knowledge-sharing practices. The often-severe public response to these omissions reflects the importance placed on this expectation. Furthermore, by looking at past egregious cases like the Tuskegee Syphilis Study,[24] we can see how knowledge suppression can erode the publics' epistemic trust in scientific communities.[25] The fraught relationship between Black Americans and institutional medicine continues today as a part of the legacy of Tuskegee[26] and other failures to meet the ethical expectations that the publics place on medical institutions (Grasswick 2010, 404). On the flipside, through recurring practices of responsive communication, scientific bodies build their reputations as concerned for public interests, thereby gaining and maintaining public trust (Grasswick 2010, 394; see also a more sustained discussion of this issue in this book's chapter 5).

Yet there will be those critics who find these "fashionable" appeals to public engagement, democratic science, and engendering trust to be a distraction from science's ultimate aim: to create reliable knowledge (see Taverne 2005, 214–18; Levitt 1999). This view misunderstands public health science's additional outreach mandate and fails to appreciate the damage that has already been incurred by not taking this communicative route. When parental concerns over the safety of the newly introduced MMR triple vaccine in the UK started to foment, those apprehensions called for a hypothesis-building science of clinical case histories of individual children. Yet parents faced a medical establishment and government organizations that were reticent to entertain parent-driven concerns for fear that doing so would lend credence to the dissenting view (Leach and Fairhead 2007, 90). The British parent groups reached out to the scientific community against all odds and found an ally within the medical establishment willing to entertain their concerns and take their insights and experiences seriously. This ally was Andrew Wakefield.

Without this willingness for engagement from the scientific and governmental institutions mandated to pursue public health and the public good, parent groups mobilized their own research agenda, opening the door to Wakefield's insidiousness and opportunism. Wakefield deserves blame for inciting vaccine hesitancy and lowering vaccination rates. But the scientific and policy establishment also contributed heavily to the problem they are trying to fix by trivializing public hesitancy and framing the debate as a conflict of science versus ignorance. As a result of the failure to shore up public confidence in both vaccines and the institutional apparatuses that promote them as a safe and effective public health measure, the stage was set for the conflict and controversy that continues, unrelenting, to this day.

## COUNTERING THE KNOWLEDGE DEFICIT MODEL WITH A CONTEXTUALIST PUBLIC UNDERSTANDING OF SCIENCE

My analysis of the dominant narrative of vaccine hesitancy, as well as the failures to remedy the problem thus far, join a familiar line of criticism found in the science communications and public understanding of science literature. This literature has largely rejected the "knowledge deficit model" underlying the framing of public resistance to science-backed policies (Wynne 1991; 1992; 1995; 2006; Lewenstein 1992; Layton et al. 1993; Evans and Durant 1995; Irwin and Wynne 1996; Miller 2001; Jasanoff 2005). Vaccine concerns and resistance have been previously tied to this critical approach to public understanding of science by Hobson-West (2003; 2007) and Leach and Fairhead (2007).

The "knowledge deficit model," first identified by Brian Wynne (1991), presumes that expert forms of knowledge provide a sufficient basis for deciding the most important public policy questions. It follows that lay beliefs that run counter to this expert knowledge are unacceptable and must be corrected through education and public relation strategies. Those who disagree do so because they simply do not understand the science. Furthermore, the science is sound and comprehensive in incorporating all the values relevant to this policy decision (Brunk 2006).[27]

While scientists, bolstered by numerous science indicators surveys (see, for example, National Science Board 1981; 1983; 1986), have taken the publics' knowledge deficit as fact, sociologists, historians, and philosophers have plied their research methods to explore the interaction of science and the publics and have found a much more complex knowledge exchange. Some have highlighted the "contextual" nature of scientific knowledge—scientific facts are not as unproblematic as the deficit modellers assumed. Instead social context and lay knowledge play a significant role in how science is assimilated into public understanding (Wynne 1995; Irwin 1995; Brunk 2006). Sociology of scientific knowledge practitioners like Bruno Latour (1987) have highlighted the various social processes that precede the designation of any scientific knowledge as reliable. The "contextual approach," as Steve Miller (2001) called this response to the problematic deficit model, opened the door to more dialogical and communicative approaches to the public understanding of science.[28]

This contextualist critique has been influential in prompting some valuable rethinking at the policy level of science-public relations. The British minister of science declared the "demise of the deficit model" in a 1999 address to the British Association for the Advancement of Science, and the House of Lords shifted away from the Bodmer findings to admit that public resistance to scientific claims may not be due to misunderstanding of science but to lack of uptake regarding their concerns (Miller 2001; House of Lords 2000).[29] However, contemporary research by Brunk (2006), Wynne (2006), and others indicates that the deficit model still prevails in interpretations of public resistance to science-backed policy. My research into vaccine hesitancy further supports this claim.

## REAPPRAISING THE "IGNORANT PUBLIC"

This chapter challenged the orthodox reading of the problem of vaccine hesitancy as stemming from public misunderstanding of science and antiscience sentiments. While the lay publics do suffer from some knowledge deficits with respect to the complexity of vaccine science, it is incorrect to assume that this explains vaccine hesitancy, or that this hesitancy amounts to the publics' rejection of scientific claims. Instead, concerned parents approach the question of vaccine safety differently from the scientific establishment. This realization sheds new light on why concerted efforts to reform public attitudes toward vaccines have failed so far. By presuming the publics are ignorant of the science, and thereby directing outreach efforts at educating the publics, health outreach efforts are misdirected. The pervasive and reinforcing assumption that members of the publics only hesitate because they are ignorant shields science and government institutions from examining their own practices with respect to earning and maintaining the public trust. I share Brunk's (2006) position that those institutions and agencies demonstrate a knowledge deficit of their own when they evade this self-scrutiny. In rereading the supposedly ignorant public, I flag the importance of trust and communication for remediating allegedly intractable conflicts between science and society. We will return to these themes in part 2 of the book, which reframes vaccine hesitancy and refusal as a crisis of trust.

# 2

## THE "STUBBORN MIND"

"You Can't Change an Anti-Vaxxer's Mind" read the title of a widely circulated *Mother Jones* article by science reporter Chris Mooney in March 2014 (Mooney 2014b). The article detailed the release of a study by Brendan Nyhan and colleagues (2014) into the effectiveness of communication strategies for persuading parents to vaccinate their children against measles, mumps, and rubella. The study was highly anticipated due to a surge in public concern regarding measles and whooping cough outbreaks attributed to vaccine refusal. The "frustrating" results, as Mooney characterized them, showed that when parents read any one of four different pamphlets aimed at persuading parents to immunize, they became less likely to vaccinate their children. In other words, the pro-vaccine message was backfiring. Rather than interpret these findings as evidence that *these* four interventions do not work, or (more broadly) that a didactic educational model is ineffective for improving intention to vaccinate, the media largely concluded that vaccine hesitators simply could not be convinced, whether by facts, science, or reason. *Time* magazine ran the headline "Nothing, Not Even Hard Facts, Can Make Anti-Vaxxers Change Their Minds!" (Alter 2014), while the *Conversation* reported that "Throwing Science at Anti-Vaxxers Just Makes Them More Hard-Line" (Stafford 2015). *Slate* reported the research to show that "reason doesn't work either" (Bouie 2015). The logical conclusion of these indictments was that "The Science Is Clear: Anti-Vaxxers Are Immune to Truth" (Editors 2015).

Nyhan and his colleauges had gone against the grain by refraining from attributing vaccine refusal to information deficits (see chapter 1) and instead speculated that their results illustrated cognitive biases in how individuals assimilate information. Mooney and other media pundits quickly drew from psychology research a lexicon of biased reasoning terminology to explain the research findings: confirmation bias, disconfirmation bias, cognitive dissonance, motivated reasoning, and cultural cognition. All these terms had been previously employed to make sense of science resistance and acceptance of pseudoscientific claims, for example, in the climate change debate. This new terminology helpfully laid the foundation for a (much needed) shift in the familiar vaccine hesitancy narrative that framed it as a problem of poor scientific literacy among members of the publics. The new "cognitive turn" was understood to signal something much more deeply entrenched—an inability to think otherwise—thus making the problem of vaccine hesitancy far worse than previously thought. When news outlets ran headlines like "Study: Trying to Convince Parents to Vaccinate Their Kids Just Makes the Problem Worse" (Abrams 2014), they framed the cognitive situation as one where education can lead to understanding and enlightenment *unless* cognitive biases undermine information processing and reasoning. The knowledge deficit model was thereby retained but now had an additional cognitive dimension. Panic-inducing headlines, as well as frustrated commentary, characterized much of the media coverage of Nyhan and colleagues' vaccine communication study (for media analysis see Goldenberg and McCron 2017).

This media-spun misinterpretation of the study's findings that vaccine-skeptical attitudes are unshakable led to the corollary conclusion that past vaccine outreach efforts had not worked because outreach *could not* work. The public misunderstanding of science explanation for vaccine hesitancy was only partly challenged. If any errors had been made in outreach strategies, many reasoned, it was that too much credence had been given to the rational capacities of vaccine hesitators. The flaws did not lie in the health promotion practices themselves, a fatalistic conclusion that undercut consideration of alternative and possibly more effective vaccine communication strategies.

But vaccine advocates were wrong to draw this defeatist conclusion about vaccine communications. Rather than suggesting all efforts to be futile, the cognitive turn invites novel strategies for encouraging vaccine compliance.

Using the study by Nyhan et al. (2014), followed by the psychology literature to mark the "cognitive turn" in the war on science, I argue here that the literature on motivated cognition does not support the fatalistic conclusion that vaccine hesitators and refusers cannot be reasoned with. Instead, there are promising research-driven directions for changing attitudes and behavior in the face of cognitive barriers to information assimilation. Some of them will be reviewed here. This analysis offers the optimistic conclusion that even with cognitive biases, attitudes *can* shift.

## THE STUDY

Nyhan et al.'s 2014 study "Effective Messages in Vaccine Promotion: A Randomized Trial" tested the effectiveness of several typical vaccine-promoting communications employed by public health agencies to persuade parents. The researchers concluded that no single vaccine message effectively motivated parents to vaccinate their children. In fact, there was a measurable "backfire effect," wherein some parents became less inclined to have their children immunized after exposure to the promotional materials (Nyhan et al. 2014).

The study was novel insofar as it actually tested educational interventions (incredibly, the efficacy of decades-old didactic strategies had not been tested previously), and by doing so, revealed that the information deficit was not the problem. If it was, we would expect to see greater vaccine acceptance as a consequence of at least some of these interventions. Instead, the study demonstrated that providing accurate and reliable scientific evidence was probably not going to boost vaccine compliance. This finding was stunning to many immersed in vaccine advocacy, one of the reasons the study made headlines. The attention drawn by this finding is itself quite remarkable. We already know from chapter 1 that there had been decades of science communications theorizing and qualitative research disavowing the deficit model, yet still vaccine communications have remained firmly situated in the public misunderstanding of science framework. By directly testing archetypal vaccine interventions, Nyhan et al.'s empirical research made vaccine advocates notice that their preferred thesis was flawed.

Nyhan et al. polled 1,759 Americans with at least one child under the age of seventeen living at home for their baseline beliefs about vaccines and then randomly assigned respondents to review either one of four pro-vaccine pamphlets or a control message about bird feeding. Their vaccine beliefs were then tested again to measure for postexposure changes in attitudes and beliefs.

**TABLE 2.1.** Results from Nyhan et al. 2014

| Intervention | Belief that vaccines cause autism | Fear of vaccine side effects | Intention to vaccinate |
|---|---|---|---|
| Autism correction | LOWERED | Same | Same and LOWERED* |
| Disease risks | Same | Same | Same |
| Disease narrative | Same | INCREASED | Same |
| Disease images | INCREASED | Same | Same |

*"Backfire effect" among parents with strongest initial vaccine opposition

The first intervention, called "Autism Correction," debunked the myth that vaccines cause autism by citing multiple epidemiological studies that failed to find a link between vaccine exposure and rates of autism. The second message, titled "Disease Risks," listed the many unpleasant symptoms and serious risks associated with contracting measles, mumps, or rubella. "Disease Narrative," the third intervention, told the terrifying story of an infant nearly dying from measles, which he had contracted from another child in a pediatrician's waiting room. To increase the generalizability of the results, the three intervention were adapted from the CDC website, with source information withheld to avoid biased interpretation of the materials based on the subjects' prior views about the organization. The final intervention was "Disease Images"; it featured disturbing photos of young children suffering from measles, mumps, or rubella. Throughout the study, the researchers measured three dependent variables: 1) parents' perceptions of whether the MMR vaccine could cause autism in a healthy child; 2) parents' opinions of the likelihood of a child suffering serious side effects from an MMR vaccine; and 3) parents' intentions to have their own child vaccinated.

The results of the study disappointingly showed that none of the interventions increased parents' intentions to vaccinate their children, the third dependent variable (table 2.1). Likelihood of vaccination did not increase even when some misperceptions about vaccines were corrected by exposure to vaccine education materials. Additionally, intention to vaccinate even decreased among those with the strongest vaccine concerns.

The findings included some limited success in diminishing misperception of the dangers associated with vaccines: the "autism correction" message decreased perception that vaccines cause autism but did not alter concern regarding other serious side effects. Meanwhile, the "disease risk" message did not alter perception of the apparent risks of vaccine-induced autism or serious vaccine side effects. Some of the messages were even detrimental: both the disease narrative and the images of sick children increased parental concerns about the risks associated with vaccines. And crucially, despite the "autism correction" message's success in decreasing the misperception that autism is caused by vaccines, it also made the parents with the highest preintervention opposition to vaccines less likely to vaccinate their children. The preintervention intention to vaccinate had been about 70 percent; after exposure to the "autism correction" message, the subjects' intention to vaccinate dropped to 45 percent. Meanwhile, "disease risk" and "disease narrative" led to a negligible decrease in intention to vaccinate among the most resistant participants, while "disease images" produced no change in intention (that is, intention to vaccinate was near identical to the control group). The research team referred to the phenomenon of decreased intention to vaccinate as a "backfire effect," seeing this response as "broadly consistent with the literature on motivated reasoning about politics"; when confronted with disconfirming evidence, "respondents brought to mind other concerns about vaccines to defend their anti-vaccine attitudes" (Nyhan et al. 2014, e840).

## MOTIVATED REASONING AND COGNITIVE DISSONANCE

With this claim regarding the backfire effect, and a few citations for good measure, Nyhan and colleagues redirected vaccine pundits to a literature on the psychological propensity we all have for biased assimilation of information and arguments and the resulting polarization of attitudes. The phenomenon was well-described in Lord, Ross, and Lepper's classic 1979 study: "People who hold strong opinions on complex social issues are likely to examine relevant empirical evidence in a biased manner. They are apt to accept 'confirming' evidence at face value while subjecting 'disconfirming' evidence to critical evaluation, and as a result to draw undue support for their initial positions from mixed or random empirical findings. Thus, the result of exposing contending factions in a social dispute to an identical body of relevant empirical evidence may be not a narrowing of disagreement but rather an increase in polarization" (Lord, Ross, Lepper 1979). The literature employs the term "motivated reasoning" (Kunda 1990) as well as a few other similar terms—"biased assimilation" (Lord, Ross, and Lepper 1979; Munro and Ditto 1997), "confirmation bias" (Nickerson 1998), "disconfirmation bias" (Edwards and Smith 1996), "motivated skepticism" (Taber and Lodge 2006), "motivated social cognition" (Jost et al. 2003), "identity-protective cognition" (Kahan et al. 2007)—all working to capture this phenomenon of biased preferencing of information that confirms prior held beliefs. Motivated reasoning (and its synonyms) characterizes a cognitive process whereby a person's goal directs or motivates one or several possible cognitive mechanisms in order to generate a goal-supporting perception or belief (Kahan 2011).[1] These cognitive mechanisms include biased information search (see for example, Schulz-Hardt et al. 2000) and biased assimilation of information (e.g., Munro and Ditto 1997).

While these terms are popularly employed to explain how misinformation persists—for example, motivated reasoning has explained the persistence of "birther" and "deather" theories concerning Barak Obama's place of birth and Osama Bin Laden's demise (Vernon 2011; Mooney 2011)—we *all* engage in motivated reasoning. This is not because we do not want to know the truth—many of us do—but because that truth is sometimes too threatening to our self-identities and the values we cherish. Motivated reasoning is driven by the desire to avoid cognitive dissonance, a feeling of conflict between some aspect of our attitudes, behaviors, and beliefs. Faced with this discordance, many people confronted with disconfirming evidence of something held to be important and certain will "move the goalpost" or develop other elaborate rationalizations to justify maintaining their prior beliefs. This is not to say that we singularly strive for false understanding when the truth is threatening. We also desire accuracy in our perception of things and will at times adjust our beliefs even when it "hurts" to do so. Motivated reasoning underscores the fact that "we have *other* important goals besides accuracy—including identity affirmation and protecting one's sense of self—and often those make us highly resistant to changing our beliefs when the facts say we should" (Mooney 2011; emphasis added).

One way to relieve the tension of cognitive dissonance is to challenge the factual claim itself by bringing in counterevidence. When that is not possible, we might challenge the legitimacy of the source. Whose interests are being served? Who funded this research? Alternatively, we find new reasons to hold on to the now-threatened belief. Some of the participants in Nyhan et al.'s study reconciled disconfirming evidence about the dangers of vaccines by bringing other vaccine concerns to mind. So maybe vaccines do not cause autism, but what about the mercury and other toxins in vaccines? Or the vaccine's side effects? And so on. Vaccine hesitancy and resistance, this suggests, is about much more than disliking vaccines; it signifies a constellation of attitudes and behaviors comprising a social identity. Motivated reasoning enters because of a perceived need for maintaining a valued identity, particularly membership in a social group.

If what is being described sounds like a cult-like adherence to our prior beliefs, you would be right to the (very limited) extent that the term "cognitive dissonance" was first invoked in the context of a pseudoscientific cult. The phrase was famously coined by psychologist Leon Festinger and colleagues in their 1956 study of members of a doomsday cult the day after the anticipated apocalypse failed to materialize (Festinger, Riecken, and Schachter, 1956).

In the summer of 1954, Festinger saw a news article about a small local apocalyptic cult organized around Minneapolis housewife and alleged clairvoyant Dorothy Martin, who was said to have communicated with an extraterrestrial that prophesized the end of human civilization by massive flood on December 21, 1954. Festinger decided to infiltrate the group, posing as a true believer, to study how Martin and the cult members would react on the morning of December 22 once it became obvious that the prophesy had failed.

On the night of December 21, Martin's followers gathered in her home to wait in anticipation. The prophecy had included salvation for the believers by a man who would knock at Martin's door at midnight to escort the group to a flying saucer that would take them to a new home. As midnight passed, the group waited breathlessly and, eventually, restlessly (Festinger, Riecken, and Schachter 1956, 160–66). The next four hours were marked by periods of silence, fearful questions, needless diversions, and numerous attempts to rationalize the distressing turn of events. Festinger observed the group coming to grips with the fact that no caller had arrived at midnight. Their problem was "to reassure themselves and to find an adequate, satisfying way to reconcile the disconfirmation with their beliefs" (166–67). The group reexamined the original message that prophesized the midnight caller, in order to devise a plausible reinterpretation of its meaning (167). Surely it was allegorical, one member suggested, with the "parked cars" referring to their own physical bodies (which *had* been there at midnight) and the flying saucer symbolizing the "inner strength, the inner knowing, and the inner light which each member of the group had" (Festinger, Riecken and Schachter 1956, 167). Only some of the members were satisfied with this explanation. There were ensuing tears and confusion, until finally, at 4:45am, Martin called everyone into the living room to announce that she had received a message:

> For this day is it established that there is but one God of Earth, and He is in thy midst, and from his hand thou has written these words. And mighty is the word of God—and by his word have ye been saved—for from the mouth of death have ye been delivered and at no time has there been such a force loosed upon the Earth.

Not since the beginning of time upon this Earth has there been such a force of Good and light as now floods this room and that which has been loosed within this room now floods the entire Earth (169).

Amazingly and heroically, their powerful faith had prevented destruction. As Festinger et al. described it, "it was an adequate, even an elegant, explanation of the disconfirmation" (169). A total of two believers lost their faith and left Martin's home quietly in those tumultuous hours, but the remaining group was jubilant. The explanation was compelling; the dissonance was resolved. Although Martin's predictions had been falsified, the believers were now even more convinced of her gospel. Her acolytes spent the next two hours calling the local newspapers and national wire services to convey their important message. Soon after, they would proselytize and try to recruit new believers. The believers had responded to the painful dissonance of being wrong by becoming more assured that they were right. They had rationalized the situation in a way that maintained their sense of purpose as well as their self-esteem.

Festinger and colleagues' account was published in the book *When Prophecy Fails* (1956). It opens with the words, "A man with conviction is a hard man to change. Tell him you disagree and he turns away. Show him the facts or figures and he questions your sources. Appeal to logic and he fails to see your point" (Festinger, Rieken, and Schacter 1956, 3).

When irrevocable actions follow from one's beliefs, like quitting a job, depleting your savings, and breaking off social ties, it becomes even harder to turn back. Presented with indisputable evidence that one's action-guiding beliefs are wrong, many will, like the cult members analyzed by Festinger et al., display admirable resourcefulness in defending those convictions. As a result, "the individual will frequently emerge, not only unshaken, but even more convinced of the truth of his beliefs than ever before. Indeed, he may even show a new fervor about convincing and converting other people to his view" (3).

Yet it would be incorrect to conclude that this discussion about cults and the recalcitrance of strongly held beliefs demonstrates the failure of reason. This is not the case; rather, the lesson is that reason is not divorced from emotion. Eighteenth- century philosopher David Hume famously argued, "Reason is and ought only to be the slave of the passions and can never pretend to any other office than to serve and obey them" (Hume [1739] 1975, 415).[2] This doctrine, controversial to this day (e.g., Baggini and Jenkins 2019), separated Hume from ancient and modern moral philosophers who widely saw reason and emotion in continual conflict. Today, we still use the colloquial language of following your head or your heart. Against the dominant view that the dominion of reason over the passions is necessary for guiding good decisions and right actions, Hume understood the impulse to act ("the motivation of the will") to be emotionally driven, with reason assisting those goals. Reason can modify how we feel but cannot justify the things we value. Returning to motivated cognition, our desire to belong, the threat of exclusion, can direct the mental operations that assimilate information. We are capable of reason, but the processes involved are infused with emotion (Mooney 2011).

## CULTURAL COGNITION

Cultural cognition of risk theory investigates the tendency to base one's factual beliefs about risks (say, the risks of getting vaccinated) on cultural appraisals of the allegedly risky activity in question (Kahan et al. 2009). Similar to motivated reasoning and cognitive dissonance, cultural cognition is a term that holds up identity-protective cognition as the most salient dynamic in disputes over policy-relevant science. The focus on culture, however, is unique—cultural cognition theorists emphasize group identities, specifically how feelings of belonging to a social group affect cognition. Thus, we may engage in motivated reasoning not just to avoid dissonance between an aspect of our behavior and our personal beliefs but also to protect our ties to others (Kahan et al. 2012). The Cultural Cognition Project at Yale University investigates how the motivation guiding the processing or assimilating of information—whether scientific evidence, policy arguments, the credibility of experts, and so on—leads to conclusions that reinforce the status of, and one's standing in, important social groups (Kahan 2012). This research can explain noticeable divisions between political and cultural groups on perceived risks of complex social issues, like global climate change and vaccines.

Cultural cognition ties the individual risk appraiser to their cultural group via a marriage of cultural theory and psychology. The cultural theory of risk, as articulated by Mary Douglas and Aron Wildavsky (1982), offers an influential "cultural" account of the nature of risk perception: individuals' risk perceptions typically reflect and reinforce their value commitments regarding some preferred form of social ordering or "cultural way of life" (Thompson, Ellis, and Wildavsky 1990). Cultural cognition operationalizes cultural theory by way of psychometrics, the science of measuring mental capacities and processes. The

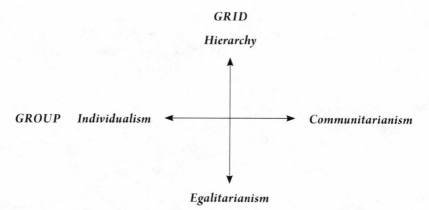

**FIGURE 2.1.** Representation of cultural theory's two-dimensional scheme of cultural worldviews. "Group" and "Grid" delineate ways of life and supportive worldviews. In this model, an individual's alignment along these two sociological dimensions largely predicts which side they will take in an argument, irrespective of the facts.

psychometric theory of risk (Slovic 2000) posits a collection of well-established social and psychological mechanisms "that dispose individuals to selectively credit or dismiss evidence of risk in patterns that fit values they share with others" (Kahan, Jenkins-Smith, and Braman 2011; for more, see Kahan 2012). Cultural cognition, then, provides the analytic means for measuring cultural influences on risk assessment.

Cultural cognition theory utilizes cultural theory's two-dimensional scheme (fig. 2.1) for measuring cultural worldviews (Douglas's [1970] "group-grid" scheme).[3] The "group-grid" refers to two crosscutting dimensions that represent cultural outlook. The x-axis or "group" spectrum captures affinity toward collective engagement and action. At one end of the spectrum, there are "individualists" with weak group inclination, while at the other end are those who value solidarity and depend on others to achieve their goals ("communitarianism"). The y-axis, or "grid," delineates affinity toward role differentiation and social hierarchy. "Hierarchical" refers to a preference for rigid social ordering based on birthright or other forms of entrenched social ranking (like race, gender, and class), while "egalitarians" prefer a society where no one would be prevented from participation in any social role. Characterizing people along these two sociological dimensions results in a fairly straightforward sociometric for determining where individuals stand on a variety of social issues. This is the case because we make decisions (and assess the risks involved) that reflect and reinforce some view of how we think society ought to be organized (Kahan, Jenkins-Smith, and Braman 2011).

For example, people who value equality and community (the bottom right quadrant in fig. 2.1), what we usually call "progressive" values, tend to support public health initiatives like mass vaccination campaigns. The science supporting these measures—for example, studies indicating the safety of vaccines and the effectiveness of mass vaccination campaigns—will be more readily accepted as sound evidence by members of this social grouping. Those who lean toward more individualistic beliefs will likely have negative attitudes toward vaccination programs and look at the same research findings skeptically if not dismissively. This explains why two people can look at the same evidence and perceive it so differently. This is also why facts, mounting evidence, and strong science are not winning over the skeptical publics on vaccines, climate change, GMOs, and so on. It is not because the naysayers are antiscience; it is because they perceive the scientific consensus to be less secure than the supporters do (Kahan, Jenkins-Smith, and Braman 2011). Those who find scientific evidence and consensus claims offering explanations and recommendations that are congenial to their general social outlook will be more accepting of the findings, while those more opposed will question, belittle, or dismiss them. Both sides do not need to have prior views about vaccines in particular; it is enough to have an understanding of how vaccines fit into one's own constellation of identity-defining values and beliefs. For the naysayer, "because accepting such information as legitimate could drive a wedge between them and their peers, they have a strong emotional predisposition to reject it" (Kahan 2010). The same pressures are put to bear on vaccine supporters to suppress any doubts about vaccines.

By adding the cultural dimension to biased assimilation and motivated reasoning, the idea of cultural cognition assists in explaining the selectivity with which individuals attend to risk patterns. It also makes cultural ways of life or worldviews psychometrically tractable (or measurable), which can inform recommendations for how anti-vaccine sentiments can be changed.

## IMPLICATIONS FOR UNDERSTANDING VACCINE HESITANCY

The media rush surrounding Nyhan and colleagues' damning findings about the efficacy of vaccine persuasion efforts focused on the allegedly forgone conclusion that nothing can be done to change vaccine skeptics' minds (Goldenberg and McCron 2017). The uptake of psychology terminology was directed toward

**TABLE 2.2.** Competing explanations of vaccine hesitancy

| Narrative | | Causal association | | How to counter vaccine misperception |
|---|---|---|---|---|
| Public misunderstanding of science | Wrong beliefs *ex. "Vaccines cause autism"* | ▶ | Negative attitudes | Correct misinformation (DIRECT MEANS) |
| Biased cognition | Wrong beliefs *ex. "Mercury in vaccines cause brain damage"* | ◀ | Negative attitudes | ~~Nothing can be done~~ Change attitudes (INDIRECT MEANS) |

justifying that claim. The conclusion that nothing could be done was frustrating, but, with the added cognitive factor, it was still congenial to the "cultural way of life" or social ordering wherein educational interventions are expected to work. The new thinking in the media reports was that educational interventions *should* have worked, had the target audience been rational agents. That education was unsuccessful was an indictment of the audience rather than evidence of a poor interventional effort. The knowledge deficit was still retained, albeit not merely because the publics misunderstood the science. Instead, biased reasoning assured that they *could not* understand it. Because of the seeming fit of the conclusion with prior thinking about the problem of vaccine hesitancy,[4] the cognitive turn was not recognized to seriously challenge the deficit model. This might explain why more investigation into the psychology of misperception, which would have shown that the fatalistic conclusion was incorrect, was not undertaken. The same literature that outlines the complex mechanisms of identity-preserving cognition also offers means for reducing those biases.

My argument is that, rather than modifying the popular public misunderstanding of science explanation with auxiliary hypotheses about cognitive biases, the cognitive turn in understanding vaccine hesitancy radically challenges the dominant narrative of public misunderstanding of science and the knowledge deficit. The cognitive explanation suggests a reversed ordering of beliefs and attitudes, where misperceptions about vaccines *are reflections of* less favorable attitudes toward vaccines rather than the cause (see table 2.2). If this is correct, then educational interventions are misdirected; successful persuasion must address the negative attitudes rather than the wrong beliefs.

The research literature on identity-preserving motivated reasoning and cultural cognition does not conclude that nothing can be done to unhinge stubbornly held misinformed beliefs; rather, it suggests approaching things differently. While direct response to misperceptions entails addressing the informational error (correcting the misperception), indirect strategies address the surrounding values and attitudes that make uptake of corrective information so threatening. Indirect methods work to lessen the threat, thereby allowing individuals to be more responsive to new information.

## "INDIRECT" STRATEGIES FOR COUNTERING VACCINE HESITANCY

Drawing from the same psychology literature into biased cognition and cultural cognition, what follows are three suggested methods for addressing biased cognition that can be applied to vaccine hesitancy. While each is distinct, they employ the "indirect means" tactic of reducing the threat associated with confronting challenging information. By lessening that threat, the target audience can be more open to considering new evidence. These strategies are:

Self-affirmation
Enlist a diverse set of experts to convey the message
Examine the values that support our beliefs

### Self-affirmation

Instead of targeting instances of false belief directly, the self-affirmation strategy seeks to validate or affirm the individual's competence and character, or some other strongly held belief (Lewandowsky et al. 2013; Lewandowsky et al. 2012; Sunstein and Vermeule 2009). Self- or values-affirmation is known to make individuals respond more openly to information or experiences that are threatening to their self-conception by strengthening their sense of self-worth.

Self-affirmation theory focuses on how people adapt to information or experiences that are identity-threatening (Sherman and Cohen 2006). After American social psychologist Claude Steele popularized self-affirmation theory in the late 1980s, the theory has been successfully applied (in experimental settings) to help individuals cope with stress and fight low self-esteem. To counteract feelings of poor self-worth, participants either write down or say aloud positive moments from their past that made them feel good about themselves (it could even be unrelated to the task at hand; see Fein and Spencer [1997]; Steele [1988]). College students who do self-affirming writing exercises before writing a final exam, for example, perform better than those who do not undergo such conditioning. Self-affirmation exercises have also been shown to diminish the negative impact of prejudice and stereotype threat, with subjects performing better at tasks where poor performance is socially expected. For example, studies show improved performance by women and racialized people engaging in mathematics and computing after undertaking a self-affirmation exercise (Logel et al. 2012; Sherman et al. 2013). Self-affirmation exercises have been shown to improve performance in a variety of demanding tasks, ranging from public speaking to weight loss (Logel and Cohen 2012).

Self-affirmation has only very recently been investigated as a strategy for false-belief correction. This new direction of inquiry has been prompted by the knowledge that persistent false beliefs stem from issues closely tied to our conception of self. As part of this research trajectory, Nyhan and colleagues have explored self-affirmation in the context of correcting political misinformation (Nyhan and Riefler 2018). As yet, experiments regarding false belief correction among vaccine hesitators have not been conducted.

The transferability of the positive findings from classroom settings to other environments is still unknown. It is also still not known how long the effect lasts. But the finding should make us mindful of how to approach ideologically charged issues like vaccine hesitancy. Instead of informational assault, which tends to make the interlocutor more defensive, health interventions should work to lessen the negative feelings that create cognitive resistance to new information.

## Enlist a diverse set of experts

Because people interpret information through a variety of cultural cues, another promising technique for mitigating public conflict over scientific evidence is to make sure that sound information is supported by a diverse set of experts. The publics are frequently guided on scientific issues by experts—for example, healthcare workers are the public face of vaccine advocacy—ostensibly because the years of training and practice make scientific experts epistemically trustworthy (they are most likely to know) and their professional roles make them morally trustworthy to provide honest assessments. But the publics need more than academic credentials. They need some assurance that the experts understand their values. (The role of expertise will be examined in chapters 3 and 6).

In a study on cultural cognition of risk regarding the HPV vaccine, researchers were able to substantially reduce polarization by exposing their subjects to advocates with diverse values on both sides of the HPV vaccine debate. People feel that it is safe to consider evidence with an open mind when they know that a knowledgeable member of their cultural community accepts it. The researchers found, for example, that giving a platform to a spokesperson who is likely to be recognized (by dress and appearance) as a more "traditional" parent with a hierarchical worldview can help to dispel associations between HPV vaccination and condoning permissive sexual behavior (Kahan et al. 2010).

This might explain the success of Katherine Hayhoe, an evangelical Christian and climate scientist, in public outreach regarding climate change to her religious community (see Walters 2016). American evangelicals are characteristically a climate skeptical cohort. Climate change communications from a person with shared religious beliefs disarms some of the resistance to climate change messaging, which is commonly thought to be antithetical to an evangelical worldview.

### Examine the values that support our beliefs

Cultural cognition theory proposes that culture is prior to facts; therefore, empirical data can be expected to persuade individuals to change their views *only after* those individuals come to see certain policies as compatible with their core cultural commitments (Kahan and Braman 2003). For example, members of the Cultural Cognition Project tested whether they could break culturally entrenched associations of factual claims on climate change with their subjects' values by tying those facts to more congenial values (Kahan et al. 2015).

Kahan and colleagues measured the responses of research subjects to reading a scientific study demonstrating the anticipated effects of global warming to be more catastrophic than had been previously thought. They primed their subjects, who represented a wide political spectrum, by having one experimental arm first read a news report featuring an expert calling for strict carbon dioxide restrictions, while the second experimental group was conditioned by reading a news article about the promise of geoengineering to counteract human-induced climate change. For those unfamiliar with this term, "'geoengineering' refers to deliberate, large-scale manipulations of Earth's environment designed to offset some of the harmful consequences of [anthropogenic] climate change" (National Research Council 2010). Geoengineering is widely seen as a necessary partner to the (still inadequate) political will required by industrialized countries to seriously address climate change (Kahan et al. 2015). Some examples of geoengineering innovations include "carbon scrubbers," towering structures (that look like smoke stacks) made to suck carbon dioxide from the atmosphere; seeding the ocean floor with iron pellets to stimulate the growth of carbon-consuming phytoplankton blooms; and deploying millions of mirror-coated nano-sized flying saucers into space to form a stratospheric solar reflector (Kahan et al. 2015; Kahan 2015). The final group, the control, read about a topic unrelated to the environment, namely municipal funding for new traffic signals in Broomfield County, Colorado. All three group then evaluated the scientific study on climate change impact.

When the participants were asked about the climate study, cultural cognition was evident in the parsing of who accepted and who dismissed its findings. The control group demonstrated the same spread of climate change views known to exist along the political spectrum. Specifically, hierarchical individualists responded more skeptically than egalitarian communitarians to the study's conclusions. The cultural cognition of risk framework can explain this: citizens who prize individual ingenuity and self-sufficiency (individualists) tend to dismiss claims of environmental risk because accepting these claims would license restrictions on free markets. Also, those with hierarchical preferences, that is, favoring stable and clearly defined social rankings, will also respond negatively because "they tend to see environmentalism as an implicit indictment of social elites" (Kahan 2015).

Members of the first intervention group, having first read an argument for increased environmental regulation, exhibited the most dramatic polarization. Hierarchical individualists were extremely dismissive of the study findings while egalitarian communitarians were more accepting than like-minded subjects in the control group. Reading a news article titled "Scientists: Even Stricter Anti-Pollution Regulations Needed to Fight Climate Change" triggered "antagonistic associations between climate change and free markets," which resulted in the measurable increase in polarization among people with different cultural outlooks (Kahan 2015; Kahan et al. 2015). The geoengineering group, in contrast, demonstrated an encouraging convergence of responses to the factual claims proposed in the study. What was different?

The researchers proposed that the central idea, that human ingenuity can resolve environmental problems (which were themselves created by human ingenuity), resonated positively for people with individualistic-hierarchical outlooks as well as communitarian-egalitarians (Kahan 2015). For the former group, notably, environmental action did not require market restrictions and increased government regulations. For both groups, part of the appeal could be the aspirational language of the geoengineering news story—in marked contrast to the usual doom-and-gloom tone of environmental reporting. For instance, the geoengineering news article quoted a Harvard professor saying, "Human beings have faced challenges from nature throughout history; we've never succumbed to these challenges—we've always overcome them with ingenuity" (Kahan et al. 2015). The resulting non-necessity of limiting commerce and industry was mentioned in the article, but this socially divisive issue was not a central focus of the climate-related narrative. The researchers had accurately predicted that "substituting this identity-affirming 'yes we can' narrative for the denigrating 'we told you so' one" would mitigate responses to climate change evidence (Kahan 2015). By replacing the negative value associated with the scientific fact with a positive value instead, the identity-preserving cognitive apparatus was not invoked. The cultural cognition thesis indicates that we *can* shift the dial on even our most trenchant controversies.

## ON FACTS AND VALUES

Because cultural cognition theory posits that culture is prior to facts, and the climate change intervention was described as tying facts to congenial values, the project (probably unwittingly) instantiates an indefensible fact-value distinction. I highlight this point not to challenge the experimental findings but to suggest that something else is happening here other than prioritizing values over facts. This position, that values precede facts, incorrectly assumes that values and facts *can* be disentangled. Correcting the theoretical explanation will strengthen the rhetorical strategy for vaccine and other outreach efforts that might follow from this research.

Much has been written in the philosophy of science literature about the demise of the fact-value distinction. (For a good historical review, see Putnam's (2002) "The Collapse of the Fact-Value Distinction.") Whereas scholarly attention has been focused on facts as value-laden and the impossibility of value-free science due to the normativity of experience, far less attention has been given to the facticity of values.[5] Yet, some scholarship in this direction does exist.

For example, Elizabeth Anderson (2004) recognizes that the resistance many might have to the entry of values into scientific reasoning stems from the (uncritical) belief that value judgments are mere preferences or whims. But value judgments, if they are judgments at all, need some standards. Anderson follows John Dewey's classical pragmatism to argue that value judgments should be arrived at by reflective decisions based on good reasons. Furthermore, value judgments are even open to empirical testing of a sort, because they connect a valued state or course of action with the desirability of the consequences of pursuing and attaining them (Anderson 2010). The evidence by which we test value judgments can include the emotional experiences that follow from adopting and acting on those values (Anderson 2004). We test our value judgments by living in accordance with them and "if we find life in accordance with the value judgment satisfactory, we stick with it; if not, we seek new judgments that can better guide our lives" (Anderson 2010, 96). Specifically, we want to know if living with those value judgments can result in actions (in accordance with the value judgment) that solve the problem those judgments were intended to solve. Does living in accordance with those value judgments result in actions that bring about worse problems? Might our goals be better met by adopting different value judgments? (Anderson 2010, 96).

Thus, scientific reasoning is not harmed by the value intrusion that follows from the collapse of the fact-value distinction, providing that value judgments are held to standards of empirical examination akin to those used to interrogate scientific facts. Furthermore, just as facts were understood to be value-laden, values can now be understood to be fact-laden (for more, see Clough 2003a; 2003b; 2014).

Returning to the Cultural Cognition Project, I propose that what is happening in the climate change intervention is a critical testing of the cluster of values that define climate denial and acceptance. To what extent are the desired outcomes of a hierarchical individualist achieved or thwarted by climate change mitigation efforts? Are other efforts more congenial to the desired outcomes? To ask these questions is to interrogate the links between facts about climate change and the facts underlying the identity-defining values of hierarchical-individualists. As a rhetorical strategy, climate change discussion can and should move beyond the facts about climate change to include the facts that inform the social and cultural identities of public stakeholders that hold climate skeptical views. The values, commitments, and lifestyles associated with vaccine hesitancy and refusal can similarly be interrogated, as the example in the next section demonstrates.

## WHAT WOULD A PROMISING VACCINE INTERVENTION LOOK LIKE?

The "I Immunise" social marketing campaign that ran in Western Australia in 2014 serves as an exemplar of indirect means for changing entrenched negative attitudes toward vaccines. It captures numerous features of the three strategies just discussed. "I Immunise" (see fig. 2.2) was run by the Immunisation Alliance of Western Australia, the country's first health promotion nonprofit organization founded to advocate for the community benefits of vaccines. "I Immunise" was created by Alliance member Katie Attwell, a political scientist at the University of Western Australia and a resident of a progressive eco-ethical lifestyle community with lower-than-average national vaccine coverage. Attwell understood the low coverage to stem from the natural-living ideology shared by many of her neighbors, a lifestyle that she also supports. Consistent with cultural cognition theory, the campaign organizers recognized that geographical clustering of like-minded families contributed to how individuals will think and act on vaccines (Attwell and Freeman 2015). Unlike the vaccine promotions examined by Nyhan and colleagues, the Australian campaign notably focused on identity rather than vaccine facts to improve vaccine perception and behavior, invoking many of the community's shared values and behaviors and working to remove vaccine hesitancy from that cultural cache.[6]

Community members, including Attwell (fig. 2.2d), appeared in the ads and in the more detailed story lines on the "I Immunise" website. They were all residents of Fremantle, Western Australia, a city with demographics similar to those of Portland, Oregon. As seen in other communities with highly educated residents maintaining "eco-friendly" lifestyles, many Fremantle parents place high value on organic food, homebirthing, cloth diapers ("nappies"), and alternative medicine; as a corollary, they exhibit high rates of vaccine hesitancy and refusal, to the point where Fremantle (or "Freo") has some of the lowest rates of vaccine compliance in the country.[7]

The "local experts"[8] deployed by the "I Immunise" campaign included "Andrew" (fig. 2.2a) carrying a baby in a sling, with the message "I use cloth nappies, I eat whole foods, and I immunise." The ad denies the trope of the "whole foods" or "natural living" vaccine refuser—a characterization that resonates across continents, for instance, in the international press's scornful appraisals of vaccine-refusing coastal Californians during the 2015 Disneyland measles outbreak—and suggests, instead, that you can be an "eco-parent" and still vaccinate your children. The ads not only affirm the local lifestyle and value-set but

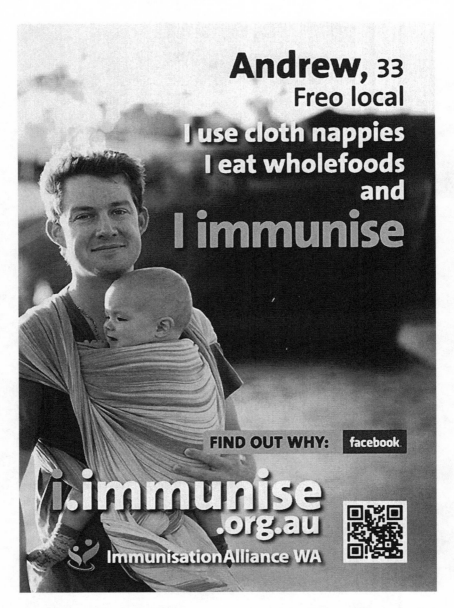

**FIGURE 2.2A.** Sample of ads that appeared in newspapers and on billboards in Fremantle, Western Australia, as part of the "I Immunise" campaign.

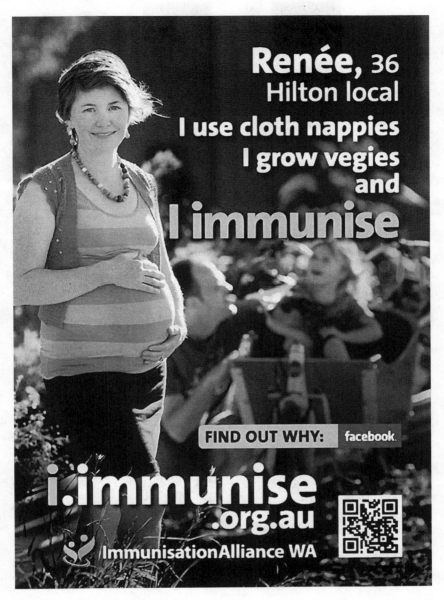

**FIGURE 2.2B.** Sample of ads that appeared in newspapers and on billboards in Fremantle, Western Australia, as part of the "I Immunise" campaign.

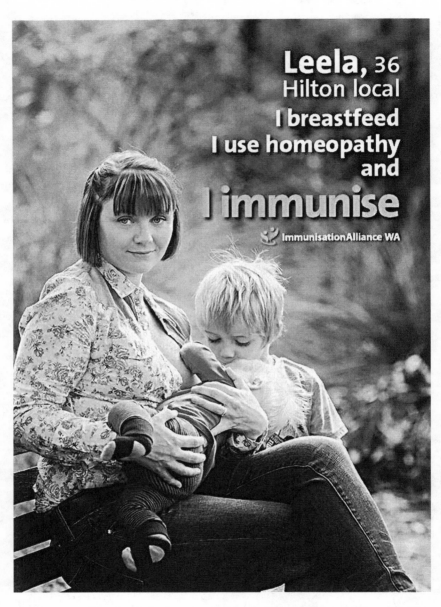

**FIGURE 2.2C.** Sample of ads that appeared in newspapers and on billboards in Fremantle, Western Australia, as part of the "I Immunise" campaign.

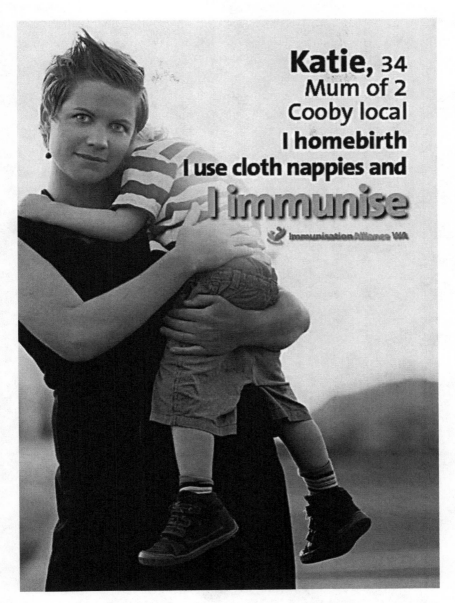

**Katie,** 34
Mum of 2
Cooby local
I homebirth
I use cloth nappies and
I immunise

Immunisation Alliance WA

FIGURE 2.2D. Sample of ads that appeared in newspapers and on billboards in Fremantle, Western Australia, as part of the "I Immunise" campaign.

propose importantly that there is no cognitive dissonance in those choices, that lifestyle. To strengthen this proposition, viewers are introduced in this ad series to a new community that shares those values (fig. 2.2). Here the vaccine-supporter can sustain feelings of belonging and acceptance.

The "I Immunise" campaign thereby carries many elements of the indirect strategies discussed earlier to confronting vaccine hesitancy. It focuses on identity instead of vaccine facts[9] to challenge ideologically loaded beliefs and break their ties to other social values—in this case, the purported negative association between eco-lifestyles and vaccination. The campaign also affirmed the lifestyle, values, and group identity of its target audience, thereby making the challenge to common attitudes and practice among community members more palatable. For instance, in the web entry by Renee (fig. 2.2b), she explains: "Some parts of modern society aren't great. Plastic packing and convenience food are too pervasive, and our suburbs should be designed for people instead of cars. We resist this by growing our own food and keeping chickens who eat our scraps. It's important that my daughter Saskia has some link to where our food comes from, so she collects the eggs and helps in our vegie patch. Her placenta is buried underneath our mulberry tree."[10] Renee continues with a recollection of good medical care that her daughter received for a serious health incident (which was not vaccine preventable), and how that experience engendered her own trust in medical advice, including the advice she received to immunize her children. Thus, we see how Renee incorporated vaccination into her eco-friendly worldview. While the campaign did not rely on conventional experts like nurses and doctors to convey the message, preferring peer interactions instead, it capitalized on cultural tropes (dress, activities) that made the information providers seem trustworthy insofar as they shared the values of the viewer. Both community-based peer interventions and the practice of using a diverse set of experts draw from research into behavior change that finds attempts to influence are more effective when the message comes from trusted and like-minded sources (Attwell and Freeman 2015).

In a coauthored paper evaluating the campaign, Attwell and Immunisation Alliance colleague Melanie Freeman (2015) conducted an online survey to gauge community members' responses to the ads and website. Respondents were asked whether the images and narratives improved feelings about vaccines and whether they increased intention to vaccinate. There was a general increase in positive attitudes toward vaccines among all respondents, even minimally so among those most opposed to vaccines. There was a slight increase in intention to vaccinate in all respondents except for a slight decrease in intention among that subset of highly opposed individuals. While the results were not dramatic, they demonstrate success in changing attitudes and behaviors by at least opening up the possibility of vaccine acceptance for those committed to an alternative lifestyle. When identity is no longer threatened by the factual claim in question, there is less inclination to resist the claim.

## CONSIDERING THE ETHICS OF PERSUASION

All of the strategies suggested by the cognitive turn in thinking about vaccine hesitancy are persuasion efforts, that is, they aim to change the beliefs or actions of others without coercion. Persuasion raises ethical concerns insofar as it can be associated with deception and propaganda. Many public relations scholars and practitioners actively avoid use of the term "persuasion" for that reason, even though changing beliefs and behaviors is exactly what public relations is tasked with doing (Fawkes 2007; Messina 2007). There is general agreement that persuasion efforts are unethical when they are manipulative, deceptive, and work against the interests of the target audience (Baker 1999). Some theorists object that actions so described do not qualify as persuasion but rather propaganda (Messina 2007). Pushing back against what they see as an unfair conflation of terms, those scholars now employ the term "ethical persuasion" to delimit acceptable forms of communication intended to change attitudes and behaviors (Messina 2007; Fawkes 2007). Ethical persuasion is not propaganda, coercion, or deception. It *is* a practice of influential communication that respects the autonomy of the audience by presenting truthful and relevant information. It enables audiences "to make voluntary, informed, rational and reflective judgements" (Messina 2007). Guidelines for ethical persuasion have been proposed; Messina (2007), for example, instructs that attempts at influential communication must

(1)   Allow audiences to have adequate information to make voluntary, informed, rational and reflective decisions;
(2)   Be truthful, respectful, authentic and equitable;
(3)   Withstand the test of "reversibility," where you put yourself in the other person's shoes, as well as the test of public scrutiny (what would others think?)

This complements Baker and Martinson's (2001) "TARES test," which establishes moral boundaries for persuasive communication:

Truthfulness
Authenticity (sincerity)
Respect
Equity
Social Responsibility

Why the effort to salvage persuasion? Because persuasion is intrinsic to communication (Miller 1989). It is how we communicate with others to achieve preferred outcomes. To set limits on acceptable communication practices is justified; to dismiss all persuasion as insidious is too extreme. As socially situated individuals, we need modes of information exchange, value considerations, and collective decision-making and action. Persuasion is part of the communication toolbox.

Ethical persuasion serves as one of the pillars of governance for achieving public policy goals, meaning that it serves not only to direct individual behavior but also to legitimize government action through representation. The other of modes of governance are hierarchy, markets, and networks (Bell, Hindmore, and Mols 2010; Mols et al. 2015). "Hierarchy" refers to legislative or executive constraints on the citizenry's freedom of choice or action, for example, legislative bans and penalties to discourage undesirable choices and actions. "Markets" employ financial inducements like tax breaks and subsidies to encourage desirable behavior. Governance through "networks" involves informal social systems (rather than bureaucratic structures), wherein stakeholders negotiate collective behavior to further individual and group interests (Börzel and Panke 2007). All these modes of governance have been employed to increase vaccine uptake—for example, tying vaccine requirements to child benefits, tax breaks, and access to schools and daycares.[11] Persuasion is distinct from the other modes because it does not seek to alter the individual's choice set. This "softer" approach instead works to change behavior by targeting the underlying preference ranking of the choice. Effective persuasion makes the desired choice more attractive to the decision-maker rather than modifying incentive structures.[12] Persuasion can impact both individuals and peer groups. These efforts are directed toward augmenting "people's beliefs about the social world, thereby modifying their understanding of what represents their (personal and/or collective) best interests" (Mols et al. 2015, 81).

All the modes of governance discussed above raise some degree of ethical concern regarding freedom of choice, because they all aim to direct or augment public behavior. Fear of penalty, ranging from small fines to jail time, severely restricts the freedom to choose. Financial incentives can be unfair in that they disproportionally dictate the actions of people with limited financial means; one's standing in a social group is governed by peer acceptance, which can direct and constrain individual action. The acceptability of any of these constraints on individual choice will typically require some consequentialist calculation of whether the overall social benefit sufficiently outweighs the harms of limiting personal choice. Persuasion, in contrast to the other modes, is nonintrusive insofar as it keeps the choice-set intact. Limiting consideration to "ethical persuasion" upholds that belief- and behavior-augmenting efforts must be honest in the information conveyed, respectful of the values of the target audience, and conducive to rational choice. Freedom of choice is supposed to be maintained.

Perhaps, like nudge techniques, the concern lies in the disrespectful characterization of the decision-making publics. The now-popular "nudge" approach (which may earn a place as a fifth mode of governance, see Mols et al. 2015) has proved to be effective and efficient in encouraging behavioral modification, including vaccine behavior (Brewer et al. 2017). Nudge techniques create non-forced compliance by not incentivizing an unwanted behavior; they add time and effort to achieving undesirable goals, thereby capitalizing on the tendency of individuals to put the lowest possible cognitive effort into decision-making and to adjust behavior in response to minor inconveniences (Mols et al. 2015). Putting fruit and healthy snacks at eye level at the grocery store, for example, "nudges" people to make healthier food choices.[13] Nudge techniques have been successfully enlisted to improve vaccine compliance. American states that have added minor administrative obstacles for parents pursuing nonmedical exemptions for their children's school-entry vaccines (i.e., requiring a letter from the child's pediatrician or having the paperwork notarized) have seen reduced numbers of opt-outs (Omer et al. 2006). The effectiveness of nudge techniques needs to be considered against the distribution of harms. Nudges are frustrating for the target audience when they perceive the "red tape" burden as manipulative, even if the burden is minor. This is not conducive to building good relations between the publics and government institutions. The strategic purpose of eye-level healthy snacks may go unnoticed by a rushed shopper, but the extra work to sign a vaccine exemption form will surely not. Nudge tactics can be discriminatory if they assume that the inconvenience is experienced equally by all. It is harder for low-income people with less flexibility in their daily lives to make the extra visits to their physician, if they have one, or to a notary.[14]

Critics think public engagement will suffer in the long term from overuse of nudge techniques, since they influence behavior by routinely targeting flaws in individual decision-making (Hausman and Welch 2010) and "take human failings as a starting point (e.g., inertia, loss aversion, and unthinking conformity)" (Mols et al. 2015). Successful public engagement, I have proposed, requires building and maintaining trust between expert/elite and nonexpert groups. Any disrespectful regard of the general publics is not a good starting point for meaningful exchange (see chapter 6).

Persuasion, its supporters maintain, is a morally preferable goal-directed decision-making framework; it targets its audience's authentic beliefs, specifically those governed by our social identities, to encourage positive change in beliefs and behaviors. It avoids the deceptiveness of propaganda that objectionably limits rational choice by its target audience. If we take seriously the designated criteria of voluntariness and informed, reflective judgment, ethical persuasion *encourages* rational choice in its service to inform and motivate the target audience to realize and actualize their authentic desires. Effective persuasion efforts, like the "I Immunise" campaign, are successful because they are able to capture identity-defining values and beliefs and to reframe them in such a way that new norms can be integrated into the (new) shared identity. Rather than being manipulative, persuasion capitalizes on the self-satisfaction individuals derive from enacting identity-affirming behavior. We derive meaning and direction from the social groups whose norms we embrace and enact. Persuasion techniques encourage reviewing new and established norms for consideration as to how they tie into other deeply held convictions.

Yet there is reason to be suspicious of these claims of self-actualization through persuasion in a world organized with significant structural inequality. To be ethical, ethical persuasion must include ongoing critical evaluation of the communications and how they impact preference ranking and careful attention to unintentional intrusions on choice-sets. While straightforward informational exchange still strikes many as the most honest form of communication, it fails in practice because it invokes numerous cognitive defenses when dealing with sensitive topics. If meaningful consideration of alternative viewpoints is our goal, then persuasion efforts are indeed the preferred mode of communication.

What remains in this investigation into the ethics of persuasion is consideration of whether persuasion efforts are being channelled to encourage the right social goals. We rightly balk at the notion of policy elites setting the social agenda without democratic consultation. Policy is limited in its legitimacy and efficacy without democratic public approval. Public consultation and buy-in are important parts of the policy-making enterprise. So while persuasion might be morally acceptable, even morally commendable, as a mode of communication, the content of those communications must be equally legitimated. The solution lies in a democratic and pluralist approach to setting and achieving public policy goals,[15] with the important caveat that democratic representation includes diverse voices and attention to the protection of minority rights and the amplifying of traditionally underrepresented perspectives. Persuasion techniques can only be morally acceptable when executed in concert with meaningful deliberation about issues of public concern. I put this out as a challenge for policy makers, with the hope that the new framework focusing on trust in part 2 of this book can and will inform policy efforts.

## REEVALUATING THE "STUBBORN MIND"

This chapter challenged the media-driven conclusion that appreciating the impact of cognitive biases on vaccine decision-making showed the problem of vaccine hesitancy to be unsolvable due to stubbornness. The focus on cognitive biases is helpful because it better directs how one can create change. The "cognitive turn" that entered media discourse in the wake of Nyhan et al.'s 2014 publication has helpfully provided a new way to think about vaccine hesitancy, thereby unseating the familiar public misunderstanding of science framework's intellectual stronghold. What filled the void, however, at least in the early media frenzy described in this chapter, was an incomplete understanding of the implications of this research. Not only was the fatalistic conclusion espoused by the media wrong, but it obscured the ingenuity of the cognitive turn. The focus on cognition productively offers a new causal account of vaccine hesitancy, which in turn invites alternatives to the education model to change perception and behavior regarding vaccines. These new directions for vaccine communications research and public health outreach deserve further exploration.

Nyhan et al.'s study (2014) and corroborating science communications research strongly suggest that the beliefs of strong vaccine skeptics will not be altered by countering misbeliefs with corrective factual information. This is uncomfortable in the context of science denial; facts and evidence are precisely what science can usually offer to heated science-policy debates. The psychology of misperception instructs that individuals are all deeply motivated to hold onto their strongly held beliefs. But changing the conversation so that those facts are not so threatening is possible.

Following the argument made in the previous section that persuasion techniques are only acceptable if they are accompanied by democratic and publicly accountable processes regarding policy initiatives, the issue of trust—the theme of this book—returns to the investigation. It has already been argued that the framing of vaccine hesitancy as a problem of cognitive biases was appealing initially because this alternative still places blame on the publics and leaves untouched the credibility of the institutional apparatus tasked with protecting public health. But the inevitable need for legitimate public engagement means that trust between governmental institutions and the publics they serve is an inescapable issue. This important point will be taken up in part 2 of the book, where I offer a framework for reconfiguring vaccine hesitancy as a problem of public mistrust of science rather than public misunderstanding of science.

# 3

## THE "DEATH OF EXPERTISE"

I wonder if we are witnessing the "death of expertise": a Google-fueled, Wikipedia-based, blog-sodden collapse of any division between students and teachers, knowers and wonderers, or even between those of any achievement in an area and those with none at all.

— Tom Nichols

When political scientist Tom Nichols coined the phrase "death of expertise," he did not mean "the death of *actual* expertise, the knowledge of specific things that set some people apart from others in various areas." Nor did he mean the death of expert categories like "doctors, lawyers, engineers, and other specialists in various fields." Rather, what has died, he claimed, is acknowledgement of the epistemic value of expertise, and recognition that experts ought to inform nonexpert opinions and decisions. Many Americans, Nichols contended, "now seem to reject the notion that one person is more likely to be right about something, due to education, experience, or other attributes of achievement, than any other" (Nichols 2014). The "death of expertise" is the complaint that no one listens to experts anymore.

This chapter examines the third and final narrative regarding the alleged war on science: the "death of expertise," wherein expertise is said to have lost its prior standing as the means for addressing issues marked by uncertainty and/or complexity. In the *Harvard Business Review*, "the end of expertise" has been described as a shift in public opinion away from reverence of expert evaluation, *inter alia* the lost public regard for Michelin guides in favor of peer-generated Yelp reviews (Fischer 2015). Where once experts were valued for the utility that learned wisdom offered for solving complex problems, expertise has been succeeded by populist common sense (Fischer 2015; Nichols 2014; Nichols 2017a).[1] Nichols similarly chronicles the widespread dismissal of expertise, noting a "self-righteousness and fury" to this phenomenon that signals more than mere "mistrust or questioning of the pursuit of alternatives: it is narcissism, coupled to a disdain for expertise as some sort of exercise in self-actualization" (Nichols 2017a).

What is being described here is termed "epistemological populism" (Saurette and Gunster 2011) in the political science literature.[2] Whereas populism typically challenges the elite in terms of political power, epistemological populism challenges knowledge elites. Populism eschews experts in favor of "folk wisdom" (Hawkins 2010; Wodak 2015a; 2015b; Cramer 2016), and epistemological populism valorises "the knowledge of 'the common people,' which they possess by virtue of their proximity to everyday life" (Saurette and Gunster 2011, 199). When commentators proclaim the "death of expertise" and the "end of expertise," they suggest that the populist war on experts has been won. Unsurprisingly perhaps, the "end of expertise" is commonly invoked to explain public resistance to scientific claims. When patients challenge their physicians' educated pronouncements on vaccines, "expertise is dead." When Hollywood celebrities captivate parents with vaccine-skeptical views, "expertise is dead."

In this chapter's discussion of the war on science framework, the focus is on scientific experts. The culture war has been interpreted as a willful rejection of expert opinion and disdain of experts. This narrative appears in the popular press, popular science writing, and in some science studies scholarship. The death of expertise narrative is distinct from the previously discussed accounts covering public misunderstanding of science and the publics' cognitive limits, insofar as the social dimensions of science communications now get some attention, albeit insufficient. This final narrative deserves critical examination because it forces attention toward the embodied actors involved in science-publics relations, a focus that should counteract any uncritical thinking about science communication as merely transmission of established facts to a passive and (rightly) receptive publics. Examining the "death of expertise" framework highlights the sociality of knowledge generation and communication, inviting the socially situated "crisis of trust" reframing of vaccine hesitancy presented in the second half of this book.

The "death of expertise" also extends the war metaphor by identifying the casualties of war—the scientific experts—and a more insidious othering of the enemy, the supposedly expert-loathing publics. Public resistance to scientific claims is understood through this construct to be part of a dangerous ideology of anti-intellectualism,[3] rather than an unfortunate educational deficit or problematic biased psychology. The publics become the enemy and are now portrayed as fully blameworthy for the seemingly intractable problem of vaccine hesitancy and refusal.[4]

In reality, the argument that no one listens to experts anymore, or that expertise is *dead*, is flawed. I propose that expertise is not dead and that members of the publics do not think they know better than experts. Instead, expertise is being vigorously challenged, a phenomenon that stems from poor public trust in experts. Rather than the death of expertise, this is a *recalibration* of expertise by members of the publics. This is good news for vaccine advocates (including its experts), as there is now an opportunity to reestablish the role of experts in relation to a society more complex than ever. In twenty-first-century democracy, experts can be re-centered as both technically competent and responsive to public interest and concern.

## DO THE PUBLICS THINK THEY KNOW BETTER THAN EXPERTS?

Nichols followed up his widely read essay with a 2017 book by the same title, *The Death of Expertise*. Published by Oxford University Press, the book is written in a frustrated and exasperated tone, rife with bombastic assertions such as "Americans have reached a point where ignorance, especially of anything related to public policy, is an actual virtue" (Nichols 2017a). Such claims are unlikely to do much more than appeal to those already convinced of the problem, and indeed, the book's reception suggests that many *are* already convinced that expertise is dead. For example, a *New York Times* review stated, "'The Death of Expertise' turns out to be an unexceptional book about an important subject" (Kakutani 2017). In what is more of a "flat-footed compendium than an original work," Nichols covers familiar terrain to make his case, including the sociological and psychological research into cognitive errors such as framing effect, cognitive bias, the Dunning-Krueger effect,[5] how experts are created and validated, and how mistakes by or disagreements among experts are exaggerated to undercut the very idea of expertise. The premise of the book is built upon an already well-rehearsed position that expertise is in serious trouble. Nichols's bibliography includes such works as Al Gore's *Assault on Reason* (2007), Susan Jacoby's *Age of American Unreason* (2008), Robert Hughes's *Culture of Complaint* (1993), and Richard Hofstadter's 1963 classic, "Anti-Intellectualism in American Life." The death of expertise is familiar in science policy and communications circles as well, where the Bodmer Report (discussed in chapter 1), published more than thirty years earlier, expressed the same anxiety over the publics' inability to recognize science as the key to solving complex social problems.

Alternative explanations abound for why expertise has been demoted in status: members of the publics are confused, the publics are no longer interested in knowing the truth, the experts are not perceived as trustworthy, to name a few. But Nichols commits to the thesis that the general publics think they know better than experts (Nichols 2017a, 6, 166)[6] and goes so far as likening American public life to "a hockey game with no referees and a standing invitation for spectators to rush onto the ice" (2017a, 25). He laments how a little learning is a dangerous thing insofar as it can inflate one's sense of expertise—the Dunning-Krueger effect. Further elaborating his thesis in a 2017 article in *Foreign Affairs*, titled "How America Lost Faith in Expertise," Nichols wrote, "Like anti-vaccine parents, ignorant voters end up punishing society at large for their own mistakes" (Nichols 2017b). These ideas have found widespread resonance among the punditry, starting with book reviewers who were sympathetic to this view that the publics think they know better than they really do. The idea that members of the publics overestimate their expertise is widely taken up as a good explanation for why global warming is debated, GM foods are questioned, and vaccines are refused.

It is notable that the downfall of expertise in both past and present formulation is seen as a problem lying squarely with the publics, while science and its institutions require little or no scrutiny. While Nichols does lament instances of experts' overreach in pronouncing on issues outside of their sphere of expertise and recognizes that cases of misconduct erode public trust, he ultimately derides the publics both for not recognizing that science is fallible (and so even good experts can be wrong) and for failing to check their experts more diligently, thereby getting themselves caught-up in orchestrated nonsense by self-serving gurus (Nichols 2017a).

Nichols does not, however, provide empirical support or strong theoretical justification for the claim that the publics think they know better than experts, preferring instead to infer it from a confusing smattering of causal factors, including an allegedly broken higher education system, dependency on automation, and an American cultural heritage of anti-intellectualism and narcissism. He points to the downgrading of higher education that has resulted from universities pandering to high tuition-paying "clients," which, he claims, leads to the general publics thinking they know better than experts. Yet, the causal link between the alleged failures of higher education and the public embrace of anti-intellectualism is, as one should expect, tenuous. As for automation, Nichols explained in an interview that "when you're looking around the world and everything just works, you ask yourself, 'How hard can this be? Who can't fly a plane?'" (Nichols in Buck 2017). This kind of hyperbole is unhelpful to anyone who wants to genuinely assess the thesis, rather than accept the death of expertise as established fact. Nichols claims that deep societal narcissism has resulted in a culture of anti-intellectualism, where "[w]e have become so acclimated to thinking that our views on everything are as important and as worthwhile as everyone else's. Every professional in the world at this point has encountered somebody who has told them how to do their job" (Nichols in Buck 2017). These features of social life, poor education, automation, and anti-intellectualism are said to result in a culture of people who think they know better than experts.

My focus in this chapter is not on unpacking the broad claims of the demise of higher education and sweeping claims about American culture (as if it is a single entity), but rather on the charge that the publics think they know better. I argue that the publics do *not* think they know better. Rather, they are not buying what the experts are selling. Against the doomsday predictions of a losing battle or war on science and expertise, this challenge to the previously secure position of experts and expertise in democratic society is a demand for institutional governance[7] that is both accountable to, and works in the interest of, the publics. A constructive response to such public discontent cannot begin or end with insistent reassertions of truth (science) known only by the few (experts) singularly capable of directing the best social order. Public disaffection demands a robust democratic engagement rather than facile calls for trusting science and scientific experts. This view should not be understood to be creating post-truth equivalents between facts and "alternative facts." Instead it involves recognizing that there is more at issue here than science and facts (this point will be further developed in chapter 4).

## MEDIA AND POPULAR SCIENCE REPRESENTATIONS OF THE PROBLEM OF EXPERTISE

Despite the *Death of Expertise*'s scholarly and argumentative limits, the book secured a prestigious publisher, likely because the "death of expertise" is a prominent cultural concept. The familiarity and repetition of a concept can make its content seem compelling. Indeed, the sentiment that expertise is under attack is widely held, as seen in media representations and both popular science and science studies writing on this subject.

"Expertise under attack!" is a phrase that has been frequently used to describe the tumultuous politics of 2016, particularly the Brexit referendum in the United Kingdom and the election of Donald Trump as president of the United States. It is true that these "nativist" agendas, which pushed back against decades-long rise of cosmopolitanism and globalism, were defined in part by a rejection of expert opinion. To offer a few notorious examples, when asked on live television to name one economist who supported the UK's exit from the European Union, Conservative MP and Brexit "leave" advocate Michael Gove famously responded, "I think people in this country have had enough of experts" (Mance 2016). Glyn Davies, another Conservative MP, similarly dismissed lack of expert support for leaving the EU, tweeting in October 2016, "Personally, never thought of academics as 'experts.' No experience of the real world." In America, then-presidential candidate Trump echoed this view. In response to persistent criticism that he knew very little about basic issues of public policy, he told an audience in Wisconsin in in April 2016, "They say, 'Oh, Trump doesn't have experts . . . ' You know, I've always wanted to say this—I've never said this before with all the talking we all do—all of these experts, 'Oh we need an expert—.' The experts are terrible" (Gass 2016). The regime-changing populist turn away from liberalism (discussed in the introduction to this book) and globalism had been captured in the political rhetoric as a disavowing of expertise.

Nowhere are the catastrophic proportions of the death of expertise better articulated than in popular science writing, which boasts a fast growing literature on the interfaces of science and policy, and science and the publics, and which ties antiexpertise and anti-intellectualism to science denialism. Many popular science books published in the second decade of the twenty-first century have deplored populist science denialism regarding the science-based policies that matter—climate change, vaccines, GMOs—and have argued that such refusal to follow expert advice presents an existential threat to the future of our species. This is apparent in the titles chosen for these books, for instance: *Unscientific America: How Scientific Illiteracy Threatens Our Future* (Mooney and Kirshenbaum 2009); *Denialism: How Irrational Thinking Harms the Planet and Threatens Our Lives* (Specter 2010); *Reality Check: How Science Deniers Threaten Our Future* (Prothero 2013); *Deadly Choices: How the Anti-Vaccine Movement Threatens Us*

*All* (Offit 2011a), among many others. This polemical genre of popular science writing uncritically interprets public resistance to scientific claims as science denialism. In turn, this phenomenon is viewed as a kind of contagion—it spreads! (Johnson 2017)—and enforces an us/them mentality between the experts, as vigilant defenders of science, and the publics, as ill-informed and threatening the future of humanity in their propensity for misunderstanding facts and spreading misinformation.

## THE PROBLEM OF EXPERTISE IN SCIENCE STUDIES

Various narratives of science denialism and the public embrace of irrationalism have also emerged within science studies, the academic domain that studies scientific expertise in broad social, historical, and philosophical contexts. Sociologists Harry Collins (2014) and Bruno Latour (2004; 2015; de Vrieze 2017; Kofman 2018) and philosopher of science Philip Kitcher[8] (2011a) have all addressed this pressing issue. For example, in *Science in a Democratic Society*, Kitcher addresses the problem of how scientific authority has been eroded in Western democracies. He opens the book with the comment: "Many Americans do not believe contemporary evolutionary theory offers a correct account of the history of life. Europeans are skeptical about scientific endorsements of the harmlessness of genetically modified organisms. Around the world, serious attention to problems of climate change is hampered by suspicions that the alleged 'expert consensus' is premature and unreliable." By Kitcher's account, the optimistic legacy of the Enlightenment is increasingly called into question (p. 1). He regards this embrace of unscientific views as democracy run amok and is unhappy with an image of science as answerable to "vulgar democracy," that is, to unconstrained majority rule by nonexpert citizenry. He is equally unsatisfied with the alternative option that science should be answerable only to its own standards, and works to find a better middle ground with a reasonable division of cognitive labor (Kitcher 1990; 1993) between expert and nonexpert to create scientifically informed democratic choice (or nonvulgar democracy).

A 2017 interview with Latour in *Science* ran under the headline "Bruno Latour, a Veteran of the 'Science Wars,' has a New Mission;"[9] here, Latour is described as having "long been a thorn in the side of science," but now "in the age of 'alternative facts,' he's coming to its defense" (de Vrieze 2017). He was profiled similarly by the *New York Times* in 2018: "Bruno Latour, the Post-Truth Philosopher, Mounts a Defense of Science" (Kofman 2018). With seeming affection for the very battle and war language that I have been eschewing, Latour explains in the interview that he hopes to help rebuild public confidence in science, specifically concerning climate science. While he denies that the infamous "Science Wars" of the 1990s (to which his name will always be attached) constituted a "war," the current situation *is* indeed a "science war . . . run by a mix of big corporations and some scientists who deny climate change." When asked how scientists should wage this new war, he responded, "We will have to regain some of the authority of science. That is the complete opposite from where we started doing science studies. Now, scientists have to win back respect" (Latour in de Vrieze 2017).

The irony of both Kitcher's and Latour's efforts to win back respect for science and scientists is that they are both associated with the genre of critical science studies that is often said to be responsible for the erosion of scientific authority. Both Kitcher and Latour reflect on how science studies research has contributed to what they see as an absurd situation. The work of science studies, including their own celebrated works, has undermined the idealized Enlightenment image of science by revealing the nonrational elements of scientific inquiry, extolling lay expertise, and championing democracy in science. Just as their critics two decades earlier had forecasted that critical science studies would undermine public trust in science (see Gross and Levitt 1994), contemporary war on science aficionados say that the prediction has materialized. Specifically, they argue that postmodernist science studies have undermined the authority of science and contributed to the present downgrading of scientific experts and expertise (i.e., Bergkamp 2016; Pluckrose 2017; see also Hendricks 2018).

Kitcher strongly denies the causal role of social constructivist science studies in undermining public confidence in scientific expertise in the opening pages of *Science in a Democratic Society*. It is unclear whether he holds himself to be part of the scholarly group at the center of this question; he references many of his contemporaries (postmodern philosophers Derrida and Lyotard, and historians and sociologists of science Kuhn, Foucault, Bloor, Collins, Shapin and Schaffer, and Latour) but does not mention himself (15). Yet the placement of an insistent defense of critical science studies on the first page of the book suggests the author sees himself as implicated. To that supposed culpability, he offers the tongue-in-cheek response, "Skepticism about scientific authority has not grown because postmodernism has been injected into the drinking water" (16). Rather, Kitcher argues, public skepticism toward science is best understood as a reaction against scientism, which encompasses exaggerated claims about science's social benefits as well as the misguided belief that science should be entirely disinterested and free of values. He writes that the contemporary erosion of scientific authority stems from a poor argument strategy, whereby scientists involved in debate insist "on the value-freedom of Genuine Science, while attributing value-judgments to the scientists whose conclusions you want to deny" (40). When members of the publics see that science does not deliver the great benefits promised by its champions, and that science is inevitably shaped by values, they react with skepticism about the integrity of scientific practice.[10] They come to assume that everyone is "entitled to their own opinions across the board"; this is "epistemic equality" (20). Kitcher wants to restore a division of cognitive labor among experts and nonexperts that is befitting of scientifically informed democratic choice.

For my part, I dispute Kitcher's diagnosis of cognitive error or erroneous division of labor between expert and nonexpert for the very reason that expertise is *not* dead. My assessment is instead that there is a weakness in the (trust-mediated) relationship between science and the publics. However, Kitcher's downstream aim is similar to my own. Both of us seek to restore an equitable and effective relationship between science and the publics.

Latour has been more willing than Kitcher to acknowledge that science studies criticisms of science (including his own) have created a basis for antiscientific thinking. He has expressed the fear that the critical "weapons" of science studies, or at least a caricature of them, have been abused by the forces of science denialism. Corporate-funded climate skeptics have been using arguments about the constructed nature of knowledge to seed doubt regarding the scientific consensus on climate change. In "Why Has Critique Run out of Steam? From Matters of Fact to Matters of Concern," Latour wrote, in his typical imaginative style: "Maybe I am taking conspiracy theories too seriously, but it worries me to detect, in those mad mixtures of knee-jerk disbelief, punctilious demands for proofs, and free use of powerful explanation from the social neverland, many of the weapons of social critique. Of course, conspiracy theories are an absurd deformation of our own arguments, but, like weapons smuggled through a fuzzy border to the wrong party, these are our weapons, nonetheless. In spite of all the deformations, it is easy to recognize, still burnt in the steel, our trademark: *Made in Criticalland*" (Latour 2004). Some of the central ideas of Latour's most famous works, *Laboratory Life* (with Steve Woolgar, 1979) and *Science in Action* (1987), were that facts are constructed by communities of scientists, and that science's social and technical elements are coproduced. He garnered great admiration for these ideas, as well as disdain. For example, Latour's social constructivism was strongly rejected by scientists who saw the relativist implications of his framing of science and a resulting threat to scientific authority (Gross and Levitt 1994; Sokal and Bricmont 1999; Koertge 2000).[11]

Yet in his 2017 *Science* interview, Latour was more reluctant to accept responsibility for the present death of expertise, or to frame it as a consequence of social constructivist science studies. He recalls how critical social scientific study of how science is done "triggered a reaction of people with an idealistic and unsustainable view of science who thought they were under attack." As a result, he was castigated as antiscience and unfairly "associated with that postmodern relativist stuff." If any damage was done, it was due to misinterpretation of his work. He then offers the slight concession that his writing might have been misinterpreted because, although he was not antiscience, "I must admit it felt good to put scientists down a little. There was some juvenile enthusiasm in my style" (Latour in de Vrieze 2017).

To reclaim the authority of science, both Kitcher and Latour enlist the theoretical tools of science studies rather than repudiate them. They both want to upend popular misconceptions about science as value-free, which they both see as undermining scientific expertise today.[12] Kitcher focuses on the role of values in science, while Latour attends to the relationship of politics and science. Kitcher sees problems in scientists insisting on value-free science. When values are exposed, the publics become convinced that scientists are ideologically driven. This, in turn, gives an opening for dissenters motivated by religion or by their own ideologies to develop supposedly scientific counterclaims of their own (Kitcher 2011a). Kitcher's effort to resolve this problem involves drawing from his past scholarship, specifically his contextual account of science (2001) and his "ethical project" (2011b), to articulate the relationship between science and values. Latour similarly draws from, rather than renounces, past science studies scholarship, as he believes the problem of the downgrading of expertise may be resolved by insisting more strongly on the relationship between science and politics. He wants science enthusiasts to refuse the "science versus politics" bifurcation in favor of a "science *with* politics" that recognizes even good science operates in a context of values and politics (Latour 2015; Latour in de Vrieze 2017). Rather than return to archaic formulations of expertise and scientific authority, it is better for experts to be frank about science and values (Kitcher) and science and politics (Latour).

While Kitcher and Latour maintain some distance from the thesis that expertise is dead, sociologists of expertise Harry Collins and Robert Evans exhibit closer allegiance to the idea. Kitcher and Latour root the downgrading of scientific authority in the publics' misunderstanding of the nature of science (as value-free and devoid of politics), while Collins and Evans situate the problem in the publics' misunderstanding of the nature of expertise. In the introduction to their book *Rethinking Expertise* (2007), they list a confluence of contributing events: late twentieth-century technological failures and disasters like Chernobyl; challenges to the presumed social benefits of scientific progress brought on by environmental and animal rights movements; and the usurpation of science studies research by postmodern literary criticism. All of these led to a *"Weltanschauung* [or worldview] in which we no longer understand how to balance science and technology against general opinion. In today's world the scales upon which science is weighed sometimes tip to the point where ordinary people are said to have more profound grasp of technology than do scientists" (Collins and Evans 2007, 1–2). Also unlike Kitcher and Latour, Collins and Evans understand the "death of expertise" to necessitate a radical reworking of science studies scholarship. Rather than merely refine their science studies programs to address this early twenty-first-century problem, they initiate a new "wave" of science studies called "studies of expertise and experience" (Collins and Evans 2002), with the aim of reclaiming the place of scientific expertise in public life.

Collins and Evans provide a rough historical division of science studies into two previous "waves" or schools of thought (2002). The first refers to scholarship produced in the 1950s and 1960s. Mirroring the postwar confidence in scientific progress, research sought to understand, explain, and generally reinforce the successes of science. The rightful authority of science was not questioned. The second wave refers to the social constructivist turn in science studies that materialized in the early 1970s, inspired by Thomas Kuhn's groundbreaking *Structure of Scientific Revolutions* (1962), to counter the positivism of the first wave. Collins and Evans delineate these waves as a device for initiating a new and necessary "third wave" to counter what they described as the "excesses" of second wave science studies while still guarding against the naïve scientific optimism of the first. Kitcher, Latour, and Collins were part of this second wave, which brought sociologists like Collins into the lab to study what scientists actually did and highlighted the "extra-scientific factors" that often contributed to settling scientific and technical debates (Collins and Evans 2002). Undertaking such research showed that science is not entirely rational, Collins and Evans maintain, and rightly downgraded the status of scientist from godlike being to mere mortal. Yet, Collins and Evans claim, bringing science down from the heavens had a detrimental effect of dispersing expertise too widely, such that now everyone's "got a point."[13]

The third wave proposed by Collins and Evans and further elaborated in their 2007 book *Rethinking Expertise* works to stop the current political paralysis that makes governments unable to move forward on pressing science policy issues. It is meant to strike a balance between the unsavory extremes of technological fascism (rule by technocracy) and technological populism (where everybody is an expert, or there are no experts). Collins and Evans, among others, see the latter as a "post truth" problem—the "death of expertise" and the "war on science" are various articulations of the perceived fall of objectivity and truth (offered by science) in favor of emotional responses to the difficult challenges of our time. The first wave of science studies, by Collins and Evans's (2007) account, invited the possibility of fearful technological fascism and the complementary knowledge deficit model (discussed in chapter 1), by putting decision-making capabilities in the hands of scientific experts with very little need for public input. The second wave corrected this imbalance but swung too far in favor of "everybody's got an opinion," producing the mess we find ourselves in today, where we cannot properly respond to climate change and vaccine refusal harms public health.

In more recent writing, Collins, Evans, and Weinel (2017) demand that science studies recognize and reflect on how much of its scholarship enabled the current problem of post-truth: "Science studies opened up the cognitive terrain to those concerned to enhance the impact of democratic politics on science but, in so doing, it opened that terrain for all forms of politics, including populism and that of the radical right wing." Reclaiming expertise, the third wave of science studies seeks to find the right balance of expert-informed decision-making without losing the valuable public accountability of democratic regimes. This endpoint sounds similar to Kitcher's pursuit of well-ordered science (2001) and a balanced division of cognitive labor (Kitcher 2011a), but the focus by Collins and Evans on the status of scientific experts leads to different interventions than Kitcher's reaffirming of the science-values relationship.

Working to address the troubling societal trend toward distrust of experts (the motivation for writing *Rethinking Expertise*), Collins (2014) coined the phrase "default expertise," the problematic idea that everyone or no one is an expert. "Default expertise" is meant to describe "this sense of empowerment—the sense that every citizen is part of the game of science and technology" (Collins 2014). It is the feeling of having the right to judge that ordinary citizens think they possess because science and technology are so fallible. Default expertise is supposed to explain the apparent reasonableness of telling vaccine hesitant

**TABLE 3.1.** Periodic Table of Expertises (in Collins and Evan 2007)

| | UBIQUITOUS EXPERTISES | | | | |
|---|---|---|---|---|---|
| **DISPOSITIONS** | | | | Reflective ability | Interactive ability |
| **SPECIALIST EXPERTISES** | *UBIQUITOUS TACIT knowledge* | | | *SPECIALIST TACIT knowledge* | |
| | Beer-mat knowledge | Popular understanding | Primary source knowledge | Interactional expertise | Contributory expertise |
| **META-EXPERTISES** | *EXTERNAL* | | *INTERNAL* | | |
| | Ubiquitous discrimination | Local discrimination | Technical connoisseurship | Downward discrimination | Referred expertise |
| **META-CRITERIA** | Credentials | | Experience | Track record | |

parents to "do your research and decide for yourself" and the energy with which some of them take up the challenge.

In response to these armchair researchers/default experts, Collins (2014) borrows from the Periodic Table of Expertise (see table 3.1) that he had earlier developed with Evans (Collins and Evans 2007) to contrast two key kinds of expertise: "Primary Source Knowledge," the kind of informed nonspecialist expertise that comes from reading scientific papers, and "Interactional Expertise," the specialist expertise that comes from being part of the specialist community. Primary Source Knowledge expertise is a kind of ubiquitous knowledge that anyone can have, for example, a well-read parent researcher who accesses scientific papers. But this is different from Interactional Expertise, garnered only by those who are members of the relevant expert community. Only the latter, he argues, imbues one with the specialist knowledge required to pronounce on the knowledge claim in question.[14]

Reading online commentary or even reading the professional scientific literature from the perspective of an outsider or amateur will allow a person to absorb a lot of information but will never provide anyone with Interactional Expertise. This is the sort of expertise developed by immersion in a community of scientists, getting to know the members and getting a feeling for what they think (Mooney 2014a, 2014b). In an interview (Inquiring Minds 2014), Collins explained that "if you get your information only from the journals, you can't tell whether a paper is being taken seriously by the scientific community or not . . . You cannot get a good picture of what is going on in science from the literature." While surely more informative than internet blogs or articles that summarize or comment on that primary literature, reading scientific papers does not make one an expert on the topic at hand.

The periodic table's parsing of different kinds of expertise is intended to salvage the good that came from the second wave of science studies. Specifically, Collins and Evans still want to acknowledge that expertise does not only come in the form of letters next to one's name; there are lived or experiential ways of knowing, for example, that can generate salient expertise on some matters. But the periodic table importantly also works to limit what they see as unfortunate excess, in which the quest for democratic legitimacy led to everyone being an expert.[15]

Collins's answer to the question *Are We All Experts Now?* (2014) is "no." Interactional Expertise is the key concept to justifying his claim. Even if everyone is an expert at some things, that doesn't confer specialist knowledge on everyone. While vaccine skeptics will often insist that they are experts on their children (Reich 2016), Collins would posit that this does not make them experts on vaccines. Against the insistence of industrious armchair vaccine researchers, specialist knowledge arises from education, work, *and* immersion in the community of experts. For Collins, judgments of vaccine safety and effectiveness are best left to the scientists.

## RELATIONS OF KNOWLEDGE IN COMMUNITY

The argument for the special nature of Interactional Expertise acknowledges, at least implicitly, that knowledge arises in community. It is interesting that Collins and Evans describe their book, and the preceding 2002 paper, as "an important challenge to second wave *relational* theories of knowledge via a *non-relational analysis of expertise*" (Collins and Evans 2007, 143), only to land right back on the relational features of expertise. They explain that while expertise arises in community—that is, the learning and socialization into the practices of an expert group—there is more to being an expert than group membership and recognition. In contrast to the attributional accounts of expertise offered by prior sociological investigations, where expertise amounts to being labelled expert by others, Collins and Evans set out to develop a realist and substantive account of expertise. This project is normative: they want their nonrelational account of expertise to influence the process of expert attribution, so that the designation of expert or nonexpert depends on the (substantive) qualities of the individual rather than what others think about them (Collins and Evans 2007, 2). This account will allow for individuals to possess or lose expertise independently of whether others think they are experts. Experts are, instead, those who know what they are talking about. Collins and Evans insist that a new sociology of expertise is needed to "work out what it means to know what you are talking about" (Collins and Evans 2007, 1).

The proposed novelty of Collins and Evans's research is the study of expertise as an epistemic rather than a social concept. But the excising of experts and expertise from their social contexts is both unnecessary and conceptually limiting. It is unnecessary because social epistemology allows for both. Epistemology is the branch of philosophy that studies knowledge and justified belief; social epistemology conceptualizes human knowledge as a collective achievement that is largely shaped by social relationships and institutions. Epistemic concepts can be investigated within their social contexts; doing so generates a better account of the downgrading of expertise than the current diagnosis that no one listens to expert anymore or that expertise is dead (chapter 6 will offer a new reading of the problem of expertise).

Working with the thesis that knowledge is social, science has been examined by social epistemologists not as a collection of facts, a system of language, or as an assortment of methodological commitments but as a knowledge producing institution or institutions (see, for example, Longino 1990). Science is social knowledge. Collins and Evans began their analysis with a characterization of specialist knowledge that recognizes the social nature of scientific knowledge. For this reason, Interactional Expertise separated those with specialist knowledge from armchair researchers with ubiquitous knowledge (see table 3.1). Collins and Evans's acknowledgment of the social (or interactional) nature of scientific knowledge is correct but does not go far enough. Expertise should be similarly studied and appears in part 2 of this book as part of the alternative framework for understanding vaccine hesitancy.

In an odd methodological move, Collins and Evans acknowledge that expertise is acquired and validated in relation to the community of experts, but in their effort to pin down the substantive attributes of expertise, they then explain the *breakdown* of expertise (or death of expertise) nonrelationally. What is the justification for doing so? There is no claim made by the authors that the social situatedness of science no longer matters when expertise breaks down. Indeed, my argument will be that the social nature of science strongly matters and even explains the so-called death of expertise. Collins and Evans frame research into expertise as a choice between realist or relational frameworks. But social constructivists know that the real is not precluded by the constructedness of our objects of interest. Epistemic categories can be studied socially (and they should be) and realist and substantive concepts can arise in relational contexts. There is no need to choose.

It may be because of this false choice that Collins and Evans stop short of adequately investigating the social nature of science. Their nonrelational priority directs them to characterize the problem of expertise as a conceptual confusion about the nature of expertise. Collins and Evans root the problem of expertise—its "death" or "end"—in the publics' misunderstanding of the nature of expertise; specifically, the publics wrongly subscribe to the view that everyone's got a point ("default expertise"). Making the analytic distinctions of types of expertise (as seen in table 3.1) would solve the problem *if* the problem *is* conceptual confusion. But misunderstanding of the nature of expertise is not clearly the problem.

## IS EXPERTISE REALLY DEAD?

Is expertise really dead? Does no one listen to experts anymore? Against Nichol's multiple references to the anti-vaccination movement's celebrity popularizers as cases-in-point of the demise of expertise (Nichols 2017a, 13, 21, 236), the public vaccine debate is anything but an expert-free zone. Instead, vaccine controversy is characterized by a proliferation of expertise. Just as vaccine advocates point to the earned authority of physicians and scientists to pronounce on vaccines, vaccine skeptics point to their own experts. Vaccine skeptics will frequently reference scientists and physicians who hold vaccine-skeptical views because they recognize the importance of marshalling expertise to justify their claims. The status of these experts as professional insiders matters here—even as this discourse runs alongside messaging to mothers to trust their "mommy instincts" (see vanden Heuvel 2013). For example, the vaccine-skeptical blog Vienna Report published a list of physicians and medical scientists who have spoken out about vaccine risks and ineffectiveness. The eighty-two names each link to those alternative experts' videos and lectures (Vienna Report 2019). The vaccine-critical Facebook group Malaysian Vaccines

Exposed (Malaysian Vaccines Exposed ND) has a similar list of 280 doctor and scientists.[16]

Another example of the enduring power of expertise came as an open let-ter[17] to me in response to my *Toronto Star* opinion piece on vaccine hesitancy (Goldenberg 2017) from a Canadian vaccine-critical group (Kuntz 2017).[18] The letter's author mounted an argument against my use of a Statistics Canada claim about the effectiveness of influenza vaccine by offering counterevidence from mainstream medical experts who held more skeptical views about the vaccine's effectiveness. He offered direct quotes from Dr. Michael Gardam, director of the Infection Prevention and Control Unit at the University Health Network in Toronto, and Dr. Tom Jefferson of the Cochrane Collaboration.

Calling this phenomenon the end of expertise is in part a refusal to recognize alternative expert sources as legitimate. But framing the issue as a zone of ex-pert-free discourse does not capture what vaccine hesitators are doing when they, for instance, research vaccine safety and efficacy and then insist that they hold important knowledge that their physicians refuse to properly consider. These vaccine hesitators do not follow the path of appeal to populist "common sense" or experiential knowledge over expert knowledge.[19] Instead they present counter-knowledge generated by alternative inquiry undertaken by counterexperts. Counterknowledge was identified by sociologist Tuukka Ylä-Anttila (2018) as a populist tool for challenging established knowledge. In her study of knowledge claims made by participants of Finnish anti-immigrant online forums, she found in their posts a strong predominance of arguments making epistemic appeals to science, unbiased inquiry, and rationality rather than refrains to populist "com-mon sense," "working man's truths," or other experiential appeals. On vaccines and public resistance to science more generally, I make the similar claim that counterknowledge, generated by counterexperts, plays a central role in vaccine hesitancy discourse. Expertise is not dead, but its traditional boundaries are being challenged and redrawn.

Some might object that my examples are limited to the more conservative strategy used to justify vaccine skeptical views, namely demonstrating the weak-ness of the pro-vaccine position on its own terms of scientific authority. To be sure, there is no shortage of public influencers who do not have the credentials and insider credibility of Gardam or Jefferson. Additionally, those physicians and scientists listed as vaccine critics have had their credibility as experts questioned for the very reasons that they landed on the list. For example, physician-blogger Skeptical Raptor wrote about the Vienna Report's list: "But is this really made up of respected physicians and researchers? Does it really contain doctors who are experts or authorities on vaccines? Well, thanks to Zared Schwartz, a senior at the University of Florida studying microbiology, cell science and neurobehavioral, who took it upon himself to look up each of these individuals and see if they've got anything to offer in the discussions about vaccines. Guess what? It doesn't appear so" (Skeptical Raptor 2017). The evidence I present for counterexperts, indeed, barely scratches the surface. Chapter 6 will make a stronger argument for the centrality of counterexperts, even those who lack scientific credibility, in emboldening counterculture epistemic communities.

My argument that expertise is not dead is not tantamount to claiming that expertise continues as before. Instead expertise is not what it used to be. The reverence for the white coat, described by Collins (2014, 1–3) in the form of a childhood memory of science wonderment at the 1951 Festival of Britain,[20] no longer remains. But what is in its place should not be misunderstood as the end of expertise, but rather as the recalibration of its insider/outsider status (see chapter 6).

## TRUST, THE SOCIAL NATURE OF KNOWLEDGE, AND NEW WAYS OF THINKING ABOUT PUBLIC RESISTANCE TO SCIENCE

The death of expertise explanation for public resistance to scientific claims problematically puts a scientistic gloss on the political consequences of truth claims. Frustrated opponents of science denialism and antiexpertise yearn for a time before post-truth and postmodernism, when truth and facts allegedly stood outside of social meaning. But realities are consequential for political behavior, which gives facts and those who determine them enormous power (Ezrahi 1990). Even a firmly committed realist can admit that our categories and concepts reflect the focus of inquiry (i.e., Dupré 1993; Hacking 1999). Against the claim, made in Plato's *Phaedrus*, that a good theory should "carve nature at its joints," that is, expose the natural kinds and categories of the world, pluralists insist that there are many ways in which the natural world can be carved up (see Slater and Borghini 2011). This metaphysical point about plural realism has bearing on discussions about expertise. Truth claims in the public sphere are additionally normative insofar as they reduce political options and democratic engagement (Jasanoff and Simmet 2017, 753; see also Jasanoff 1990 and 2004). Democratic governance ties what we know to how we govern, and so experts wield power. Experts, then, need to justify their power. It should be no wonder that knowledge controversies reach such a feverish pitch, with the claims and their claimants contested and questioned. Those expert knowledge claims are stand-ins for open, important questions about the democratic futures we aspire to. How, then, do scientists regain their authority? By justifying their authority as consistent with, and enabling of, those democratic futures.

I want to take the picture of science as communities of knowers—something that Collins and sociologists of expertise confidently subscribe to—in different directions, whereby public resistance to science and the so-called death of expertise is not understood as a move toward irrationality, but rather as a sign of public mistrust of scientific institutions. The social nature of knowledge and expertise is key to this reframing.

Populist antiexpertise political statements heard in the UK and US during the Brexit and Trump's first electoral campaigns, in fact, already alluded to lack of trust. The anti-Brexit economics and politics experts were said to be "out of touch" with the people. They were perceived to be vested in the "remain" camp because their EU research funding depended on staying. Trump promised to "drain the swamp," that is, to remove the Washington elites from their positions of power, which they routinely abused. In both cases, experts were seen as untrustworthy because they did not have the interests of their epistemically dependent constituents (i.e., nonexperts) at heart.

Poor trust is not just a political problem. It is a problem for science—as a site of social knowledge—as well. Trust is key to knowledge building, including science. Trust is necessary for scientific knowledge creation, the management of dissent and disagreement, consensus building, and the legitimation of consensus. Vaccine hesitancy will therefore be recast in part 2 of this book as a symptom of a trust deficit, specifically poor public trust in scientific institutions. Tying trust to the social and epistemic aims of science further challenges the lines of moral responsibility for political impasses over science policy issues. Public resistance to scientific claims is no longer only a problem with the publics, but a problem with scientific governance.

## RECONSIDERING THE "DEATH OF EXPERTISE"

This chapter's focus on the "death of expertise" as the third iteration of the culture war on science framework indeed overlapped with the previous foci on knowledge comprehension and uptake in chapters 1 and 2. The focus on expertise rather than science, however, highlighted relational aspects of science and the publics, thereby inviting more consideration of the social dynamics of knowledge. This allowed me to argue that expertise is not dead, and to begin to build my argument that expert-lay relations are strained due to a crisis of public trust. The "death of expertise" also uniquely attends to science's agents—the scientific experts—rather than scientific claims. As a narrative for explaining vaccine hesitancy and other forms of public rejection of scientific claims, it highlights interactions of science communities and the publics, rather than treating science as an asocial set of established facts available for public consumption (acceptance or rejection). In short, there are people and organizations that create and communicate science, and members of the publics are not merely receptors of science but stakeholders in the knowledge claims with particular interest in how those scientific claims impact their lives and well-being. Working with an understanding of science as socially situated highlights the importance of trust and credibility in the successful operations of science—both within research communities and in relation to the publics.

# 4

## POLITICIZED SCIENCE AND SCIENTIZED POLITICS

This book's challenge to the "war on science" framing targets its philosophical assumptions regarding the nature of science and its relationship with society. In this chapter, the popular explanations for vaccine hesitancy, namely public misunderstanding of science (chapter 1), cognitive biases (chapter 2), and the death of expertise (chapter 3), will be shown to rest on a mistaken view of science and society at the heart of the war on science framework. Thinking about the social nature of science also bolsters my preferred framework, the crisis of trust, which will be articulated and defended in the remaining chapters of this book.

Rather than being a war on science, the public controversy that frames vaccine hesitancy and other highly charged science-policy controversies is a proxy for value conflicts and differing visions of democracy. While this proxy conflict has proven to be resilient, I aim to show that we lose much by narrowing political discourse to scientific debate. My analysis situates the so-called war on science in a recent history of "scientizing" political and policy debate, seen most explicitly in the evidence-based movement of the 1990s and early 2000s as well as the "linear model" (Pielke 2004b; 2007) of the science-to-policy relationship.

Scientism is the controversial ideology that science provides the comprehensive means for knowledge and understanding, in other words, that science can or will fully explain everything we experience and seek to understand. The controversy lies in whether science can really answer all questions relevant to the human condition, and indeed, critics of scientism question the completeness of scientific explanation, a view that should not be misunderstood as antiscience. One can consistently acknowledge and admire scientific pursuits but resist scientism because it seeks to usurp questions of meaning and value that are traditionally investigated in humanities scholarship, especially ethics, metaphysics, and aesthetics. Supporters of the ideology, in contrast, see scientism as the key to moving beyond the intellectual stalemates created by millennia of philosophical argumentation.[1]

There are two negative consequences of scientizing politics: (1) science becomes politicized and (2) political practice is weakened. By "science becomes politicized," I mean that science is mapped onto desired political outcomes. This practice, at minimum, underutilizes science for exploring alternative policy options. Far worse, science can be manipulated by political interest groups to achieve specific political and policy goals (what McGarity and Wagner call "bending science" [2008] and what Mooney meant by the "war on science" [2005, 17–24]). Politics suffers too. The downstream effect of scientizing normative decision-making in politics and policy has been weakened venues for political deliberation, setting the stage for the political stalemates seen to this day. The seeming intractability of the problem of vaccine hesitancy and refusal is one such example. The stalemate in resolving vaccine controversy results from an unwinnable war over science, because science is an incomplete proxy for normative and value-driven debates.

## THE NATURE OF SCIENCE AND ITS RELATIONSHIP TO SOCIETY

The divisive "us versus them" discourse of the war on science is grounded in a misunderstanding of the nature of science and how it operates in society. Science, its embattled defenders assume, cuts through partisan politics and rationalizes democratic choice by informing and directing the populace. Scientific experts are indispensable to the flourishing of the polis in a constrained advisory role, as a division of cognitive and deliberative labor is thought to balance the democratic need for both informed policy and political legitimation through public participation (Kappel 2014). In this framing, democracy needs science to ensure social stability; as a corollary, public resistance to scientific claims destabilizes the social order. Here, the lines of responsibility are equally clear: insofar as it is the publics challenging the science, the problem lies squarely with the publics, while science and its institutions require little or no scrutiny. Whether it is a war on evidence, or a war on experts, public resistance to scientific claims is similarly envisioned as a high-stakes battle between established knowledge and destructive ignorance.

The difficulty with this framing is that science, even sound science, does not work that way. Science does not cut through politics and confusion to produce optimal policies and optimal social benefit. Science and society are also far more entangled than this model presupposes. One can, in principle, agree to the scientific superiority of the majority view on vaccine safety and efficacy without supporting the presumed corollary claims that the best policies follow from the best science and that nonexperts who question the science are the problem. It is from this mistaken view of science and its relationship to society that we arrive at the supposed war on science.

High-stakes debates like the one over vaccines can easily be mistaken as a science against antiscience battleground. This is because moral and political disputes are so commonly framed as science debates. The tenacity with which opponents engage better science to win disputes or demonstrate the limits of their opponents' science speaks to the weakened avenues for political debates that have been generated by overprioritizing science in the policy setting.

## SCIENTIZED POLITICS = SCIENCE AS PROXY

Appeals to science to legitimate public action or inaction have become a rhetorical constant in debates over practice, politics, and policy. This tendency is grounded in the widely held belief that science rationalizes decision-making and practice. This is especially the case when dealing with complex social problems. Good science, it is said, should cut through the political fray and ensure the best course of action.

The aspirational belief that science directs best action has a long history. American science journalist Shawn Otto finds it in the writings of Thomas Jefferson and Enlightenment thinking (Otto 2012; 2016). Jefferson is described as a "science enthusiast" because his arguments for America's independence referenced the works of Newton, Bacon, and Locke. Jefferson reasoned that if anyone can discover the truth for themselves, then those in positions of authority (kings, popes, wealthy lords) had no right to impose their beliefs on the people. The people should decide for themselves. From science, Otto contends, "the argument for a new, democratic form of government was self-evident" (Otto 2012). Meanwhile, historians of science highlight the rigorous institutionalization of this belief in "science driving society" in post–World War II American policy. These changes initiated major public funding of scientific research as well as the expansion of government agencies tasked with protecting and promoting environmental, health, and consumer welfare (Miller 2017). The notion that science rationalizes society supported the "evidence-based" movement that swept through health and human sciences to establish itself as a professional norm in the 1990s and early 2000s. It also led to the conceptualization and broad acceptance of the "linear model" of science-policy interactions, the idea that the right science will lead to the right policy (Pielke 2007, chapter 6). As I will show, these two influential movements operationalized and institutionalized a scientistic approach to addressing social issues that created the conditions for the so-called war on science, which is neither a war nor about science. Instead, it should be conceptualized as stalled proxy politics;[2] moreover, the intractability of public resistance to scientific claims is a consequence of the conceptual limits and reductiveness of scientized politics.

## Evidence-Based Everything

Initiated in the early 1990s, the evidence-based movement swiftly transformed health and social science research, healthcare, and policy making by shifting how we think about science in relation to practice.[3] Evidence-based practices introduced classification systems (the hierarchies of evidence) to separate good science from bad science, with the idea that once the good science was determined, good action would follow. The movement began with evidence-based medicine (Evidence Based Medicine Working Group 1992), whose success was soon followed by evidence-based policy making; from there, an explosion of evidence-based approaches spread quickly throughout the social and human sciences and professions. The term "evidence based everything" was coined by Fowler (1997), a physician, and adopted by social scientists (i.e., Oakley [2002] and Mykhalovskiy and Weir [2004]) to capture the enthusiastic uptake of evidence-based practices into business management (Kovner et al. 2000; Kovner and Rundall, 2006), public health (McGuire 2005), speech pathology (Togher et al. 2011), occupational therapy (von Zweck 1999), social work (Cournoyer 2004; Howard et al. 2003; Grinnell and Unrau 2010), education (Masters 2018; Cook et al. 2012; Horner et al. 2005; Slavin 2002), bioethics (Roberts 2000; Goldenberg 2005), and more.

The rapid uptake of evidence-based medicine can be attributed to its tantalizing promise of rationalizing the medical field, which it proposed to do by prioritizing research evidence—notably evidence from randomized controlled trials over uncontrolled and qualitative methods—and challenging the profession's overreliance on "intuition, unsystematic clinical experience, and pathophysiologic rationale as sufficient grounds for clinical decision making" (Evidence Based Medicine Working Group 1992). In law, a similar aversion to case-by-case evidential reasoning was underfoot. The 1993 US Supreme Court ruling on *Daubert v. Merell Dow Pharmaceuticals* codified standards for expert testimony on admissible scientific evidence in the courts by pinning down predetermined (rather than case-specific or contextual) standards of legitimate and illegitimate science. The parallels between evidence-based medicine and *Daubert*'s implications for the admissibility of expert evidence have been examined by Mercer (2008); the key similarity for this analysis is the shared assumption that evidence could be (and should be) generated using noncontextual standards and that the results could then be applied in numerous complex situations.

Evidence-based policy evolved from evidence-based medicine, with practitioners attracted by the promise that evidence-based approaches can substitute politics and interests (or other subjective warrants like "values" and "intuitions") with universal truths. Marston and Watts (2003) capture the iconoclastic appeal of evidence-based policy making with an example from Australian politics. In 2001, former frontbench member of parliament Mark Latham said this about welfare reform: "The myths of the welfare state are based on old ideological ways of thinking, a struggle between government-first and market-first policies. . . . Welfare policymakers need to look beyond the old Left and the new Right to those evidence-based policies that can end the human tragedy of poverty" (Latham in Marston and Watts 2003). For evidence-based enthusiasts like Latham, "evidence-based policy represents a tool or policy for going beyond political ideology. [They treat] evidence-based policy as a neutral concept where 'hard facts' will speak for themselves in addressing 'human tragedy' and politicians and policymakers will act accordingly based on the available evidence" (Marston and Watts 2003). In a 2005 paper I similarly observed that the appeal of evidence-based approaches to policy making is that "evidence-based practice appear[s] to offer a means of negotiating the demands of moral pluralism. Rather than appealing to explicit values that are likely not shared by all, 'the evidence' is proposed to adjudicate between competing claims" (Goldenberg 2005).

This purported replacement of value conflicts with scientific evidence should give us pause. The evidence-based promise of moving decision-making past partisanship and personal preference, though undoubtedly appealing, is not fully realized by silencing value disputes. In *Seductions of Quantification* (2016), anthropologist Sally Engle Merry offers this cautionary assessment of quantification without qualification:

> Indeed, it is the capacity of numbers to provide knowledge of a complex and murky world that renders quantification so seductive. Numerical assessments such as indicators appeal to the desire for simple, accessible knowledge . . . Yet the process of translating the buzzing confusion of social life into neat categories that can be tabulated risks distorting the complexity of social phenomena. Counting things requires making them comparable, which means that they are inevitably stripped of their context, history, and meaning. Numerical knowledge is essential, yet if it is not closely connected to more qualitative forms of knowledge, it leads to oversimplification, homogenization, and the neglect of the surrounding social structure (Merry 2016).

Philosophers will surely recognize Merry's forewarning as an appeal to the inseparability of facts and values, an interrelationship that is still resisted in some science circles in favor of the "value-free ideal" for science (see Douglas 2009, especially chapter 3 for a history of the value-free ideal in philosophy of science). This latter is the common view that science offers unbiased "facts" about reality, and that science's fact-determining effort works best when extrascientific factors (such as social and ethical values) are marginalized. This image is rightfully appealing, as we want to know the truth while guarding against scientific claims about the nature of things reflecting the biases or interests of scientists, funding bodies, and political authority. Philosophers and the broader science and technology studies (STS) community refer to this unsavory influence of values on scientific practice and products as "politicized science," yet maintain that the antidote is not value-free science.

They do so because the notion that science can be stripped of all values and interests is untenable. While scientific claims *can* be held to epistemic standards like empirical adequacy, the assumptions, values, and interests that go into, say, designing the experiment or interpreting the data ensure that science cannot be value-free. This is an empirical point: no scientist can operate outside of their cultural framework. While scientists can and should check their assumptions and try to limit overt bias (by double blinding the study when possible and other methodological interventions), there is no "objective" frame of reference that anyone can operate from. This is why the *community* aspect of scientific investigation is so important. Scientists check their work against each other—peer review, conference presentations, replication, etc.— to legitimate knowledge via communal practices. The rigor of the critical debate is largely determined by the parameters of who is included in discussion and which voices get uptake; those parameters dictate the extent to which biases and unwanted values can be interrogated and mitigated. This is how reliable knowledge is created: not by excising all values and assumptions, but by putting those values and assumptions to trial. Thus, science is argued by philosopher Helen Longino to be *better* when it is attentive to the inescapable inclusion of values in all aspects of scientific reasoning (see Longino 1990; 1993; 2002).

Science communications scholars have taken the communal construct-edness[4] of science further than the intercommunity dialogues highlighted by Longino and other philosophers of science. They emphasize the various non-scientific actors, institutions, and forms of knowledge that participate in what comes to count as properly scientific. Activists, lawyers and judges, farmers, patient groups, policymakers, and regulators, for example, all contribute to the bounding of scientific versus nonscientific (Jasanoff 1995; Bronson 2014).

So why does this ideal of value neutrality stick despite decades of science studies scholars discrediting both its plausibility and preferability? Kitcher suggests that the motivation behind the value-free ideal is an "allergy to public value-judgment" (2011a, 40). Tying the objectivity of science to freedom from values is based on the mistaken idea that value judgments are arbitrary and subjective—in other words, value judgment are incorrectly seen as not really a form of judgment at all, but merely an expression of preferences. The defenders of value freedom refuse to give ethical standards and other social values serious weight, a position that has motivated some philosophers of science, including myself, to work to rehabilitate the epistemic status of value judgments (see chapter 2).

Another reason that the value-free ideal sticks is because it supports existing power interests. The positivist notion that claims stand or fall in light of the evidence is certainly untenable; but positivist science is still productive in enacting truths because the method quiets supposedly empirically unfalsifiable considerations like moral claims and social value judgments.[5] As a result, so-called evidence based practice "operates with the implicit normativity that accompanies the production and presentation of *all* scientific facts left largely unchecked" (Goldenberg 2005).

## Linear Model of Science-to-Policy

The captivating scientizing thrust of evidence-based protocols has been demonstrated to have limited success in fully rationalizing normative decision-making
due to the inability of value disputes to be subsumed under scientific discourse.
We can now narrow the focus of this criticism to scientistic *policy making*, what
Pielke (2007) called the "linear model" of science-to-policy, in order to see the
full ramifications of scientistic reductionism of socially complex issues like
vaccine uptake and refusal. Not only is the linear model doomed to fail but the
current state of public resistance to vaccines predictably follows from the scientistic framework in which vaccine policies are justified and enacted.

In science policy studies, the linear model of science-to-policy is criticized,
much like the evidence-based framework, for wrongly assuming that the right
science leads to right policy action. This model quiets political debate by justifying the dismissal of political concerns and value differences. In this context,
those who are identified as promoting junk science[6] can have their political and
policy concerns dismissed in tandem with their science.

STS scholars have widely criticized the linear model since the 1990s, dis-
puting its primary assumption that science can and should compel political
outcomes. This view of the relation of science and politics has been called "the
linear model" because it posits a straight trajectory between getting the science
"right" and then making correct decisions (Pielke 2004a; Sarewitz 2004). In
doing so, the linear model mischaracterizes scientific explanation as potentially
complete or exhaustive in describing empirical phenomena (scientism). The
problems with the linear model are therefore twofold: (1) it endorses scientism (a
mischaracterization of science); (2) it promotes linearity (a mischaracterization
of the science-to-policy relationship). The result is political paralysis, because
science gets politicized while politics gets scientized, thus creating the conditions
for the so-called war on science and political stalemates on important policy
issues.

### The Impossibility of Complete Scientific Explanation

Even if we grant the realist view that science can provide true descriptions of
empirical objects,[7] those descriptions will necessarily be limited by disciplinary
constraints and the interests motivating the inquiry and inquirer. Thus, there
may at any point be multiple characterizations of the same phenomenon, all

meeting methodological criteria for robustness in their own domains. This pluralism (see chapter 3) is due to the interpretive and incomplete nature (or what Waismann [1951] called the "open texture") of scientific findings. Waismann introduced the idea of science's "open texture" as a challenge to verificationism, the central philosophical doctrine of logical positivism, which maintained that only statements that are empirically verifiable (verifiable through the senses) are cognitively meaningful,[8] or else they are tautologies. The "open texture" of science challenges the presumed presence of a firm point at which a statement could be verified. Herrick and Jamieson (1995) have adopted the term to denote the inescapable incompleteness of scientific findings *in the policy context*, thereby explicitly criticizing the predominant linear model in environmental policy (see also Herrick 2004).

Waismann had argued that the "essential incompleteness" of empirical description lies in the many frames of reference that can characterize an observational event. For example,

> If I had to describe the right hand of mine which I am now holding up, I may say different things of it: I may state its size, its shape, its colour, its tissue, the chemical compound of its bones, its cells, and perhaps more particulars; but however far I go, I shall never reach a point where my description will be completed: logically speaking, it is always possible to extend the description by adding some detail or other. Every description stretches, as it were, into a horizon of open possibilities: however far I go, I will always carry this horizon with me (Waismann 1951).

Because true descriptions of empirical objects are inexhaustible, and one is not better than another for all purposes, Waismann concluded that it was impossible to provide complete descriptions of most empirical concepts. Empirical claims could therefore rarely be verified completely. What is critically difficult for policy making is that "more tests can always be demanded and additional descriptions can always be given" (Herrick and Jamieson 1995). It is because empirical concepts are open textured, Herrick and Jamieson explain, that science-based assessments of a policy-related issue are always open to charges of "sins of omission" (Herrick and Jamieson 1995; Herrick 2004), leaving the door open to political paralysis.

For example, political stalemate may be orchestrated by vested interests who insist that more research is needed to address missing considerations. Fossil fuel industry-funded climate change skeptics in the US have managed to stall carbon-reducing policy action by raising doubt about the science (Oreskes and Conway 2010). Yet, those missing pieces of scientific information persist because scientific explanation is never complete. The many ways nature can be carved out, explained, and explored guarantees that policy makers will encounter a plurality of scientifically defensible arguments with different policy implications. The sorting of possible interpretations and actions needs to be done through careful and accountable policy deliberation, a ranking of priorities that is not answerable by value-free scientific analysis. Furthermore, democratic political structures *ought* to ensure that this prioritizing of values, interests, and experiences be subject to publicly accountable processes.

To illustrate the challenges for linear model policy determinations, Herrick and Jamieson (1995) described acid rain policy analysis, where different and equally valid characterizations of aquatic damage from acid deposition are available: "If damages are stated in terms of the *number of lakes affected*, then projections of decreased deposition appear to provide a substantial decrease in damages. If the same projection is expressed in terms of *percentage of affected lakes*, then the decrease in damage appears less significant. If acidity is characterized in terms of pH rather than acid neutralizing capacity, then future gains would be smaller still. Moreover, the choice of a reference pH value can radically alter the number of acidic surface waters" (Herrick and Jamieson 1995, 108 [emphasis in the original]). The example illustrates that numerous decisions must be made regarding the framing of the problem, all of which differently impact the outcome that will then inform policy. The framing of the problem alone is enough to justify the claim that science is not value-free. There are more points along the research trajectory, however, that are value laden: methodological decisions, interpretation of data, drawing conclusions, etc. Scientific research is thereby rife with values.[9] Against the appeal of the linear model and the promise of evidence-based policy, science does not deliver incontrovertible answers; the evidence does not "speak."

To continue with acid rain policy, which measurement provides the objective numbers that could promote nonpartisan political agreement? The "open texture" once again obstructs the scientizing ideal of evidence-based policy: "A national scale assessment gives short shrift to regional 'hot spots'; a focus on chronic acidity produces a different perspective than one including short-term episodes; analyses dealing with the current situation may inadvertently miss longer-term processes threatening future degradation; and monitoring for direct effects does not preclude the possibility of indirect or synoptic effects. Still another consideration is whether chemical acidification has actually harmed aquatic life" (Herrick and Jamieson 1995, 108). The authors contend that all these measures are valid, and no single one or combination of them is intrinsically more correct than the others. Therefore, arguments over the characterization of aquatic damage from acid deposition have the potential to last indefinitely, as political opponents will always have grounds for arguing that the other side's scientific analysis is incomplete. This tells us that scientific considerations alone cannot compel closure of the political problem by rationally directing policy (Herrick and Jamieson 1995, 108). Instead the myth of singular, action-directing science does violence to democratic politics. The act of extracting a single reality from a welter of possibilities is a normative pronouncement on what matters and how things ought to be.[10]

## The Scientization of Politics and the Politicization of Science

The linear model mischaracterizes science as singular and definitive and promotes a consequent relationship between science and policy that does not hold. The linear relationship is aspirational, carrying with it many of the same rationalizing ambitions of evidence-based practices. But like the evidence-based movement, it cannot deliver without normative harm. There is ample research evidence showing that policy does not simply emerge from scientific under-standings (Jasanoff 1987; Wynne 1991). The relationship is more sinuous. Consequently, when scientists, healthcare workers, and public health officials proclaim the linear model, there is the potential to undermine both science and policy decision-making. Because resolving scientific debates is thought to resolve political conflicts, science "becomes a convenient and necessary means for re-moving certain options from a debate without explicitly dealing with disputes over values" (Pielke 2004b).

   To illustrate how the linear model's mapping of scientific findings onto policy action limits political and policy possibilities, Pielke draws from the global cli-mate change debate (as it stood circa the early 2000s). Because of the scientized nature of the political debate, scientific studies showing meaningful connections between greenhouse gas emissions and actual projected climate changes are quickly interpreted to be supportive of actions to reduce emissions. Similarly, studies that cast doubt on the significance of such connections are interpreted as challenging the need for action (Pielke 2004a; 2004b). By mapping scientific findings onto policy action, the linear model limits consideration of policy al-ternatives and possibilities for action.

Indeed, the model frames political debate around climate change such that both sides argue about science as a proxy for actually discussing the worth and practicality of possible alternative courses of action, of which the Kyoto Protocol is but one of many. Opportunity is lost here for consensus at the policy level, as many critics may accept the science but not the terms of the protocol. Where do these concerns get voiced? Such an airing of unease could reasonably inspire new policy options that could gain wider approval than Kyoto. Climate science research would be crucial for this policy exercise, as climate science can offer meaningful outcome projections on various policy actions. This resource does not get utilized; instead, climate science is used to *limit* policy options. Thus, in addition to limiting practical action, the linear model ensures that the science is underutilized in the policy context, thereby undermining the social value of science.

This mapping phenomenon helpfully explains why popular environmentalism (i.e., blogs and other environmental awareness and activism media) pays such close attention to individual studies and technical debates over, say, the significance of surface versus tropospheric temperatures: the scientific conclusion is supposed to *compel* action. Action is then narrowly defined as the Kyoto Protocol (the Paris Accord was only signed in 2015, years after Pielke conducted this research) and the political stakes are understood as victory in either securing or denying its implementation.

Even if science *did* provide "just the facts," those "facts" would still operate normatively in policy contexts. The open texture of science guarantees that the facts that enter policy deliberation are selected based on the priorities of the decision makers. The vigorous public debates over scientific facts are therefore warranted insofar as these are embedded in prior choices about what experiences and points of view matter. The presumed firmament of value-free facts allows facts to function as "arbiters of which issues are open to democratic contestation and deliberation" (Jasanoff and Simmett 2017). In the present day "war on science," the fights over facts (now impudently called the "post-fact" era)[11] occur because facts are "vehicles through which polities imagine their collective futures" (Jasanoff and Simmett 2017). No wonder we fight over science and no wonder those battles are so feverishly pitched. Science has become the language of political victory and defeat.

Thus, the scientization of controversy comes at the expense of political activity by trying to sidestep the important work of sorting out competing values and building consensus through compromise. Writing on the politics of climate change, Sarewitz (2004) has provocatively claimed that "science makes environmental controversies worse." By this he means that the value disputes hidden behind the scientific claims and counterclaims do not get proper airing in democratic deliberation. Until that happens, he warns, "the political system will remain in gridlock, and everyone will be convinced that they are on the side of truth" (Sarewitz 2010).

Political stalemates are therefore a product of the confines of the linear model and the promise of evidence-based everything. Under the linear model, science matters because it dictates which policies are acceptable and which ones are not. However, policy decision-making does not require the convergence of science and policy action; there are ample examples where general agreement on science has failed to generate consensus on political action (Sarewitz and Pielke 2000). The currently unfolding COVID-19 pandemic is one example, with the chain of causation from virus to illness firmly established but the political response for mitigating infection and reducing mortality remaining deeply contested.[12] There are also instances where disagreement on the science has not precluded consensus on action (Sarewitz and Pielke 2000). Policy decision-making can happen even in the face of scientific uncertainty; science can assist in mapping out contingencies—what could happen, how likely, and what action should follow if the hypothetical future scenario actually materializes. There are numerous decision supports and multi-criteria assessment techniques available for policy purposes. All similarly identify different criteria of relevance to the decision in question and some methods additionally assign weights to these criteria to arrive at a score or ranking for various decision options.

Andy Stirling's multi-criteria mapping (MCM) is an example of such decision support techniques (Stirling 1997). MCM assists policy makers by "mapping" the issue in question—outlining the relevant issue, identifying different perspectives and priorities—and ranking different policy options according to the priorities attached to various criteria derived from different stakeholders' perspectives on the policy question. MCM can provide two sets of insights for policy makers. By drawing from a wide pool of respondents, policy makers are less likely to overlook points and perspectives. MCM can also reveal surprising points of agreement between what at first sight might seem like very different and opposing perspectives. Stirling illustrated this surprise convergence in a deliberative exercise on electricity supply options (1997) and in a study of alternative views about GM crops (Stirling and Mayer 1999). In the former case, Stirling found that respondents largely agreed that the UK's small proportion of renewable energy in its electricity supply mix (about 3 percent) was insufficient. Only respondents who assigned low priority to environmental costs and to diversity in electricity supply sources found the current low proportion of renewable energy to be acceptable. Thus, there was room for political movement in increasing renewable energy sources despite the seeming impossibility of resolving conflicting views on environmental issues. In the latter study, the authors found widespread dissatisfaction with conventional agricultural systems across all perspectives, and a generally positive attitude toward organic agricultural systems, suggesting room for a consensus-based decision moving forward.

These multi-criteria evaluation techniques can be used by a variety of stakeholders to ensure that a broad representation of perspectives is available to policy makers. Indeed, the marshalling of science to generate scientific certainties paradoxically reveals an underutilization of science in the policy domain. Scientific utility is undermined by the linear model of policy decision-making. Policy analysis is similarly underutilized, as reductive policy decision-making does not permit nuanced integration of various stakeholders' concerns, interests, and assessments of risk in a robust and democratic way. Rather than bypassing politics by way of science, the technocratic approach to policy making shuts democratic discourse down. Rather than a war on science, it is a war on democracy (Jasanoff and Simmett 2017).

It is when science fails to settle the political debate—and past experience and science communications research have afforded us the well-grounded expectation that science *will* fail to do so—that the strategies move from *scientize* to *politicize*. This is evident in the areas of both vaccine criticism and vaccine advocacy. Vaccine-skeptical positions have long been politicized, as the minority position inevitably needs to fight for legitimacy against the scientific weight of the orthodoxy. The techniques used to gain legitimacy do not follow the accepted practices of dissent and disagreement within scientific communities. Instead, vaccine critics select scientific studies that support their views while ignoring the majority that do not, play up minor risks associated with vaccine use, use poor logic to support their views, and enlist dubious experts on vaccines (CBC Radio 2017). Vaccine critics have largely waged a public relations effort targeting the publics and policy makers to gain traction for their views. In recent years, vaccine advocates have likewise shifted to explicit politicization; facing frustrating pushback from vaccine refusers, many have endorsed a "hardline strategy" for promoting vaccine uptake (Rainford and Greenberg 2015), which includes physicians refusing to take on unvaccinated patients and calls for severe restrictions or elimination of nonmedical exemptions for vaccines. Some want to take the hard line further, to include isolation (restricted access to public spaces), fines, and jail time (Kayyem 2019).

## A PROXY FOR WHAT?

The promise of science-driven practice and policy has failed to engender peace and prosperity and has instead generated conflict and political paralysis. Vaccine and public health advocates are uncomfortably aware that the twenty-plus years of concerted effort to correct the damage to public confidence in vaccines created by Wakefield et al.'s notorious paper and the concurrent thimerosal controversy in the USA has not been very successful. Instead, political controversy around the science that lies at the center of the debate has *grown*.

There has been little willingness to challenge that central place of science in political disputes. The recently coined terms "post-truth" and "post-fact" are now popularly used to explain our tumultuous times (Davies 2016; Fukayama 2017). The war on science will end, embattled defenders of science insist, only with the rightful reestablishing of scientific expertise and a return to "truth." Yet there never was a reign of "truth" and "science" to which we can return. "Facts" have never been uncontested entities that unilaterally dictate right action. More importantly, the heated public conflicts over vaccines, climate change, and GMOs are not about science, despite the many interests that have insistently framed the conflicts as such. The war over science therefore predictably exacerbates conflict rather than minimizes it, as the values that are at stake in science-policy debates cannot get proper consideration, and policy alternatives are narrowed to map onto supposedly decisive science. This scenario has been damaging to science, policy, and democracy.

Scratching beneath the surface of the evidentiary disputes, one finds those critical of the science consensus trying to say something about how science and technology are incorporated into our lives. To illustrate, Bronson's (2013) insightful ethnographic work on Saskatchewan farmers' conflicts with agro-corporation Monsanto over seed biotechnology captures how, despite the courts and regulators failing to see otherwise, the farmers' resistance to the new technology was not about the science or the technology per se but about the broad social impact on their livelihoods and the food supply.

Where regulators, steeped in the deficit model, perceived farmers to be ignorant of the complex science, the farmers instead viewed crop biotechnology more holistically—that is, with consideration of a wide range of social, political, and cultural implications. They described, in detail, the limitations of the current working conception of risk within biotechnology regulation, specifically, a reductionist framing of biotechnological risk that focused on the safety and efficacy of gene transfer. They also resisted the normative implications of seed patents, namely the social cost of designating food sources as "intellectual property." The farmers held an ecological view of risk that included the impact on the quality of food produced, seed and food biodiversity, and community relationships (i.e., what would happen if farmers could no longer share and save seeds) (Bronson 2014). One farmer explained that "the problem is not gene transfer, but the domination of a crop biotechnology 'value system' over the agricultural research and regulatory agenda at the expense of alternative ways of organizing life." She elaborated: "Biotechnology is a different value system. The whole value around clean fields, monocultures, maximizing production, not a weed in sight . . . the thousand apples all looking exactly the same way . . . it's part of a general cultural bias which permeates the whole agricultural system from research to implementation towards privatizing, standardizing and industrializing everything" (Interviewee in Bronson 2013; 2014). This alternative view has not successfully entered the Canadian legal and regulatory framework, as was seen in the unsuccessful countersuit by Saskatchewan organic farmer Percy Schmeiser against Monsanto in 2004 (see Bronson 2014).

Vaccine-hesitant and -refusing parents harbor safety and efficacy concerns about vaccines, but those concerns stem not so much from scientific ignorance (indeed, parents know what the consensus is on vaccines) but from higher order concerns and cultural anxieties that do not receive airing in regulatory and policy contexts. Concerns about the how technology shapes our lives, regulatory capture, increased privatization of essential services, loss of the natural, family autonomy, health justice and inequalities, and historical public health injustices in relation to racism and colonialism rest on the margins of debates over vaccination safety and efficacy. These issues are not captured in the regulatory frameworks around risk and are surely unnoticed by those who insist that public resistance to scientific claims stem from ignorance about science. The dispute was never about the science alone.

In short, these criticisms are not "antiscience," because the science in dispute is only a placeholder for the values we hold dear. Even when the opposition is wrong about the science, it is still not necessarily the case that the opposition is "antiscience." It is instead indirect acknowledgement that science is not only a rational process but also a social and political one. Science, then, "is persistently vulnerable to contingencies that some critics might think they foresee more reliably than others" (McWilliam 2015).

Additionally, the legacies of evidence-based everything and scientized politics have made the language of science the currency of political discourse. Thus, the opponents have little recourse for expressing disapproval other than by challenging the science. To get past scientized politics and political stalemates, we need an alternative language for framing the debate (as something other than science) and venues for genuine normative debate. That effort will now be explored with the development of a new framework for understanding and addressing vaccine hesitancy.

# PART II

## A CRISIS OF TRUST

# 5
## TRUST AND CREDIBILITY IN SCIENCE

After virtually eliminating many serious and sometimes deadly infectious diseases, the US public health system has seen a recent increase in vaccine preventable diseases. Growing numbers of parents are either delaying or selectively administering these vital immunizations—and a few are choosing not to vaccinate their children at all. These trends reflect diminished public trust in the system that protects all of us against the timeless threat of communicable diseases—and the result is dangerous and costly outbreaks that are poised to grow worse in the future.

— **American Academy of Arts and Sciences**

While it is not uncommon to hear that vaccine hesitancy and reduced vaccine uptake stem from poor public trust (American Academy of Arts and Sciences 2014b; MacDonald et al. 2015; Dubé et al. 2016; Siddiqui et al. 2013; Yaqub et al. 2014; Corben and Leask 2018), it *is* uncommon for the implications of this widely accepted claim to be rigorously studied. In broad discussions of vaccine hesitancy, poor trust typically appears on the laundry lists of the multiple causes of this phenomenon. But this finding does not get carried into strategies for addressing the problem, which are still largely fact-based interventions aimed at addressing perceived knowledge deficits.[1] How do we address poor public trust as a determinant of vaccine hesitancy?

The empirical research into trust and vaccines is limited in both quantity and quality. A 2018 systematic review (Larson et al. 2018, "Measuring Trust") uncovered only thirty-five papers that used the concept of "trust" in their vaccine-related research question or aim, and within that sample, trust was often ill-defined and loosely measured. Most studies left as implicit the definition of

trust, and methodologically weak single-item measures were commonly employed despite the easy availability of more rigorous multi-item validated psychometric measures for health-related trust. A 2013 systematic review identified and
evaluated forty-five such measures (in Larson et al. 2018, "Measuring Trust"). So
why was a key concept left undefined, and why were the best measurement tools
underutilized by researchers? The 2018 review concludes that the prevalence of
methodological weaknesses "indicates that a thorough understanding of trust
as it relates to vaccine acceptance is currently underresearched." Lying beneath
the poor framing and execution of the research, I would add, is poor theorizing
about trust.

Interest in opening up research into trust and vaccines seemed to have
motivated the publication of the American Academy for the Advancement of
Science's (AAAS) 2014 report on vaccine hesitancy, *Public Trust in Vaccines:
Defining a Research Agenda* (2014b). The report did not convey the usual "war
on science" trappings, offering instead more sensitive attention to the contexts
in which vaccine hesitancy and refusal can arise, persist, and grow. The paper
was premised on the belief that increased numbers of American parents delaying or refusing vaccines reflected diminished public trust in "the system that
protects all of us against the timeless threat of communicable diseases" and
that providing accurate information about vaccines is not enough to engage
and persuade vaccine hesitant parents (AAAS 2014b, 1). The proposed research
agenda was directed toward building an evidence-based toolkit for communications with anxious parents regarding vaccines. Those communications were,
importantly, meant to be dialogical, rather than didactic. The communications
toolkit would need to be informed by research into (1) parental attitudes and
knowledge about vaccines; (2) optimizing the medical encounter; and (3) identifying and intervening in communities with high risk of disease outbreaks.This
public trust research agenda also required the theoretical grounding for empirical research to employ, yet the *Public Trust* report did not adequately provide
such theorizing.

Indeed, despite having "public trust" in its title, the AAAS report said very little about trust. No definition of trust was offered, nor was there reference to the
trust, public trust, or health-related trust literatures. Minimally, the definition of
trust appeared to be implicit in the report's agenda-setting effort to address the
publics' "vaccine confidence gap" (7).[2] Addressing the vexing question motivating the report, "Why do parents say no?", the authors offer a "myriad of reasons"
why parents request personal belief exemptions. They are:

Belief that vaccines are unnecessary due to unfamiliarity with the diseases
     they prevent
Broad vaccine safety concerns
Concerns regarding rare vaccine side effects
Questioning of the efficacy of providing vaccines to healthy individuals
Concerns about overloading children's immune systems
Preference for "natural immunity"
Desire to "hide in the herd" (or "free ride" on the collective immunity of
     the highly vaccinated community)
Preference for alternative medicine practices
Distrust of the medical system, science, and government recommendations

Here, distrust was listed as only as one reason why parents may choose not to
follow recommended vaccine schedules (7). Yet it is incorrect to think that the
problem of trust is only endemic to those with broad suspicions of science and/
or medical and governmental institutions—a line of thinking often disparaged
as "conspiracy theories." Instead, all but one[3] of the items listed as reasons for
vaccine hesitancy suggest a problem of trust, specifically a lack of confidence
in those experts and institutions conveying the message that vaccines are safe,
effective, and part of a broader public health strategy worth supporting. Expert
scientific testimony does not satisfy many people's vaccine concerns, and vaccine hesitators address those points of uncertainty by incorporating alternative
testimonies from unorthodox sources.

   Why is it that public trust only appears as a last bullet point on the listed myriad reasons why parents refrain from vaccination? My thesis is that this compart-
mentalizing of the problem of trust, rather than centralizing it in characterizing
vaccine hesitancy, stems from underappreciation of how trust pervades science,
its institutions, and relations of expertise both within scientific communities
and in relation to the publics.

   This chapter resists such a deflated analysis of trust, which merely cycles
back to the problem of biased reasoning discussed in chapter 2. Such reductive
accounts of the problem of public trust misconstrue the nature of science, whose
successful operations rely on the consonance of trust and credibility (the *perception* of trustworthiness). Here, I investigate the extensive relationships of trust
in science, seeking thereby to add theoretical substance to the understanding of
trust operating in empirical vaccine hesitancy research and research agendas.

## DEFINING TRUST

The exploration of public trust in scientific institutions, and its link to vaccine hesitancy and refusal, must begin with an articulation of what is meant by trust. The concept is heavily theorized across multiple disciplines, especially ethics, philosophy of science, and social theory. Ethics emphasizes how trust underscores interpersonal relationships, social theory stresses trust as precursor to society, and philosophy of science attends to the necessity of trust for knowledge formation and acquisition. Notable scholarly attention to trust has been offered by feminist theorists in all these domains, due to the long-standing feminist focus on relational aspects of morality, knowledge production, and social structures, especially relationships involving imbalances of power between participants.

These multidisciplinary investigations generally converge on the definition of trust as *having confidence in someone or something*. Trust in the context of science may be directed at a variety of actions or behaviors, like trusting a colleague to store their harmful chemicals properly, but most of the discussions about trust in and within science refer to *epistemic trust*: "To invest epistemic trust in someone is to trust her in her capacity as provider of information" (Wilholt 2013). When we trust a person, organization, or institution, that is, deem them to be trust*worthy*, we are judging them to be dependable and worthy of our confidence. Moral theorist Annette Baier (1986) made the influential distinction between trust and mere reliance on another, explaining that when I trust you, I exercise a kind of relying that makes me *dependent on your good will*. This distinction highlights the vulnerability that comes with trusting others. Philosopher of science Torsten Wilholt (2013) adopts Baier's distinction for considerations of scientific practice and argues that epistemic trust is not mere reliance; instead, the trustor is dependent on the trustee's goodwill. And just like the interpersonal relationships that Baier and other ethicists were more interested in, Wilholt maintains that this epistemic dependence on other people's good will makes the trustor vulnerable to being misled or harmed. In science, vulnerability arises because this trust requires deferring to others "about something beyond our knowledge or power, in ways that can potentially hurt us" (Whyte and Crease 2010, 412). It can be difficult to trust the judgments and actions of others that directly affect our own welfare (Crease 2004, 18).

Trusting others requires a careful negotiation of vulnerability and confidence. To trust is to hold the optimistic attitude, or confidence, that the trustee will competently perform the task with which they are entrusted;[4] even more, we expect the trustee to be favorably motivated[5] to do the task well because they know we are counting on them (Jones 1996, 4). With that confident expectation of the trustee's moral and epistemic character (to demonstrate good will and competent work) in place, we trust a friend or professional with something important to us. Yet there is no guarantee that they will do it, which makes the trustor vulnerable.[6] The trusted expert has the power to abuse that trust and to exploit those who trust them. It is with this risk in mind that trust is widely thought to be rightly hard-earned. Those who want to be trusted must convince others of their trustworthiness, and those who must trust are reasonably skeptical of strangers as well as those who have previously betrayed their own or others' trust. Even when trust is conferred it may need to be continually reaffirmed.

This account best describes trust between participants who are in a direct, or one-to-one relation to each other. When considerations of trust expand to community-wide trust and trust in institutions, such as a marginalized population's trust of health systems, the relations of trust become more complex. Even if patients trust their physicians, they may not trust the medical system that their healthcare provider represents. This can be due to current or historic injustices experienced by their own communities or by other populations. Trust might falter even among witnesses of healthcare injustices who are not themselves members of communities that have suffered them.

The risks associated with trusting others are inescapable. Everyone finds themselves in situations where we lack adequate information to know for ourselves, and so we must take the risk of trusting others. Those risks can be managed and minimized, but never eliminated. Philosopher Onora O'Neill explains that "elaborate measures to ensure that people keep agreements and not betray trust [such as contracts and professional codes] must, in the end, be backed by—trust. At some point we just have to trust" (O'Neill 2002). This is more than a transactional limitation. Nineteenth-century sociologist Georg Simmel argued that "without general trust that people have in each other, society itself would disintegrate." Yet very few relationships, he explained, are "based upon what is known with certainty about another person, and very few relationships would endure if trust were not as strong as, or stronger than, rational proof or personal observation" (1900/1978, 191). While there can be penalty for betraying trust, the harms experienced by those who were betrayed may never be fully compensated. Trust cannot come with absolute guarantees that those who are trusted will fulfill their commitments. According to O'Neill, "trust is needed precisely because all guarantees are incomplete. Guarantees are useless unless they lead to a trusted source, and a regress of guarantees is no better for being longer unless it ends in a trusted source." Trust cannot guarantee proper behavior by those we trust. In fact, "Where we have guarantees or proofs, we don't need to trust. Trust is redundant. We don't need to take it on trust that 5 x 11= 55, or that we are alive, or that each of us was born of a human mother or that the sun rose this morning" (O'Neill 2002). This statement is not a restating of the assumption underlying the war on science metaphor, that scientific facts speak for themselves and therefore are outside of the purview of trust. Trust enters into knowledge transactions when, and because, issues are more complex. When seeking information and advice, the expert (discussed in chapter 3) is thought to be valuable for their advanced skillset for solving complex problems. Their ability to decipher, or make meaning, despite indistinctness or obscurity is supposed to be more sophisticated and informed than that of nonexperts. There is, then, a prima facie argument for following expert advice, that is, trusting experts. The risk of betrayed trust, however, is still a problem.

The tension between the unavoidability of trusting despite the risk makes trust ripe for ethical analysis. When we find ourselves in situations where we lack adequate information to know for ourselves—and this happens often—we must trust others. Knowing the risk that our trust might be betrayed requires what has been described by some sociologists as "leaps of faith" (Lewis and Weigert 1985; Mollering 2006; Brownlie and Howson 2005).[7]

This "leap" refers to the necessary bridging of an information gap in situations of risk, where any perceived knowledge gaps are filled with "a kind of suspension or bracketing-off of uncertainties" (Brownlie and Howson 2005). Trust is thereby in large part an affective commitment to something or someone, as cognitive understanding is unavoidably incomplete in the face of future unknowns (Giddens 1990). Knowledge is both generative and interpretive, and knowledge experts are trusted (or not trusted) for their interpretive skills. Qualitative research into the reasons parents give for their vaccination choices have highlighted multiple "leaps" taken in the face of incomplete knowledge, and anxiety over those future-directed uncertainties. Parents take a trusting leap or withhold it based on advice from relations of familiarity such as peers, family members, and health professionals; the leap also depends on perceptions of the trustworthiness of scientific bodies or institutions.

Importantly, it is not the growing mountain of data that are leading parents to vaccinate their children, but their willingness to "leap" in favor of the scientific consensus. Similarly, vaccine hesitators and refusers situate themselves in communities and social circles that disqualify the majority view on vaccines. There is symmetry in the decision-making processes of both vaccine accepters and refusers. It is not the case that vaccine accepters are scientifically literate while refusers are not; nor does the former group demonstrate more critical thinking while the latter is more prone to biased reasoning. Instead the calculations these parents make aim for in-group belonging, much in line with the cultural cognition thesis for information processing discussed in chapter 2. For example, Elisa Sobo's (2015) anthropological research on vaccine-refusing parents at US Waldorf schools highlights a cultivated value-set, identity, and lifestyle among Waldorf parents that includes vaccine rejection; there are similar findings among vaccine refusing parents in Southern and Western Australia (see chapter 2) (Ward et al. 2017). Parental decision-making on vaccines is not merely a cognitive exercise; it is historically informed and culturally situated. It is along similar lines that Baier describes trust as cognitive, affective, and conative (Baier 1991), whereby trust is rationally determined to some extent but also emotionally and purposefully assigned.

Trust arises in community and operates as a means of social cohesion—"the willingness of members of a society to cooperate with each other in order to survive and prosper" (Stanley 2003). This conceptualization of trust as social cohesion (see Misztal 1996) is useful when contemplating the operations of trust in scientific communities as well as for understanding the role of trust in public controversies over scientific claims. Cohesion, in the form of shared understanding of issues, assessment of risk, or agreement on actionable policy is notoriously difficult to achieve. It is trust that builds the necessary bridges.

## TRUST WITHIN SCIENCE AND IMPLICATIONS FOR EPISTEMIC RIGOR

"It seems paradoxical that scientific research, in many ways one of the most questioning and skeptical of human activities should be dependent on personal trust. It is intensely skeptical about the possibility of error, but totally trusting about the possibility of fraud. Without trust the research enterprise could not function. . . . Research is a collegial activity that requires its practitioners to trust the integrity of their colleagues" (Relman in Schechter et al. 1989). Trust and skepticism are typically understood to be opposing factions in the pursuit of secure knowledge. Skepticism is thought to underscore the epistemic superiority of scientific modes of inquiry—seen, for example, in Popper's laudatory "critical attitude" for scientific investigation (Popper [1963] 2002)—while trust is counterproductive for rigorous research. Thus, former *New England Journal of Medicine* editor Arnold Relman's comment that "without trust the research enterprise could not function" offers a paradoxical provocation. How can science be both epistemically rigorous and lax? Furthermore, isn't intellectual temperance something we want to avoid?

Popular histories of the scientific revolution and the birth of modern science extol the iconoclastic heroes of science, such as Copernicus and Galileo, who eschewed the dogma of the day—specifically the beliefs of the Catholic Church regarding planetary motion—and let the evidence "speak" (Kuhn 1962). Kuhn described this "fable" of strictly rational science, that is, science proceeding by dispassionate reasoning from observation to theory, as the "textbook image of science" in the first of his 1951 Lowell lectures (Marcum 2005; Galiston 2016). He was referring to the brief histories of science that appear in the opening pages of science textbooks. In this narrative of science, trusting the word of another offers no epistemic merit and potentially undermines rigorous efforts to know.

The venerable Royal Society of London, established in the 1660s by Sir Robert Boyle and other "natural philosophers" interested in the new empiricist philosophy of observation and experiment that we now call science, maintains the motto *"Nullius in verba"*—"on the word of no man"—to capture this iconoclastic sentiment. Today, the society's website describes the motto to be "an expression of the determination of Fellows to withstand the domination of authority and to verify all statements by appeal to facts determined by experiment." This phrasing evokes independent skeptical inquiry as fundamental to reliable knowledge acquisition. This image pervades much philosophical thinking in the Western tradition on models of rationality and intellectual responsibility—Descartes's methodological doubt, for instance, and Kant's ([1790] 2016) maxim "think for *oneself*" in order to avoid error.[8] It should be no surprise that many of us find it intuitive to think that studying for oneself is a better means for gathering reliable knowledge than accepting the word of another person.

Despite its initial appeal, this model of rationality ("epistemic individualism"), and its accompanying solitary or solipsistic thinker whose knowledge claims are reliable insofar as they are based on their own examination of the issue, has been strongly criticized. Social epistemologists argue that atomistic epistemic frameworks fail to acknowledge the social nature of knowledge production and acquisition. Even science, which allegedly utilizes the most objective methodologies for knowledge inquiry, is argued to rely on relationships of trust and epistemic dependence between scientists. In "The Role of Trust in

Knowledge," philosopher John Hardwig (1991) rejects the presumed knowledge/ trust antithesis of epistemic individualism and argues instead that trust is endemic to modern scientific knowledge (693). He writes, "In most disciplines, those who do not trust cannot know; those who do not trust cannot have the best evidence for their beliefs" (694).[9] He had similarly argued in a previous paper, "Epistemic Dependence" (Hardwig 1985), that without deferring to epistemic authority, we would have to suspend judgment on most things. The case for a social account of knowledge, which makes room for trust in the testimony of others as part of legitimate knowledge acquisition, becomes compelling, as sticking with epistemic individualism would require the "unpalatable" concession that much of science is not knowledge, as it relies heavily on claims made by other people (Hardwig 1991, 696–97).

The large research team, now ubiquitous in scientific research, serves as a case study in epistemic dependence and undermines the prima facie appeal of epistemic individualism and its accompanying solipsistic thinker as a model of rationality. In 2015 a scientific paper was published in *Physical Review Letters* with a record breaking 5,154 coauthors (Castelvecchi 2015).[10] The wide body of contributors suggests that no single person could have the knowledge or work hours required to conduct such a large-scale and complex experiment. Similarly, no single scientist has the knowledge to oversee the experiment and test the experimental findings in their entirety. Yet, barring methodological problems, we are inclined to accept the resulting research findings as science. Knowledge production thereby requires relationships of trust between collaborators: I trust my colleagues to do their work rigorously and to report it honestly, and they similarly trust me to do the same.

Because collaborative research and the knowledge it generates rely on trust, it is cooperation, rather than self-reliance, that is "the key virtue in any scientific community" (Hardwig 1991, 706). Epistemic cooperation builds knowledge on the testimony of others rather than limiting its acquisition to self-study. In science, Hardwig similarly writes, "scientific propositions must be accepted on the basis of evidence that only others have . . . because the relevant data and arguments are too extensive and too difficult to be had by any means other than testimony" (706). Knowledge is built collaboratively, with the ideas of others undergirding new ideas. Much of the supportive data is taken on trust because limits on time and the demands of highly specialized knowledge inhibit anyone's ability to figure it out on their own.

One need not limit consideration of trust in science to the contemporary

context of large research teams; historical research suggests modern science has
always operated this way. Historians Steven Shapin and Simon Schaffer (1984)
highlight the epistemic role that trust played in the formation of experimental
science in seventeenth-century England. Even in the hands of archetypical epistemic individualist and modern scientist Robert Boyle and his colleagues in the
*Royal Society*, considerations of trust dominated the intellectual environment; indeed, they were central to the rise of the new experimentalism. Specifically, trust
defines the boundaries of the peer group, which allows the science produced
within this community to be regarded as objective[11] and thereby trustworthy.
The Royal Society membership at that time was comprised of English aristocratic men. It was only a person of means that could fund his own experiments,
but Shapin and Schaffer argue further that the *social and economic circumstances*
of the gentleman rendered him trustworthy.[12] It was thought that the gentleman's privilege made him independent, and that by being beholden to no one
save the monarch, he had little compulsion to lie. Furthermore, truthfulness
and trustworthiness were considered basic to the identity of the gentleman—a
gentleman really was as good as his word. Because the members of the Royal
Society characteristically upheld these gentlemanly virtues, these trust relations
between members were able to operate invisibly beneath the guise of objective,
empiricist methods (see also Shapin 1995). Like the collaborative scientists today,
the gentleman's methods, measurements, and findings were presumed to be both
epistemically sound and truthfully shared with the rest of the community.

This argument for trust in science might strike some as counterintuitive, as
Enlightenment thought disrupted hierarchical knowledge. The concurrent rise
of modern epistemology—Descartes and the rationalists as well as the British
empiricists in seventeenth- and eighteenth-century Western Europe—and
experimental philosophy (as science was called at the time) were motivated
by a desire to unbind the individual knower from dependence on forms of authority, especially religious doctrine. The political climate was inching toward
democratic principles of rule and egalitarianism, a trend reflected in the strong
epistemic individualism of early modern philosophy. Thus, modern science arose
out of a crisis of trust—"the need to find foundations for knowledge that would
survive [these] challenges to authority" (Scheman 2001, 34). The solution was
found in the novel conceptualization of an individual generic knower who could
come up with the same answers as others by use of proper method. The epistemic
individualist detailed in Descartes's *Meditations* ([1641] 1993) and *Discourse on
Method* ([1637] 1998) could pursue knowledge in solitude with the confidence

that careful compliance with epistemic principles and methodological rules would produce universal results.

Surely then, one might object, modern science is grounded in objective methodology rather than trust among peers. But Shapin and Schaffer's analysis strongly suggests, and elsewhere Naomi Scheman (2001) has argued explicitly, that *trust lies at the center of discussions of objectivity*.[13] We can accept that proper use of the same method will lead you and me to arrive at the same conclusion, but I need to trust *you* to exercise that methodology without error or willful bias in order to obtain that same result. These worries about the trustworthiness of others were what made epistemic individualism attractive. Checking one's colleagues' methods and results is meant to ensure objectivity, that is, to *rationally ground trust* in the work of others. Yet this ideal is rarely met. In Boyle's time, and even more so today, replication of experimental results has been impractical. New knowledge builds on previous knowledge. We would rarely be able to create new knowledge if every knower replicated every experiment in which the results contributed to something they took themselves to know. Thus, the trust scientists take in the testimony of others is, to some degree, a leap of faith. Even those findings vetted by peer review or replicated by others do not pass the test for "true knowledge" for the epistemic individualist. The researcher is now placing trust in others' testimony that the knowledge claim is credible. The reader would not know for themselves to any degree suitable to epistemic individualism.

This finding, that considerations of trust pervade experimental science (both past and present), is troubling for the strong tradition of epistemic individualism, as this epistemic framework understands the use of any such "leap of faith" modes of belief acquisition to be inferior cognitive processes that result in something other than knowledge (even if we generate true beliefs). Returning to Hardwig's damning challenge that the tenets of epistemic individualism discredit the epistemic strength of scientific inquiry and practice, we might save science (as Hardwig hopes to do) by considering our dominant epistemic model to be flawed. We have mischaracterized how we come to know things and should accept instead that trust is a legitimate part of knowledge acquisition.

The cases made for trust and epistemic dependence provide a rational grounding for an epistemology of expertise (Hardwig 1985; 1991; 1994), that is, for establishing good reasons to trust the testimony of experts rather than rely on one's own limited knowledge base. Hardwig appears to force the hand of the epistemic individualist regarding the rationality of accepting expert opinion. Even those who believe that the best way to formulate reliable knowledge is to inquire diligently into the subject matter must recognize that there will be occasions where we have good reasons to trust others in possession of the necessary evidence to justify a belief more than we trust ourselves (Hardwig 1994, 84). There is far too much knowledge available for any one person to know. To study any issue for ourselves often requires consideration of extensive amounts of evidence, much of which is only accessible to those with advanced skills cultivated over years of study and practice. Someone who has invested the time and energy into a particular area of scientific pursuit will likely have better understanding and judgment than those who have not been similarly committed to that area of study. It is prudent to rely on the expertise of others rather than to rely on one's own often inadequate self-study or to suspend judgement on just about everything. The large research team example demonstrated how hearsay evidence is often the best evidence *anyone* can have, rather than being a poor second-best substitute for direct first-person evidence (Hardwig 1994).

This account of scientific knowledge production and acquisition has undermined the idealized account of evidence linearly guiding scientific belief (see chapter 4). Instead, scientific knowledge is marked by the social: the people who do science and their interpersonal dynamics, the social forces that deem some voices credible, and so forth. This is not to say that there are no reliable scientific findings, or that method is secondary to in-group politics; the claim is rather that reliable science is established within the everyday of social dynamics. The reliability of science may still hold, but our accounts of how they are established require rethinking—away from objective in the sense of "value-free" accounts of science in favor of something more grounded in the social (see, for example, early and agenda-setting investigations into social epistemologies of science by Fuller [1987; 1988], Goldman [1997], and Longino [1990]).

## MISPLACED TRUST WITHIN SCIENCE

So far, we have established that there can be good reasons to trust others' knowledge claims rather than rely exclusively on our own investigations. There are rational grounds for epistemic trust for the purpose of knowledge acquisition. But acknowledging trust within scientific communities is still unsettling because trust is so often misplaced. Misplaced trust threatens the integrity of science. Fraud, for instance, can go unnoticed for longer than it should. Indeed, when research misconduct makes headlines, pundits will usually lament the problem of trust in science. For example, in an interview with CNN following his exposure of Andrew Wakefield's research fraud, journalist Brian Deer responded to the question of how Wakefield managed to get away with fabricating data in the following way: "Well, that's one of the great weaknesses of medicine and medical publishing, is that people can publish things that are false. People talk about peer review and such like. And they imagine [there's] some kind of safety system. But, in fact, the whole system works on trust . . . And so, it is actually possible for a determined cheat to get away with the kind of behavior that Dr. Wakefield has been involved in" (CNN Transcripts 2011). How do we determine trustworthiness? Because it is a presumption of goodwill and competence that warrants trust in another, the reliability of the trustor's belief depends on the reliability of the expert testifier's character (Hardwig 1991, 700; Smolkin 2008). An expert is trustworthy if they are: *honest* (truthful in their claims); *competent* in their domain of expertise; *conscientious* (careful and thorough in their work); and *capable of epistemic self-assessment* (recognizes the extent of their own knowledge, its reliability, or its applicability) (Hardwig 1991, 700.) The first quality, honesty, or the effort to be truthful, is part of the testifier's moral character, while the latter qualities—competence, conscientiousness, and self-reflectiveness about one's knowledgeability—speaks to their epistemic character.[14] Character judgments are made via personal interactions with the expert in question or from assessments by others of the individual's qualities (Hardwig 1991).

Yet misplaced trust stemming from poor character judgment is not limited to the occasional misfire where a cheat gets away with it but is arguably built into our everyday cognitive apparatuses. Psychologists and social epistemologists have pointed to gender and racial biases that position people to overestimate the epistemic and moral character of some people, while underestimating others. Kristina Rolin (2002) takes the underrepresentation of women in science to stem from such explicit and implicit biases. In a critical response to Hardwig, she argues that trustworthiness and credibility (the *perception by others* of your trustworthiness) often do not line up. Hardwig discusses only trustworthiness, that is, the qualities of the testifier's character and assumes that those qualities are transparent to others—either by familiarity with the testifier or by way of accurate character assessments offered to us by others. But investigations into pervasive cognitive biases seriously challenge the accuracy of such character assessments. Therefore, "[Hardwig's] criteria of reliable scientific testimony need to be revised. A reliable testifier is distinguished not only by honesty, competence, conscientiousness, and epistemic self-awareness, but also by properties that indicate to others that the testifier has these virtues" (Rolin 2002, 112). Hardwig had demonstrated that trust relations in science were not damaging to science's status as a knowledge-seeking enterprise so long as the trust was allotted reasonably. Rolin demonstrates that assignments of trustworthiness will often be misplaced. Both the problems of scientific misconduct and implicit bias follow from poor judgments of the epistemic and moral characters of others, resulting in a mismatch of (actual) trustworthiness and credibility. This finding should highlight that the effort to match trustworthiness and credibility is an underappreciated task when it comes to ensuring the success of scientific communities. The rationality of science depends on it.

## PUBLIC TRUST IN SCIENCE

When members of the public consider action or policy on science-based questions—is this water safe to drink? Will reducing the speed limit on city streets save lives? Is the recommended vaccine schedule safe for children?—the publics are arguably well advised to defer to scientists with expertise in the specific area in question (Hardwig 1985; Collins and Evans 2007; Goldman 1987; Anderson 2011). Their specialized knowledge makes it likely that their judgments will be better than our own (Hardwig 1985). But epistemically dependent members of the publics have many of the same vulnerabilities as scientists involving relations of trust.

Whereas, within scientific communities, trust operates behind the scenes in establishing and legitimating knowledge as universal (true for everyone), trust plays a more visible role in the science-publics exchange. This is the site where vaccine controversy takes place. When the channels of knowledge transfer, translation, and mobilization work well, this move from expert advice to nonexpert action can go smoothly. We are talking about vaccine hesitancy because relations between experts and nonexperts are not so secure.

While the publics benefit from well-placed trust,[15] the challenge is knowing when trust is well-placed. Where nonexperts lack the capacity to check the scientific claims for accuracy—if we could comprehensively check those claims, we would arguably not need expert advice—nonexperts *can* evaluate the character of the scientific expert or the integrity of the institutions they represent. The character determinants are the same moral and epistemic qualities that scientists look for in each other. The publics need to determine that the expert is properly motivated, that they have the interests of the publics at heart (Mollering 2001), and that they have the knowledge and professional competence to act on that good intention. In short, the rationality of following expert advice hinges on trust and credibility: experts must be trustworthy and nonexperts must recognize them as such. Relations of trust mediate successful exchanges between scientific institutions and the publics.

The publics need additional trust beyond confidence in the epistemic and moral integrity of the individual expert; trust is also needed in the integrity of expert institutions to work in the publics' interest rather than in the further-ance of alternate agendas that are oppressive or unjust. Public trust in science demands socially responsible science that is transparent about the interests it serves and aware of its own histories of power and privilege. This demand harkens back to the discussion of facts and values in chapter 2, specifically the relationship of epistemic values and social values in science. Insofar as science is not value-free, public trust hinges on the value set that influences scientific research (but does not determine scientific conclusions). Those values include not only epistemic rigor but also equity and social responsibility. Several models of socially responsible science have been offered by philosophers of science, in-cluding Janet Kourany's (2010) "ideal of socially responsible science" and Long-ino's (1990; 2002) "social values management." There are numerous accounts of how rigorous science and equitable social values intersect offered by feminist empiricist philosophers of science (e.g., Antony 1993; Solomon 2001; Wylie and Nelson 2007). Discussion and evaluation of these models are beyond the scope of this investigation (see Kourany 2010, chapter 3 for a comparative review of these models; see also Brown 2020).

The charge of death of expertise (chapter 3) is tantamount to saying that the publics are not good judges of character. Indeed, everyone suffers from lapses in judgment. Members of the publics are, again like the scientists within a research community, also prone to misjudging the trustworthiness of scientific experts. We may dismiss the research and recommendations of diligent and honest sci-entists, or we may follow the advice of a so-called expert unworthy of our trust (see chapter 6). Members of the publics also harbor memories of false assurances by scientists and public officials that reasonably inform current decision-making and make the provision of trust in experts exceedingly difficult. Some examples include insistence by government officials about the safety of eating British beef during an outbreak of Bovine Spongiform Encephalitis (BSE or "mad cow dis-ease") (Carrington 2000) or drinking tap water in Flint, Michigan (Clark 2019). Put simply, trust and mistrust travel (Grasswick 2018). That skepticism might lead to better nonexpert decision-making but can also fuel wholesale rejection of the scientific establishment or poorly placed trust in persuasive charlatans. Indeed, "whether scientists actually are trusted by ordinary citizens is a different issue than whether scientists should be trusted" (Whyte and Crease 2010). As Rolin has argued, trustworthiness and credibility do not always line up.

Here again, the moral and epistemic tensions surrounding trust are visible. While trust is still ineliminable, and sometimes suspect, the public context is slightly different than intracommunity trust insofar as trust relations are maximally visible due to the outsider status of the publics. The publics are not scientists with specialized insider knowledge, thus making the vulnerabilities associated with epistemic dependence more apparent.

## SCIENTIFIC CONSENSUS

It is shocking to many vaccine advocates that the scientific consensus on vaccines does not settle public concern. The scientific consensus represents the position generally agreed upon at a given time by most scientists specialized in the field. It does not suggest unanimity among the community of experts, and it does not terminate further investigation into the area where consensus has been achieved (although there may be a momentary "closure" [Pinch and Bijker 1984]). The rigor and reliability of the scientific consensus is grounded in its methods for building consensus and its openness to further review and revision in light of new evidence. Through communal and communicative practices, which include communication at conferences, peer review and publication of papers, replication of reproducible results by others, and scholarly debate (Laudan 1984) collective agreement and consensus can arise. These methods not only catch error and fraud but invite an airing, and sorting through, of points of disagreement and dissent. Engaging with criticism and alternative points of view can strengthen collective knowledge and consensus claims (see Longino [1990; 2002] on "transformative criticism"). The consensus is the best approximation of scientific truth, offering a testament of the current state of knowledge, an accounting of the scientific community's relationship to that knowledge claim, and, at times, public directives for guiding good political choices and policy action with informed scientific assessments.

Much is made of the scientific consensus in publicly charged science policy debates. This is most visible in climate change debates, where the 97 percent consensus claim is a particular flashpoint. The 97 percent consensus, popularized by science communicators John Cook and colleagues (2013), is heavily debated by proponents and opponents of climate mitigating measures. Both sides of the climate change debate are invested in the measure because public perception of and action on climate change are thought to be influenced by the degree to which the publics accept the claim that 97 percent of climate experts[16] agree that climate change is anthropogenic (Cook et al. 2018). There is ample evidence that "manufacturing doubt" is an effective means of stalling political action (Oreskes and Conway 2010), and so casting doubt on the degree to which scientists agree on climate change is fodder for environmental inaction. To counter misinformation about climate change, the *Climate Consensus Project* (Cook et al. 2018) uses the clear and numeric message of 97 percent consensus, and the now-ubiquitous pie-chart graphic, to rally public support for climate action. This effort builds on the tenet that effective science communications require simple and clear messages, repeated often, by a variety of experts (Cook et al. 2016). The expectation is that convincing the publics that 97 percent of climate experts believe in anthropogenic climate change will lead to public acceptance of the position as well as motivate political action to mitigate the phenomenon's damaging effects.

This expectation is grounded in some of the scientistic thinking that was criticized in the previous chapter regarding the linear progression from science to action and does not fully acknowledge the role that trust plays in both building the scientific consensus and in promoting public uptake of consensus claims. To appreciate the connection between the scientific consensus and trust, science must (once again) be understood socially. Knowledge building, including the generation of consensus, is a socially managed exercise.

Because knowledge is produced in communities, disagreement between members are to be expected. Science even encourages it: dissent and disagreement are widely understood as signs of healthy epistemic enterprise. The avenues for managing dissent and disagreement in science follow from a generally accepted democratic orientation toward truth-seeking and consensus building: one that is public and accountable. Social epistemologists view these mechanisms favorably and even make recommendations to *improve* the democratic tenor of science, for example, by increasing diversity in scientific communities to make dissent and criticism more robust (Longino 1990; 2002). They also suggest measures to limit spurious dissent that is meant to be obstructionist rather than knowledge seeking (de Melo Martin and Intemann 2018). With these communicative practices in place, a robust scientific consensus can arise on some issues, while points of disagreement can still respectfully endure without rupturing community cohesion.

In marked contrast, science controversies on the public stage are not as well-managed. Here there are no comparable shared rules for the management of disagreement and for consensus building. There are no shared frames of reference; instead, we have facts and alternative facts, disagreement about which side offers legitimate science or junk science, and which of the opposing experts are credible. The consensus does not motivate public solidarity around scientifically informed directives, neither neutralizing political partisanship nor rationalizing democratic decision-making. Instead, the consensus gets positioned as one side of a debate, where scientific experts must jockey for legitimacy against seemingly disreputable opponents who claim to have science (and moral credibility) on *their* side.

We should appreciate the scientific and policy establishments' surprise and frustration regarding equivocal public uptake of strong consensus claims. The consensus functions to settle debate, not invite it, by representing the majority view of those most suited to pronounce on the issue. Consensus claims can also educate the publics and promote personal and political action. The failure to achieve these aims is no doubt frustrating. Doesn't the consensus deserve more deference? It is the best approximation of scientific truth, because it is produced by the best of science's truth-seeking procedures and practices. The universal applicability of the findings presented to the publics rests in the methods of consensus building. For members of the publics to question the consensus is to reject an elaborate set of epistemic, methodological, and institutional mechanisms meant to ensure reliable knowledge and public benefit from that knowledge. Science isn't something you are supposed to "believe" in or be against. To say otherwise is to say that science depends on trust.

But it does.

My key claim is that much of what members of the publics know about vaccines pivots on epistemic trust.[17] Tied into the scientific consensus is a claim to the epistemic and moral legitimacy of its authors and their institutions. Vaccine hesitators question those claims and more strident vaccine refusers reject them.

What is the appropriate response when the consensus does not fulfill its function of engendering public trust? This is what happens now: vaccine hesitators and refusers are ridiculed for raising concerns, questioning expert testimony, and taking seriously minority dissenting opinion. Against the democratic tenor of science, science journalists write articles like "This is Why You Have No

Business Challenging Scientific Experts" (Mooney 2014a) to convey sincere disgust over the current state of affairs. Why, vaccine supporters ask incredulously, would anyone take the word of a media-savvy celebrity mom who attributed her knowledge of autism to the "University of Google"[18] over *many* expert scientists?

We know that the consensus is an expert-generated directive for epistemically dependent outsiders: it is meant to offer the scientific information that we need to know. Yet the mechanisms used to ensure the trustworthiness of that information—the negotiation of conflicting views in academic conference settings and in expert journals, replication of findings, peer review, and so on—are internal to the scientific community and are therefore largely shielded from public view. Thus the final step in the expert-lay exchange, where (if all goes well) the publics accept the scientific consensus view, requires some degree of a trusting "leap of faith" that the scientific experts have done their due diligence and reported responsibly. The trust requirement places the outsider in a vulnerable position. There is no sympathy for this challenging predicament. The publics are implored to *trust science*: trust in a process where trustworthiness lies in it being shielded from public opinion or other nonexpert contributions (Scheman 2001, 34). Without an eye on or participation in the innermost practices of scientific knowledge and consensus building, with various threats of sanction for *not* accepting the findings, the publics are instructed to trust. But trust is not built upon threat or mockery, and some people are not willing to trust in these circumstances.

## SOURCES OF MISTRUST

There are many reasons why members of the publics may not trust the scientific consensus on vaccines. Here, I focus on three serious sources of public mistrust that are known to impact public attitudes regarding vaccines: (1) social media, (2) medical racism, and (3) commercialization of biomedical science. The first, social media, is widely recognized by vaccine promoters as a serious threat to vaccine confidence. The latter two deserve more attention and response than is currently given.

### Social Media

Despite vaccine hesitancy being recognized as multicausal, social media is widely regarded as central to the problem. These platforms host easy-to-find sources of vaccine misinformation and spread the content effectively by targeting forums for new parents. A December 2018 report by the Royal Society of Public Health (2018) suggested that half of all surveyed parents with small children have encountered vaccine misinformation through social media. The thinking seems to be that since people do not understand the science, they are easily misled by vaccine misinformation. Research does show that online anti-vaccine messages have a negative impact on vaccine-related attitudes and behaviors. For example, parents who search vaccine-related information online tend to regard health professionals and organizations as less credible, perceive vaccines as less effective, and vaccine-preventable disease as less contagious than parents who do not use the internet for health-related information (Jones et al. 2012). A study of several thousand German internet users reported that five to ten minutes of exposure can heighten viewers' perception of risk associated with vaccine commission and lower the perception of risk associated with vaccine omission (Betsch et al. 2010). Parents who view vaccine misinformation are more likely to seek nonmedical vaccine exemptions for their children (Jones et al. 2012; Salmon et al. 2005). Furthermore, these media platforms allow vaccine skeptics to find each other, form community, and create noxious echo chambers that amplify vaccine misinformation and harden vaccine critical sentiments (Chiou and Tucker 2018).

As of 2019, many popular social media sites, including Instagram, Facebook, YouTube, and Pinterest, had bowed to pressure to exclude anti-vaccine content (Ortutay 2019; Tran, Alter, and Flattum-Reimers 2019). This is a positive measure, because online vaccine-critical content is so visible and so influential. But technical solutions like scrubbing content and flagging questionable sources will not solve all challenges. When parents make vaccine decisions, the trusting leaps or refusals they make are surely influenced by the misinformation peddled on the internet; however, those dubious claims only gain traction because they fit with a broader narrative of perilous healthcare. Informed news consumers are well-aware of problems in health research and practice. The replication crisis, the weaknesses of the peer review system, profit-driven disease mongering (Payer 1992; Moynihan and Henry 2006), and lawsuits against pharmaceutical companies are part of health consumers' background knowledge. Parents draw on these narratives when they evaluate new information about vaccine risks. Prior trust will impact whether the consensus view on vaccines is accepted.

Informed news consumers are also well-aware of the uneven quality of online information. This invites the question, why do parents seek information outside of the standard expert sources like professional medical bodies and public health agencies? More specifically, why is it that the clear and simple scientific consensus claims on vaccines, repeated and reproduced in official communications, are not satisfying the information needs of parents to make a confident decision about their children's vaccinations?

## Medical Racism

Trust in systems of expertise is known to vary among communities given historic and contemporary interactions. The WHO's SAGE Working Group on Vaccine Hesitancy acknowledges that trust in vaccines varies across populations (SAGE 2014). Research exploring lower rates of influenza vaccination among Black American adults compared to white American adults has highlighted lower levels of trust that are a result of historic racial injustices (Freimuth et al., "Determinants of Trust," 2017; Freimuth et al., "Role of Risk," 2017; Quinn et al., "Exploring Racial Influences," 2017; "Determinants of Influenza Vaccination," 2017; Lindley et al. 2006). Friemuth et al. ("Role of Risk," 2017) have found that "while factors including poverty and insurance status were important factors in vaccine decisions, participants were more likely to cite barriers to care as a secondary reason for not getting vaccination, while issues related to vaccine confidence and vaccine trust were a more immediate concern." Quinn et al.'s ("Exploring Racial Influences," 2017) examination of attitudes regarding influenza vaccines found the clearest racial divide in vaccine confidence between white and Black participants' different levels of trust in government's role in vaccination. This finding is consistent with the broad sociological literature demonstrating Black American adults to be significantly less trusting of government than white adults due to historical and contemporary experiences of discrimination and racist social norms (Smith 2010). In healthcare, the distrust in the system stems from a long history of medical racism and abuse and is reinforced through experiences of discrimination that continue to this day (Freimuth et al. 2001). Studies have confirmed the impact medical racism and events like the Tuskegee Syphilis Study have had on trust in medical research (Corbie-Smith et al. 2002; McCallum et al. 2006), trust in physicians, and on trust in the healthcare system more broadly (Alsan and Wanamaker 2017).[19] Minority status and high levels of distrust also are associated with increased acceptance of conspiracy theories (Quinn 1997; Corbie-Smith et al. 1999).

There is also a long history of violence against minority groups in the name of public health. For example, in late nineteenth-century San Francisco, Chinese

immigrants were scapegoated for smallpox, leprosy, and malaria and subject-
ed to harsh quarantine measures after city officials incorrectly attributed the
outbreaks to Chinatown's "vapors" and overcrowded conditions (Trauner 1978).
Minority groups have frequently been targeted for public health and social reform purposes. Examples include: early twentieth-century eugenics programs
aimed at "race betterment" (in Canada, see McLaren 1990; in the United States,
see Engs 2000; 2003, 275–78);[20] the destruction of neighborhoods deemed
"unsanitary" (e.g.,. Bacher [1993][21] and Swope [2018] [22]); coerced sterilization
of Indigenous women in Canada (Stote 2012); and child apprehension policies
regarding mixed-raced Aboriginal children in Australia (McGregor 1997). These
policies were considered, at the time, to be progressive public health reforms.
The most extreme application, Nazi racial purification policies,[23] incited a global
rethinking (but not entire elimination) of those ideas and practices (Kuhl 1994).
Public health, medicine, and health science institutions must continue to reck-
on with this dark history in its current practices. People today remember those
past abuses, and scientific and medical racism still persists (Frakt 2020). Many
public health practitioners know their discipline's history, including many of the
problematic elements that I have highlighted. Public health practice must, however, constantly affirm the commitment to redress this injustice. Knowing that
much of the public skepticism encountered today is historically rooted requires
accepting that there are reasons why some members of the publics do not regard
public health measures as progressive or benevolent.

    The greatest difference between white and Black participants in the influ-
enza vaccine focus groups was attitudes regarding government's motives in vaccination programs (Quinn et al. 2016; see also Jamison et al. 2019): "A common
refrain from black focus groups was, 'You don't trust a government vaccine' or
'don't trust the government for nothing' (AAFNT-FG). This distrust extended into
conspiracy theories including beliefs that the government was experimenting on
minorities as 'guinea pigs,' that the vaccines were being diluted and distributed in
Black communities, or that vaccines were a form of population control. Additionally, the legacy of the Tuskegee Syphilis Study emerged in every focus group as
a justification for distrust." The historical injustices and harms experienced by
marginalized communities at the hands of health and government institutions
informs contemporary distrust (Grasswick 2010; Scheman 2001). Knowledge
or experience of these fraught histories make it reasonable to demand more evidence of goodwill and honesty from the experts, as well as of the reliability of
the research in question.

If vaccine conversations were approached with the understanding that members of the publics, especially members of historically and currently marginalized communities, have reason for skepticism, the discussions could certainly go differently. Research into vaccine hesitancy shows that parents are uncomfortable accepting expert advice on vaccination without proper information and discussion (Evans et al. 2001, 907). Consideration by health providers of the historical and social contexts of the people and communities they serve can help calibrate the levels of information and kinds of discussion appropriate for different patient populations.

Rather than leaning on the strength of science for justification, a more careful treatment of parents' and patients' concerns could (and should) be undertaken. This is a mild strategy in comparison to addressing the structural issues that undermine trust but could nonetheless be an effective way to build trust in order to improve vaccine compliance.

More substantive efforts to rebuild trust involve bringing equity, antiracist justice, and access to the forefront. The health of populations depends on rebuilding trust for historically oppressed people. Priority must be placed on expanding representation in meaningful positions in science and public health at every level, including the highest. *Equity is paramount to making public health impactful.*

## Commercialization of Science

There is ample research into financial conflicts of interest in health research (Sismondo 2018; Goetzsche 2013; Moynihan and Cassells 2005), healthcare education and practice (Lexchin 2017; Elliott 2004), and health technology regulation (Lexchin 2013; Piller 2018). The research details many past and present cases of those conflicts of interests being poorly managed by industry, academia, and regulatory bodies, with scandalous harms to patients (Welch 2011; Lenzer 2017). Efforts to counter these so-called "pharmascolds"[24] (Shaywitz and Stossel 2009) by arguing that critics make overly emotional and unsubstantiated claims regarding the harms from financial conflicts of interest (Rosenbaum 2015a; 2015b; 2015c; Stossell 2015) are comparatively weak.[25] So is the insistence that critics of industry-funded biomedical research fail to appreciate the public benefits that come from the pharmaceutical sector (Rosenbaum 2015a; Stossell 2015; Shaywitz and Stossell 2009). The critical scholarship into financial conflicts of interests in biomedicine provides ample evidence in support of the need and viability of conflict-of-interest regulation and does so with the aim of maximizing the public benefits that biotechnology industries offer. The charges of overemotional "scolding," "outrage" (Rosenbaum 2015a), and "pharmaphobia" (Stossell 2015) are ad hominem attacks rather than serious engagement with the issues. Profit-driven pharmaceutical and medical device companies have indeed produced life-saving technologies, but they have also perpetuated the current opioid crisis (Armstrong 2019) and medical device scandal (Bowers 2018) amid lax regulatory oversight (Goodnough and Sanger-Katz 2019; Lenzer 2017).

Vaccine-hesitant parents have made it abundantly clear that their uneasiness about vaccines stems in part from distrust of commercialized health science and healthcare. The issue comes up repeatedly in social scientific research on vaccine-hesitant parents (many sources are cited in chapter 1).Vaccine-promoting media pundits tend to dismiss those concerns. One common refrain is that unlike pharmaceutical blockbusters, vaccines are not profitable, and therefore people need not harbor "Big Pharma" safety concerns. However, vaccines are profitable (Lam 2015).[26] Another common response is to minimize the risks associated with commercialized medicine. In a *Chicago Tribune* op-ed titled "There is No Other Side to the Vaccine Debate" (Caplan 2015), bioethicist Arthur Caplan swiftly dismissed the spurious vaccine-autism link, and then treated public concern about industry-influenced medicine with similar disdain. He wrote: "Then there is fear of Big Pharma. People think vaccines are some sort of conspiracy on the part of the pharmaceutical industry to make money by injecting us all. As a proponent of vaccines and a fierce critic of anti-vaccine claptrap, I constantly get told that I must be in the pocket of pharma (I am not), on the payroll of pharma (nope) or support organizations that take pharma money to promote vaccination (guilty)" (Caplan 2015). Why treat a fabricated theory and a well-documented problem as two of a kind? It is an interesting sign of these us-versus-them times that the pharmaceutical industry has been placed on the side of angels and public distrust of pharmaceutical companies attributed to the machinations of conspiracy theorists. Meanwhile, the publics have seen huge class action settlements and recalls of blockbuster drugs like Vioxx and Celebrex. Inquiries into serious adverse events and even deaths, thoroughly detailed by the media, have revealed such unethical industry practices as hiding data, failure to publish negative results, stealth advertising, political lobbying, and financial conflicts of interest (Sismondo 2018).

The media has also reported on the far reach of pharmaceutical influence on medical research and educational grants, medical schools, and continuing medical education programs. This has raised concerns about bias in physicians' prescribing practices and knowledge base. These biases are well known within medicine. They are disliked by the general publics. Yet the offensive practices remain commonplace. It is not off-the-grid conspiracy theory blogs and websites reporting these findings. Instead, these criticisms are coming from within academic medicine, where insiders like Drs. Marcia Angell (2005), Peter Goetzsche (2013), and Ben Goldacre (2012) are calling for change.

We can accept Caplan's point that the pharmaceutical industry has done a lot of good for human health and well-being; the industry, as he points out, invented aspirin, cancer drugs, and of course, vaccines. While most us do not want to give up on lifesaving and health-promoting medications, healthy skepticism about the industry that produces them should *not* be shut down. Instead, more ethical and regulatory oversight is needed to counter influence and lobbying. This is a public trust and safety issue that demands action.

## IMPACT ON VACCINE DECISION-MAKING

Anthropologist Sharon Kaufman (2010) describes parents as "bricoleurs" in their sorting and selection of information (as well as fragments of rumor and folklore) in order to build a coherent narrative of vaccines and to be good parents.[27] The "myriad of reasons" (AAAS 2014b) why parents hesitate regarding vaccines reflect the incorporation of alternative epistemologies of health regarding vaccines into parents' thinking about the issue. Scientific claims are often present in these curated understandings of health, but they do not fully define parents' understanding of vaccines in relation to good parenting practices.

The current climate of parental decision-making regarding vaccines is difficult. The AAAS report on vaccine hesitancy nicely describes the noisy public stage on which vaccine controversy plays out: "A welter of voices—in medicine, government, politics, media, churches, schools, and among one's family and friends—can confuse well-meaning parents who want to do the best for their offspring. Online forums, where appeals to emotion often drown out thoughtful discussion, also play a role in vaccination decisions" (AAAS 2014b, 3). While those dissenting, questioning, and confusing voices do make the decision-making process more difficult, it is due to poor trust that the institutions tasked with protecting the public good are not able to carry out their mandate. The consensus does not fulfill its function of guiding parents' understanding and behavior, steering well-intended parents out of the fray by offering the definitive directive on vaccines.

There is general agreement that the publics need science, but my point is that it goes both ways. Science needs the publics too. The fulfilment of many institutional mandates hinges on positive public relations. Science strives to create universally applicable knowledge, and this knowledge is universal only insofar as it is accepted by various stakeholders. This places a demand on scientific communities to earn and maintain the trust of the publics.

Research institutes and agencies rely on stable relations with the outside, at minimum to ensure access to public research funds and to enjoy little interference with their work. When that minimal level of public trust is in place, science can operate smoothly. In policy-relevant science—research motivated by practical goals like furthering human, animal, and environmental welfare—there are more elaborate ties to the publics. These practical goals require scientific claims to be accepted by stakeholders outside of specialized epistemic communities (Scheman 2001; Wilholt 2009; Whyte and Crease 2010). Policy relevant science can only provide those public benefits if its institutions are regarded as trustworthy by members of the publics.

For example, public health science can only improve population health if the general publics largely accept and follow its recommendations. Health recommendations and consensus statements bank on the publics' trust in these institutions' conscientious and honest efforts to inform and protect. Political scientists refer to this as "social capital" (see Bjørnskov 2006; Gilson 2003; Rothstein and Stolle 2008). Offering the best science and the most carefully considered action-directives are not enough. The science must be trustworthy, but also trusted by public health stakeholders. Persistent vaccine hesitancy indicates institutional failure to engender and/or maintain public trust. This warrants self-reflection on trust-building practices by these institutions.

## TRUST IN SCIENCE

The evidence that most members of the publics accept regarding vaccines turns crucially on epistemic trust. Poor trust in the expert sources engenders vaccine hesitancy. What if focus shifted to building that trust rather than educating the misinformed publics or puzzling over their moral and epistemic failings? Doing this would not discount that public health agencies have the science on their side. Instead it means that we must recognize that the best science is not enough. This is not a war with the publics or a war over science. I have offered a different picture of science in relation to the publics than that of science singularly steering rational political organization. Science should still be understood to hold firm ground,[28] but the idea that the *evidence speaks*, or dictates right policy, is a fiction. All evidence is subject to interpretation, and political and policy decision making requires numerous nonscientific considerations. The language of "evidence-based" is misleading in that respect. Scientific evidence operates within a constellation of social and historical influences that guide personal decision-making and policy formation. Good trust relations ensure that science stands prominently within policy frameworks. The current tendency of criticizing the skeptical publics for failing to appreciate the primacy of scientific reasoning and the rightful authority of experts does not address the problem of public mistrust of scientific institutions. If anything, it exacerbates the mistrust by entrenching a polarizing us-versus-them mentality.

# 6

## THE SCIENTIFIC EXPERT
## AS HERO AND MAVERICK

The account of trust in science, especially public trust in science, developed in the last chapter invites a recasting of the problem of expertise first described in chapter 3. In characterizing the problem of expertise, all discussants agree that experts are not venerated like they used to be (although the reverence was never absolute), and that the shift in status has been recent and swift. But where I disagree with most of the commentaries is in the conclusion that expertise is dead. Instead, I argue that expertise has proliferated, albeit to encompass unorthodox sources. Current public scientific controversies do not arise within, or due to, an expert-free zone. Instead public resistance to scientific claims arises within the space of a trust deficit.

In this space, alternative expert voices emerge, often powerfully, capitalizing on public uncertainty or ambivalence and stoking those sentiments. When members of the publics are reluctant to take the "leap of faith" (see chapter 5) in favor of the scientific consensus view, some will energetically pursue alternative expert sources instead. Others remain somewhere in the middle, unsure of whom to believe. Where the orthodox scientific experts' word was once seen as authoritative,[1] the current state of science-publics relations does not afford them this kind of reverence. This downgrading of expert authority, and concurrent ascent of unqualified opinion influencers, is not due to conceptual confusion regarding the

nature of expertise (the position of Collins and Evans [2007]). Instead, the shifting of who is seen as holding expert authority is due to inattention by traditional
expert institutions to two of the three sources of mistrust in science discussed
in the previous chapter: 1) scientific racism, discrimination, and injustice and 2)
financial conflicts of interest in health research and practice. The third source,
social media, was described in chapter 5 as both a generator of mistrust and itself a
product of poor trust in conventional sources of scientific and health information.
In a reinforcing cycle, people pursue unconventional sources of health information because they are not satisfied with official expert communications. That
initial mistrust may then be strengthened by persuasive online misinformation.
I had posed the question in the previous chapter as to why people seek health information from unconventional online sources at all, and pointed to the other two
sources of mistrust, discrimination and financial conflicts of interest, as causative.

Yet expert response to vaccine hesitancy focuses mostly on social media and
not on discrimination and conflicts of interest. Vaccine proponents use their
scientific expertise to debunk vaccine myths while communicating the message
that online sources vary in quality. These efforts are not enough, because they
miss the pressing question of *why* social media is seen by many media-savvy
users to be a good resource for health information. My thesis is that the answer
to this question lies largely in the neglected sources of mistrust. Furthermore,
the advice offered by public health communicators to concerned parents to limit
their searches for health information to expert-sanctioned resources may further
alienate the skeptical publics who are unsatisfied with those expert sources, as
it doubles down on the increasingly unpopular and condescending idea that
experts know best.

Health injustices and financial conflicts of interest increase public perception
that science does not always operate in the public interest. Scientific institutions
and agencies have not made adequate progress in addressing those sources of
mistrust, and the publics notice this. Health sectors continue to be nonrepresentative demographically and slow to address ongoing discriminatory attitudes
and practices. In American healthcare, for example, only 6 percent of physicians
self-identify as Black or African American (Tweedy 2015). Medical schools are
complicit in the poorer quality of healthcare received by Black patients compared
to white patients, by not prioritizing antiracism training and aggressively recruit-
ing trainees from diverse cultural, racial, and economic backgrounds. Studies
show that many American-trained physicians uncritically hold onto racist myths
about Black people's higher pain tolerance, which they bring into their clinical

practices. The same nineteenth-century pro-slavery myths perpetuated by physicians (Tidyman 1836; Cartwright 1851; Haller 1972) about African slaves' high pain tolerance to justify strenuous labor and corporal punishment practices persist in health practice today, where pain is undertreated in Black and Hispanic patients, including pediatric patients, compared to their white counterparts (Wyatt 2013; Goyal et al. 2015; Hoffman et al. 2016). A 2016 survey of 222 white American medical students and residents showed half of them to endorse at least one myth about physiological differences between Black and white people, including Black skin being thicker and nerve endings being less sensitive, thereby making Black people more resilient to pain (Hoffman et al. 2016). At issue is not just that harmful ideas and practices continue but that politically powerful professional bodies and medical schools have done so little to change the culture (Williams 2018).

The second major source of mistrust, industry influence on health research, continues unabated. The justifications typically offered are that health research is too expensive to carry out without corporate support and that the pharmaceutical and biotechnology industries are unfairly criticized. Public concern is thereby dismissed as unrealistic and uninformed. This discounting only reinforces the public sentiment that science and healthcare are elitist institutions that are just as capable of harm as they are of help. Any efforts by scientific bodies to counter those beliefs by insisting on their own legitimacy due to their good science misses the point. The "alternative" experts who are the focus of this chapter, however, understand this missed opportunity for public engagement and capitalize on public unease about organized science's goodwill.

Contrary to the death of expertise thesis, public science controversies unfold as a *clash* of expertise rather than a dearth thereof. Chapter 3 ended with a challenge to the claim that expertise is dead by way of the empirical observation that vaccine skeptics refer to their own experts and frame their arguments around expert opinion. The credibility of these alternative figures seems questionable to vaccine advocates, but it is still not the case that no one listens to experts anymore. Instead, the field of expertise has become more competitive, as it has enlarged to include nontraditional or alternative forms of expertise. Relied-upon experts may not hold the traditional credentials of established science, or they may be establishment figures promoting minority views. While orthodox experts tie their claims to rigorous science, alternative experts challenge the integrity of establishment research and introduce questions of power and privilege in regard to scientific discourse. This is jarring to many scientific professionals,[2] but it is salve to members of the publics who feel that their concerns about the goodwill of science are finally being recognized. The previous chapter highlighted the many similar trust concerns that arise between scientists and between science and the publics to show that trust permeates all facets of science—but I also noted some differences. Where scientists need to trust the epistemic and moral integrity of their colleagues in order to ensure the rigor of science, the publics cannot trust science on the basis of rigor alone. As outsiders, the publics cannot see the inner workings of science, which would presumably enable them to confidently know that it is performed rigorously. The goodwill of scientific enterprise—to improve lives and promote public interests—needs to be trusted as well. Scientific practice can proceed with methodological and empirical adequacy even when the broader ethical framework is unacceptable.[3] The publics want assurance that vaccine science is both epistemically and morally sound.

In order to explain the reconfiguration of expertise that has followed from the "problem of expertise," I will introduce a new character to the narrative of trust in science undertaken in chapter 5: *the maverick*. This scientific antihero contrasts the scientific hero, a familiar trope in science studies. The scientific hero has figured crucially in explaining the trust relationships that constitute modern scientific practice (see Shapin and Schaffer 1984). I propose that where the supposed death of expertise signals the demotion of the scientific hero, public mistrust advances the new antihero, the maverick, thereby creating a clash of experts on the public stage. The maverick is a reconfiguration of the scientific expert in the current crisis of trust in science. Andrew Wakefield, originator of the debunked autism-MMR thesis, serves as an exemplar of the maverick. Despite persistent attempts by the medical establishment to discredit him in an effort to calm public fear, Wakefield has a dedicated following and continues to influence public response to childhood immunization practices. To understand his appeal and why he is trusted by so many, we must look at institutional science's own credibility problem. With that, we complete the effort to reframe the problem of vaccine hesitancy by shifting the focus (and moral derision) away from the intellectual failings of the supposedly scientifically ignorant publics in favor of institutional failures to ground public trust. This new focus is useful for addressing the problem of poor public trust in scientific institutions.

## TRUST AND THE EXPERT/HERO IN SCIENCE

Trust was characterized in chapter 5 as both *invisible* and *ubiquitous* in the workings of science. But how does this complex picture of trust relations remain latent, obfuscated by a robust and seemingly compelling account of science as characteristically skeptical and untrusting? Shapin and Schaffer (1984) argued that trust relations operate quietly and pervasively in science by being tied to the Enlightenment-era image of the *scientific hero*—the trustworthy scientist whose observations reflect true or objective representations of nature. The scientific expert qua hero is central to trust in science.

Shapin and Schaffer saw the idealized figure of the scientific hero as underwriting objectivity in science, that is, science's unique epistemic ability to discern matters of fact. The birth of modern science came with new technological innovations that worked to justify science's elevated epistemic status. One of those technologies was scientific writing. Its stipulations were heavily formulated by Boyle in the late seventeenth century, and it is still employed today to convey the results of an experiment to an audience much wider than those who were physically present to bear witness to scientific advancement (see also Lareo and Reyes 2007; Shapin 1984). But with that social distance between the scientist and his[4] audience, "it was the burden of Boyle's literary technology to assure his readers that he was such a man as should be believed. He therefore had to find the means to make visible in the text the accepted tokens of a man of good faith" (Shapin and Schaffer 1984). Boyle promoted a sober style of writing that contrasted the rhetorical flourish of the philosophical tracts of the time. This terse literary style promoted a nobility of character in the author, permitting the writer to be seen as more interested in the advancement of "natural philosophy," as science was then called, than in furthering his own reputation. This added to the perception that the accounts were truthful (Shapin and Shaffer 1984). When coupled with the trust already afforded to the new experimentalists due to their status as gentlemen (see chapter 5), the objectivity of the scientific claim could be accepted. The author was trusted to describe nature faithfully—both as an honest reporter and an unconflicted observer. The confluence of new technology and class-driven expectation of virtuous character firmed up an image of a scientific hero and "modest man": a " man whose narratives could be credited as mirrors of reality was a 'modest man'; his reports should make that modesty visible" (Shapin and Schaffer 1984; Shapin 1984). Haraway (1996; 1997) similarly characterized the hero as a "modest witness," noting the reversed gendering of a traditionally feminine virtue (modesty) that was now uniquely *un*available to women. Women did not possess the ability to truthfully witness matters of fact, not due to inferior intelligence[5] but because they lacked the independent status of aristocratic men (Haraway 1997, 27). Only gentlemanly circumstance permitted cultivation of the strength of character required to do the important act of modest witnessing.

Modest witnessing was seen as one of the "founding virtues" of modernity (Haraway 1997), because it allowed the scientific hero to access immense knowledge. This virtue "guarantees that the modest witness is the legitimate and authorized ventriloquist for the object world, adding nothing from his mere opinions, from his biasing embodiment" (Haraway 1997, 24). With that, he was able to establish the facts by erasing his subjectivity: "He bears witness: he is objective; he guarantees the clarity and purity of objects. His subjectivity is his objectivity. His narratives have a magical power—they lose all trace of their history as stories, as products of partisan projects, as contestable representations, or as constructed documents in their potent capacity to define the facts. The narratives become clear mirrors, fully magical mirrors, without once appealing to the transcendental or the magical" (Haraway 1997, 24). The trusted and trustworthy scientific hero underwrote the objectivity of science. This is not to say that method and practice did not matter, or that scientific findings could not be challenged. The argument is that without the prima facie trust in the integrity of the scientist-hero (by other scientists and by the publics), modern science could not have gotten off the ground and established its epistemic dominance. Furthermore, this presumption of trust continues today.

The paradigmatic scientific hero, Robert Boyle, is thereby noteworthy in the history of science not only for his scientific research and pioneering work in experimentalism but also for his virtuous character. Boyle's successful influence in shifting science toward the new experimentalism was not merely because of the quality of his scientific work and the merits of experimentalism over field research for some areas of scientific investigation, but equally because of his reputation as a virtuous (and therefore truthful) gentleman (see chapter 5). In addition to this reputation, Boyle had the additional qualities of being pious and celibate and was therefore admired by many. His strength of character allowed him to be trusted in accurately describing natural phenomenon. His social standing permitted him to personify objectivity in science.

This focus on character undercuts the modern scientific norms of shunning appeals to authority in favor of empirical verification, highlighting once again modern science's paradox of trust and skepticism (chapter 5). Boyle's experimentalism demonstrated skepticism by introducing new social technologies to encourage transparency: the public witnessing of experiments, the scientific write-up, and replication of experiments. But the insufficiency of these techniques for reliably establishing matters of fact was obvious. The public experiments so strongly advocated by the Royal Society were rarely witnessed by more than a handful of practitioners (Shapin 1995). Even with a larger audience, eyewitness accounts are notoriously unreliable—a problem we still struggle with today in criminal court cases.[6] This makes the social technique of corroborating multiple eyewitness testimonies a tenuous means for establishing matters of fact. Scientific writing can mask deception, even when exposed to peer review,[7] and expensive and complicated machinery made replication a rarity even in Boyle's day (Shapin and Shaffer 1984).[8] Mechanical failure and the complexity of the experimental setup often did and still does serve to explain the inability to reproduce results.[9] And so, the gap between transparency and credibility in making universal claims was filled by trust in Boyle and other gentlemen scientists to report findings accurately. Experimentally produced phenomena became part of the stock of collective knowledge largely through the testimony of trusted authors. Those trust relations were rendered invisible, and experimental findings objective, precisely because those authors were so trustworthy.

And yet, the gentleman hero is an unsatisfying expert, for several reasons. His trustworthiness is tied to his birthright, rather than demonstrated merit, and the exclusivity of expertise (not everyone can be an expert) is not tied to meaningful demarcation. Instead trust in science is, by this account, unacceptably tied to power and privilege. How relevant is the scientific hero to contemporary science? This early modern figure seems anachronistic to contemporary scientific thought and practice. The scientific hero must be contemporized, and I do this by borrowing from feminist cultural theorist Maureen McNeil's (2007) analysis of genetics pioneer James Watson (of double helix fame) as the twentieth-century scientific hero.

## TRUST AND THE CONTEMPORARY SCIENTIFIC HERO

Although significantly modified, the image of the scientific hero persists today. McNeil's (2007) literary analysis of Nobel-winning geneticist James Watson's best-selling 1968 memoir, *The Double Helix*, offers a refiguring of the scientific hero in the later twentieth century. In her demonstration of how this text influenced subsequent scientist biographies, McNeil suggests that Watson normalized a few key tropes that characterize the modern scientific hero. The contemporary hero of science is now an "ordinary guy," heroic in his race for scientific knowledge, admirable for his scientific research contributions, but quite normal in his everyday life. Employing the popular literary genre of youthful adventure in memoirs, readers were invited to identify with Watson and encouraged to see his youthful mishaps and misdemeanors as amusing and even endearing. This counteracted popular images from literature and film of the scientist as "mad or bad" (McNeil 2007). Furthermore, it made science and the scientist accessible and appealing, which was conducive to gaining public admiration and support for scientific enterprise. The scientific hero qua "ordinary guy" also cast off the "vestigial clerical legacy" of the seventeenth-century scientific hero and displayed robust heterosexual activity characteristic of Britain's "swinging '6o's." Watson's memoir includes ample if not excessive evidence of this, with recurring references to his collaborator Francis Crick's attraction to young women, Watson's envy of those extramarital flirtations, and other ostensibly amusing or embarrassing encounters with other colleagues while they were engaged in heterosexual activities.

Heroic scientific enterprise took place in a "man's world," where cutting-edge science occurred against a backdrop of all-male fraternizing and collegial collaboration and competition. The few women characters that appeared in Watson's text were personified in relation to men either as (1) potential or actual conquests, (2) nurturers, or (3) feminist adversaries. The first group included attractive women who enticed and entertained the male scientists. There were numerous unnamed undergraduate "girls," and Watson's sister, Elizabeth, who was admired by Watson's more senior colleague, Maurice Wilkins. Watson hoped a union of some sort would result in his own career advancement. The "nurturer" was captured in the domestic and pleasant nature of Francis Crick's wife, Odile Crick. Lastly, the feminist antagonist role was played by Watson's colleague Rosalind Franklin, the one female scientist in the text. She was described as purposefully unfeminine and unattractive in appearance, difficult and uncooperative, and only redeemed when she, after some initial resistance, purportedly agreed with Watson and Crick's account of the double-helix structure. At this point Watson offered a redeeming reappraisal of Franklin: "Her past uncompromising statements on this matter thus reflected first-rated science, not the outpourings of a misguided feminist." In the end, Watson's memoir sketched an image of the modern, secular scientific hero conveying masculine and heteronormative attributes that became associated with late twentieth-century science (and can be reasonably assumed to persist today). This image, McNeil argues, appears in subsequent scientific biographies and autobiographies. Even the popular biographies of women scientists—Ann Sayre's biography of Franklin (Sayre 1975) and Evelyn Fox Keller's biography of Barbara McClintock (Keller 1983)—both utilize Watson's characterization of the modern scientific hero in order to explain the difficulties that women have had advancing careers in science. Women, by virtue of their gender and oppressive patriarchal norms surrounding it, are less likely to be deemed trustworthy and properly disinterested for scientific work (Rolin 2002).

There are two narratives at play in the depictions of gentleman and contemporary scientific heroes. First, trust has always been part of science, as discussed in chapter 5. Second, trust in science has relied upon the largely unchecked privilege and power of scientists. The gentleman hero of early modern Europe eventually became unsatisfactory because his stature as an expert rested on his birthright as much as his scientific training. Yet, the trustworthiness of the "ordinary guy" contemporary scientific hero still rests on privilege and exclusivity. Watson's culture of cutting-edge heroic science denigrated women, including women's contributions to science (McNeil 2007), while the absence of people of color in this hero narrative was (and still is) built into the structure of England's elite universities (Reay 2018). The histories of science are rife with stories of women scientists whose professional contributions were underappreciated by male colleagues. Rosalind Franklin, for example, is often forgotten as an equal contributor to Watson, Crick, and Wilkins in determining the double-helix structure of deoxyribonucleic acid (DNA). The three men shared the Nobel Prize for that discovery, with Franklin notably excluded from the honor (Sayre 1975). Computer science, now a male-dominated field, has a quiet history of women pioneers in the field, such as Ada Lovelace, Grace Hopper, Margaret Hamilton, Dorothy Vaughan, Mary Jackson, and Katherine Johnson (Abate 2012; Hicks 2017). Obscuring women's contributions to science permits a persistent image of science as better suited for men. Indeed, women are still widely believed to be ill-suited for STEM (Carli et al. 2016). Yet female scientists report that it is not the cognitive demands but the gender-hostile working environments that make science inhospitable to women (National Academy of Sciences et al. 2007; Carli et al. 2016). Today there are efforts to flip the script by amplifying the stories of women scientists, for example, in the book and film[10] *Hidden Figures* (Shetterly 2016) and the podcast *Lady Science,* as well as in children's books such as *Women in Science: 50 Fearless Pioneers Who Changed the World* (Ignotofsky 2016), *Black Women in Science: A Black History Book for Kids* (Pellum 2019), *Who Says Women Can't Be Computer Programmers?: The Story of Ada Lovelace* (Stone 2018), and *Goodnight Stories for Rebel Girls* (Favilli and Cavallo 2016). These "herstories" and "people's histories" of science (see Connor 2009) are told because the power and privilege of science have come to be understood as problematic. Along with the "hidden figures" whose stories are now being revealed are the hidden experiences of those who never got the opportunity to pursue and participate in science due to its inaccessibility. That trust in science is built upon problematic footings should make it unsurprising that the situation needs reexamination and redress.

What sustains this scientific hero as conduit of trustworthy science to the present day? The scientific hero as ordinary guy suggests that we do not expect our scientists to have upstanding moral characters comparable to Boyle's. They are as flawed as everyone else. But the role of trust remains a necessary part of scientific progress. Trust still fills in the credibility gaps of empirically generated knowledge, while the strong expressions of public outrage witnessed when cases of scientific misconduct surface suggest the moral harm of *broken* trust (rather than lesser feelings of disappointment discussed chapter 5). "Scientists Behaving Badly" was the bold headline that appeared in *Nature* in 2005 (Martinson, Anderson, and de Vries 2005), ahead of an article detailing a study demonstrating the high frequency of scientific misconduct among government-funded scientists. The study's authors decried the "striking level and breadth of misbehavior" among three thousand voluntary respondents to an anonymous ethical conduct survey. The data "formed a spectacle of ethical transgressions," in which respondents admitted to a host of misdeeds, ranging from minor to egregious. The most-commonly cited misbehavior came from the 15.5 percent of respondents who admitted to changing how they conducted experiments or adjusting their results upon pressure from funding sources. The *Boston Globe* was harsh in its assessment that these findings "threaten the fundamental working of science," while the *Wall Street Journal* denounced the "brazen culture of lawlessness" in too many scientific research communities (Kidder 2010).

If virtuous character no longer sustains trust in science, what are the new norms that keep trust in place? Strong public reaction to flagrant cases of scientific misconduct like the one just described suggests that scientists are still held to moral standards. Furthermore, the standards used to explain what went wrong in cases of scientific misconduct are not the same standards placed on the general publics. Rather, they are moral expectations uniquely placed on practicing scientists. These professional standards are captured in sociologist Robert Merton's ([1942] 1973) canonical characterization of the modern scientific ethos. Merton posited four institutional norms for scientific governance that have been subsequently read as behavioral norms for individual scientists[11]:

Universalism
Communalism
Disinterestedness
Organized skepticism

Universalism requires that contributions to scientific discourse be judged on their merit, without regard for the contributor's nationality, race, religion, gender, class, or any other social marker. Communalism makes imperative the free and open communication of methods and results. Disinterestedness requires practitioners to disclaim any personal or material stake in the outcome of their research. Finally, organized skepticism (sometimes simply called "skepticism") refers to the duty to question any and all dogma. Merton's norms represent an ideal, a popular view of how science *should* work. Indeed, it has been demonstrated, through surveys of scientists and members of the publics, that these norms capture how many scientists and publics think science should work (Ranalli 2012). Therefore, the norms are shared and have moral force.

This contemporary ethics of science relies on shared norms of conduct, rather than the individual virtue of solitary practitioners, to ground trust in science. Trust must be maintained, both between practitioners in collaborative work environments and between scientists and the publics. Within science, the norms of cooperation and communalism render trust relations even more important to science now than during Boyle's time. As discussed in chapter 5, the networks of cooperation and trust are now more complex, with the now-common phenomenon in experimental science of large research teams involving highly specialized contributors working on multiple sites. This often makes singular oversight impossible. As for public relations, the publics afford scientific institutions a great degree of independence with the expectation that this freedom will procure public benefit (see chapter 5). The publics presumably agree to this social contract with science because we trust that most scientists will follow correct norms of behavior most of the time. Ensuring this trust means that the moral character of practicing scientists is still implicated. Mertonian norms can be located in institutional arrangements and practices that influence and constrain scientists, like blind peer review and disclosure of financial arrangements. But knowing that there are those gaps where misbehavior can and does creep in, the credibility of scientific institutions is best buoyed by the creation of professional cultures where those institutional norms are internalized by the scientists themselves. In other words, those norms can be sought in the *character* of the scientists as well.

It is with the expectation that most scientists will adhere to a moral code of scientific practice that trust relations can continue to play an important invisible governance role in science. With the presumed normalcy of well-behaving scientific heroes, cases of transgressive behavior are not supposed to destabilize the integrity of science. Instead, those misbehaving scientists can serve as rare and self-contained problems that can be removed from the community and leave scientific enterprise otherwise unscathed. This is what we have seen in response to notorious misconduct cases such as those of Hwang Woo Suk (Resnick, Shamoo, and Krimsky 2006),[12] Jan Hendrik Schön (Cassuto 2002; Vogel 2011),[13] and Marc Hauser (Gross 2011).[14] The offenders are named and blamed. Yet, turning to analysis of the maverick role amid strained expert-lay relations shows that public mistrust is *not* so easily contained.

Despite being well-known, Merton's norms have sustained criticism in science studies for insufficiently accounting for how power interests shape scientific knowledge production and enterprise. Other scholars appreciate the norms for adequately conveying how power interests are effectively obfuscated from narratives of science (e.g., Ranalli 2012). I agree with the criticism as well as the approval, both of which inform my reading of the problem of expertise. Merton's norms for scientists do not include inclusion, representation, and public service. Public distrust in experts and expert institutions, the so-called problem of expertise, pivots on those missing norms. On the one hand, Merton's four norms speak to some of the publics' expectations from science—the publics *are* outraged when norm infractions occur, for example, industry meddling in scientific research that results in poor demonstrations of disinterestedness by scientists (Johnston 2010, 28). Yet the four norms do not capture all public expectations from scientists and scientific institutions. The ascendancy of the maverick as scientific expert can be explained by those missing norms.

## THE SCIENTIFIC EXPERT

Despite this more contemporary framing of the scientific hero, the hero figure in science is typically spoken of as a historical artifact or well-worn cliché. Certainly, the heroic status of the scientist remained fairly constant through to the post–World War II technological innovation boom. The socially transformative 1960s invited questioning of this view; in response, sociologists of science entered the laboratory to reveal what scientists actually *do*. As a result, scientific work came to look much more mundane, and public resistance to the products of science—notably atomic energy in the 1970s—challenged scientists' once-presumed authority to pronounce on social and policy matters (Collins 2014).

Yet the expert voice was never lost, and there has yet to be a good substitute for expertise for navigating the complexities of social life. Governments and private citizens want to make informed choices and need guidance to do so. A necessary (but not sufficient) condition of informed choice is good understanding of the relevant scientific evidence. Scientific advisors work at all levels of government and engage regularly with the publics in order to assist with this task.[15] The normative language of "hero" no longer seems fitting; the better term is "scientific expert," a more democratic and putatively accountable mouthpiece for scientific truths. The expert's status is purportedly grounded in merit—education, publication record, and regard by their peers—rather than upbringing as gentry. The expert's expertise is also more circumscribed than the hero's, typically limited to their area of advanced research.

Still, the discussion of the supposed death of expertise in chapter 3 makes clear that both expertise and experts have become highly contested categories in this online age of democratic knowledge acquisition. That so many thinkers are wedded to the dispiriting idea that no one listens to experts anymore speaks to a redrawing of lines of authority, but I characterize the revision differently.

Whereas the social constructivism of second wave science studies usefully undermined the 1950s view of scientists as heroes and science as a purely rational enterprise, Collins reports regretfully that the critical turn in science studies was then captured by radical elements who took these findings to mean that science is not special or trustworthy (Inquiring Minds 2014). Collins insists that there was no antiscience aim in trying to figure out how science actually works; nor was there any implicit or explicit undermining of scientific progress in these investigations. Instead, he counters, the heroic stories of instant discoveries and eureka moments obscured the hard work that goes into science and the development of knowledge and expertise. Rather than relying on luck or random strokes of genius, scientific experts *earn* their epistemic superiority through years of study and practice. This is what makes experts epistemically trustworthy, he argues, and it is for this reason that only those with specialist expertise should be able to pronounce on issues like vaccine safety and efficacy (see Collins on Interactional Expertise in chapter 3).

Is this a satisfying account of scientific understanding and expertise? Science writer John Horgan, for one, does not think so. In response to a news article endorsing Collins's (2014) book, titled "This is Why You Have No Business

Challenging Scientific Experts" (Mooney 2014a), Horgan provocatively penned, "Everyone, Even Jenny McCarthy, Has the Right to Challenge 'Scientific Experts'" (Horgan 2015). In this piece, he insisted on the *duty* of nonexperts to challenge scientific experts and institutional power. Horgan's language of the "right" and the "duty" mischaracterizes the argument, however, as the right to think and speak is not the issue, and he offers no argument for an obligation to do so. Horgan instead wants to make the case for the reasonableness of challenging expertise. Science and scientists, he explains, are not infallible to error. They can be unwittingly influenced by (1) "groupthink"—the uncritical acceptance of others' views, (2) political pressure, and (3) financial and political interference. Scientists also (4) make mistakes and (5) can be distracted by their own values and biases. These issues are well-known and well-documented in science. Dissent is seen by Horgan as countering these problems and serving both professional and public interest by catching errors and "speaking truth to power."

Steve Fuller (1988) has also defended nonexpert challenges to expert testimony, arguing (against Hardwig's [1985] defense of the authority of experts) that expertise is limited in terms of generalizability. According to Fuller, experts hold expertise in their ability to systematically control and manipulate a closed system consisting of a prescribed set of variables (Fuller 1988, 280). Hardwig errs, according to Fuller, by extending that expertise too far. Fuller argues that experts' mastery of such systems does not afford them the expertise or capacity to successfully address people's actual concerns. For example, while economists can derive laws from an idealized model of the market, they are not necessarily in a good epistemic position to advise people on where to invest their money. Laypeople, then, still need to think for themselves (Fuller 1988, 283), and are, following Horgan, reasonably positioned to challenge expert opinion.

Philosophical research into the relationship of values and science gives us reason not to "leave it to the experts"—even upstanding, free-thinking experts who guard against conflicts of interests and recognize the bounds of their expertise when applying their knowledge to practical matters. The presence of values in science is reason enough to challenge expertise (Douglas 2017; Irzik and Kurtulumus 2018). While experts demonstrate epistemic superiority with respect to "knowing the science," scientific decision-making is imbued with values, including social values, and scientific experts are neither uniquely qualified nor politically authorized to determine which ones ought to shape public policy. Because no hypothesis is ever verified with certainty, the decision to accept or reject it depends on whether the evidence is sufficiently strong. But this determination depends upon the consequences (including moral ones) of mistakenly accepting or rejecting the hypothesis. Rudner (1953) and Hempel (1965) raised this issue over a half century ago to highlight the presence of values in scientific assessments of hypotheses. While it may be reasonable and practical for scientific communities to determine the appropriate values, Longino (1990), Intemann (2009), and other social epistemologists have strongly argued for more diversity within those communities in order to ensure better assessment of those social values. But when scientists enter the policy arena as scientific advisors, their pronouncements are reasonably governed by wider democratic account-ability. When, for example, scientific experts are asked to weigh the evidence regarding a policy proposal to ban a commonly used industrial chemical due to concerns regarding toxicity, there are interpretive elements regarding this assessment that go beyond what the research tells them. When is there enough evidence to make a claim? The determination of "enough evidence" will be dic-tated by the perception of risk involved. A mistaken judgment that could, say, seriously harm human and animal welfare, suggests that we should err on the side of caution (the precautionary principle). A low or reasonable risk suggests a lower evidentiary standard could be tolerated. What is a reasonable risk for the publics to take on? How does the risk of harm weigh against purported benefits of, say, maintaining current industry practices? These are value questions that are not best determined by scientific experts but by democratic and publicly accountable means (see, for example, Douglas 2000).

Contemporary scientific experts, while still afforded respect and consider-able recognition, do not stand above public scrutiny and opinion; nor should they. This means that they will have to work to maintain their authoritative status, not because everyone has an opinion, but because scientific expertise does not entitle one to pronounce definitively on all matters. Pronouncements on unsettled science, for instance, will encounter dissenting views. Dissent is generally welcomed (at least in theory), as critical debate is supposed to fur-ther and improve scientific understanding. Pronouncement on policy issues and the science that informs policy will similarly encounter dispute and dis-agreement. While the science might very well be secure and settled, and the scientific opposition spurious, the impact of the science on contentious policy issues and the lives and well-being of diverse stakeholders reasonably invites public response (both positive and negative). Scientific experts and institutions wield considerable power to shape and sway politically controversial debate due to the demands and expectations of "evidence-based" policy (see chapter 4).

While stable democracies need science to inform policy, the practice of science informing policy is characteristically undemocratic. Expert communities are necessarily exclusive in terms of training and professional involvement,[16] and science is supposed to be unswerving in the face of the (circumscribed) majority interests that define democratic decision-making.

With this prima facie tension between expertise and democracy,[17] the maverick enters as a populist counterforce to the power interests that expert elites are thought to represent and reinforce. Because the language of science holds currency over moral and political language, ethical and political objections are framed as scientific disputes over the evidence (see chapter 4). The maverick as *scientist*, wielding *outsider* expertise, therefore powerfully counters the once-presumed warrant of expert-driven decision-making on scientifically informed policy.

## THE MAVERICK'S OUTSIDER EXPERTISE

Andrew Wakefield is exemplary of the maverick—the free-thinking and unorthodox eccentric. He capitalized on the important role of dissent in science (Crease 2000) and hereticism in the discipline's history (Ridley 2011a) in order to gain notoriety and public admiration as the David figure against the Goliath of institutionalized science. Wakefield's credibility in the eyes of vaccine resisters appears to have been bolstered by efforts to discredit him. Wakefield is admired by followers for speaking truth to power, while the scientific establishment looks suspect in what is interpreted as an organized effort to suppress "inconvenient truths." The appeal of the maverick lies in his antiestablishment persona.

The maverick has a glorified place in the history of science, which has a long list of ridiculed discoverers who were later vindicated (see Beatty 2002). Those historic scientific heroes like Galileo and William Harvey were mavericks, insofar as they allegedly opposed the religious and/or scientific dogma of their day in order to stand up for truth. Today's maverick stands up against another hindrance to the pursuit of knowledge: conventional thinking. In 2014 thirty prominent scientists published an open letter in the *Guardian* titled "We Need More Scientific Mavericks" (Braben et al. 2014), which lauded the history of nonconformists whose unconventional ideas radically progressed scientific thought. The objective of this nostalgia was to encourage granting agencies to change their review structure. The writers argued that conventional research trajectories building on established ideas were favored over radical, intellectually risky, and exciting new pursuits.[18]

The emotional draw to the maverick hero should, however, be circumscribed. This glossy history of vindicated mavericks in science only shines in hindsight. At the moment of pending rupture, when the maverick proposes to dismantle secure scientific thought, it may be difficult to tell if the dissenter is a genius or a dangerous heretic. Still, resistance by scientists to novel ideas is certainly unsettling given science's status as a mode of inquiry that is supposed to follow the evidence and eschew ideological thinking. It is reasonable to be troubled by stories like that of Daniel Schechtman, the 2011 Nobel prize winner in chemistry, who spent much of his career being shunned by colleagues for his radical proposal regarding the existence of quasicrystals. He reported being removed from his research group for bringing "shame upon them" (Ridley 2011a). Linus Pauling allegedly denounced Schechtman's theory by saying, "There is no such thing as quasicrystals, only quasi-scientists" (Ridley 2011b). Schechtman's unconventional thinking was eventually exonerated and rewarded with the Nobel Prize. He came to be admired and celebrated for his cutting-edge thinking and research, thereby transforming him from a crannk into an exemplary scientist.

The same goes for Barry Marshall, who proposed (along with Robin Warren) a bacterial theory of peptic ulcers in place of the conventional theory that excess stomach acid causes gastric ulcers. He was similarly mistreated by his research community until he proved his theory by intentionally infecting himself and then curing his gastric ulcer with antibiotics instead of antacids (for analysis of this case, see Thagard 1999). For this, Marshall and Warren won the Nobel Prize in Medicine in 2005 (Ridley 2011a).

Further, we may also mourn the loss of life of new mothers from puerperal (childbed) fever due to an obstinate medical establishment in nineteenth-century Vienna that refused the radical wisdom of Ignaz Semmelweis. He correctly hypothesized that physicians were spreading infection when delivering babies due to poor handwashing and sanitary practices (see Semmelweis 1983; Hempel 1966).[19]

Science writer Matt Ridley has provocatively proposed "that 90% of great scientists start out as heretics. The problem is that 90% of scientific heretics are talking nonsense" (Ridley 2011b). Unfortunately, it is quite difficult to tell who the great ones are. Our greatest minds were and still are not purely rational heroes. Even respected scientists are prone to confirmation bias, and even Newton was an alchemist (Ridley 2011a; 2011b).

Will Wakefield be vindicated like the other redeemed mavericks popularly celebrated in the histories of Western science? Only time will tell. His power has been whittled away over the years since the notorious publication, but he has reemerged recently. After being terminated from the Royal Free Hospital in London for refusing an internal request to duplicate his findings from the *Lancet* paper, he was brought to Austin, Texas, in 2004 by supporters to help found Thoughtful House Center for Children, an unconventional treatment and research center for children with autism (Dominus 2011). When Britain's General Medical Council revoked his medical license in 2010 due to a finding of ethics violations in his MMR study, Wakefield resigned from Thoughtful House. He also stopped speaking at the popular Autism Research Institute conference, for which his speaking engagements were once a major draw. Yet this closing of his professional world is arguably much like the experience of the maligned mavericks just discussed, and Wakefield still emerges, albeit less frequently, in the media spotlight, proving he has staying power. In 2016 alone, he was a headliner on the Conspira-Sea Cruise,[20] sold the film rights to his 2010 memoir, and produced a documentary on the autism-vaccine link that was slated to be featured at the 2016 Tribeca Film Festival until organizer Robert DeNiro heeded to public pressure to remove it. He was sighted in black tie at Donald Trump's inaugural ball; this prominent invitation suggested to many that his star was once again rising. Wakefield is also credited with influencing vaccine skepticism in Texas and with stoking fears of vaccine-induced autism among Somali-Americans in Minnesota (Glenza 2018; Boseley 2018).

"Why Won't the Andrew Wakefield Nightmare End?," read a 2016 blogpost for the American Council of Science and Health (LeMieux 2016). In the comments section, "Judy Harvey" offers an explanation: "He has offered to debate but has been denied. He has suffered constant vilification and punishment for questioning the holy grail of vaccinology." Another response by "Goldy750" added: "I do not understand why mainstream news is so frightened of allowing Andrew Wakefield to tell his side of the story. We are being told incredible misinformation by media whose source of income is very much attached to pharmaceutical advertising. When you read [Wakefield's memoir] Callous Disregard you realise how Andrew Wakefield has been treated in the worst possible manner—losing his license, his career, his country." Wakefield's boosters support him fiercely. Whether Wakefield is sustained because the autism-vaccine theory still endures (it is described as a "zombie theory"[21] by detractors), or whether his charisma helps keep the theory alive is unclear. Either way, the maverick is seen as a brave fighter against both orthodox knowledge and institutional power. He is also framed as a martyr for enduring so much personal and professional disparagement. No doubt the financial and emotional support Wakefield receives from his followers allows him to stay on course with his conviction, possibly even requiring of him to maintain it resolutely.

Wakefield is trusted by his supporters not merely for his scientific training, which provides him technical expertise to challenge the orthodoxy on vaccines, but for his perceived virtuous character. Because he stands up against the powerful establishment, he is exalted by J. B. Handley, cofounder of the vaccine-skeptical group Generation Rescue, as "Nelson Mandela and Jesus Christ rolled into one" (Dominus 2011). In her foreword to Wakefield's 2010 memoir, Jenny McCarthy explains that he "did the sort of thing most of us expect out of our doctors . . . he listened closely to the stories of parents and he told the truth" (Wakefield 2010, iii). His supporters regard him as brave and caring. Denounced by, and expelled from, the medical community, Wakefield has found a new home in far reaches of the public sphere, where he is admired and trusted. Wakefield has been restyled as a maverick and a courageous dissenter against the corrupt forces of institutional medicine.

Further, Wakefield speaks directly to the needs of his supporters by listening closely to the stories of parents, mainly mothers.[22] Women have a long history of being ignored, patronized, and harmed in the context of medical care. Women are also the primary healthcare decision makers in most households (Ranji et al 2018) and feel enormous pressure to make the right choice regarding vaccines for their children (Reich 2016). While some of the patriarchal and paternalistic norms that inspired the women's health movement of the 1970s have subsided, women's concerns are still frequently downplayed and their complaints are often not believed by healthcare practitioners (Pagan 2018; Fetters 2018). Gender disparities have been documented in pain management, where women receive less treatment than men (Fenton 2016a; 2016b), and cardiac care, where women's heart attacks are underdiagnosed (Pelletier et al. 2014; Stamp 2018). In both contexts, women's complaints of pain and discomfort do not receive the same uptake compared to men, as their testimonies are not seen as comparatively credible. Women's health scholars describe this phenomena as "testimonial injustice," when bias against the credibility of certain social identities results in discounting of their contributions to discussions and deliberations (Carel and Kidd 2014; Carel 2016, chapter 8; Narruhn and Clark 2020).[23] For example, women patients' descriptions of pain and signs of a cardiac episode are less likely to be investigated and addressed by physicians because of cultural tropes associating women with weakness, confusion, and overreaction.

The term *testimonial injustice*, the unfair refusal to trust someone's word, was coined by philosopher Miranda Fricker (2007) in her investigation of "epistem-ic injustice," the phenomenon of being wronged in one's capacity as a knower. Fricker parsed epistemic injustice into two forms, "testimonial injustice" and "hermeneutical injustice," both of which are shaped by different kinds of bias. Hermeneutical injustice occurs when someone's experiences are not well under-stood—by themselves or by others—because these experiences do not fit with any concepts known to them or to others. For example, many women struggled to make sense of their experiences of sexual harassment prior to the introduction of the term in 1975 and in the years it took for the concept to be more fully devel-oped and widely known (Fricker 2007; see Blakemore [2018] on "the menace with no name"). This and other missing concepts that are so important for allowing people to interpret their lives and experiences (hence the *hermeneutical* injustice) are not missing by accident. Instead, key interpretive concepts are missing due to historic exclusion of some groups of people from activities that shape which concepts become well-known (e.g., scholarship and journalism) (Fricker 2007).

Under patriarchy, women suffer from a "gap in collective interpretive resourc-es" that prevents the dominant culture (men) from making sense of many of women's social experiences (Anderson 2017; Fricker 2007).[24] This lack of shared understanding, and lack of trust in the testimony of women, leads to doubting the credibility of survivors of domestic abuse, sexual assault, and workplace harass-ment (Epstein and Goodman 2019; Fricker 2007). Those disempowered victims may eventually come to doubt themselves (Nelson 2001). The recent political movements #MeToo and #WhyIStayed target those very gaps in understanding by amplifying the narratives of marginalized voices, thereby highlighting the context in which decisions like staying in an abusive relationship are made. These acts of "narrative repair" (Nelson 2001) educate outsiders and embolden the narrator to trust her own judgment. In healthcare, stories of women patients pleading for care but having their urgent demands dismissed as "crazy" have sim-ilarly been amplified in the press. As Ashley Fetters (2018) wrote in the *Atlantic*, "Physicians have long dismissed or downplayed women's sexual- and reproduc-tive-health concerns—but in 2018, stories about 'health-care gaslighting[25]' are consistently breaking through to the mainstream."

Returning to vaccines, new mothers frequently report silencing and shaming when they attempt to raise concerns about childhood vaccinations with their healthcare providers (Kirby 2006; Navin 2015). Healthcare workers, who are rushed to get to their next patient due to stress on the system, lack of resources, and poor remuneration models, may not recognize the historic and cultural harms that they are perpetuating when they refuse to engage with these mothers. It also harms the collective vaccination effort, as these women will likely then find the information and support that they need from vaccine-hesitant peer groups.

The women's health movement of the 1970s that originated in the USA and inspired grassroots women's health activism throughout the world worked to empower women by letting them take health into their own hands. *Our Bodies, Ourselves* (Boston Women's Health Book Collective 1973) was more than a book; it was a rallying cry. The women's health movement aimed to take women's bodies back from oppressive institutions of medicine and reframe women's knowledge and experiences of their bodies in ways that were not configured by sexism and androcentrism (Goldenberg 2008). The goal was to empower women by providing them with comprehensive health knowledge that was rarely shared with female patients, and which had limited their participation in healthcare decision-making. In a 2004 interview marking the Boston Women's Health Book Collective's thirty-fifth anniversary and the publication of a new edition of the iconoclastic book, cofounder Nancy Miriam Hawley recalled the rationale and political urgency of the book's first edition: "At the time, there wasn't a single text written by women about women's health and sexuality. We weren't encouraged to ask questions, but to depend on the so-called experts. Not having a say in our own healthcare frustrated and angered us. We didn't have the information we needed, so we decided to find it on our own" (Hawley in Ginty 2004).

American vaccine skepticism has historical roots in the women's health movement (Conis 2015a). Women's health activists felt justified to resist medical orthodoxy and to pursue new sources of knowledge on health matters, including vaccines.[26] Today, vaccine-skeptical communities are epistemically and politically progressive insofar as the thought leaders are for the most part women, and because they take women's concerns and actions seriously (Navin 2015). Women, as the primary healthcare decision makers in most households, are valued for asking questions about vaccines rather than belittled or silenced. Jenny McCarthy's popular memoir recounting her fight against the system to (allegedly) heal her son's autism is tellingly titled *Mother Warriors* (2009). The community surrounding vaccine skepticism is inviting to women who want to be taken seriously; it is appealing to mothers who have had their vaccine questions and concerns shut down by their healthcare providers. This common experience leads many unsatisfied parents to search online and find alternative epistemic communities to learn from and create solidarity and resistance. Wakefield has been able to meet the needs of vaccine-hesitant parents in ways that conventional healthcare practitioners and the institutions they represent have unfortunately failed.

Wakefield challenges the power of institutional medicine by inviting a missing scientific norm that many members of the publics want: a voice for those who have not been encouraged to speak. While it is far from clear that his challenges are directed at strengthening science in the public interest—he scores low for moral integrity because of his financial conflicts of interest and his evasiveness about the findings of the infamous 1998 study—his defiant criticisms of the integrity of expert institutions are enormously appealing to people with low trust in those institutions. Here, again, we see a weak point in science-publics relations, upon which outside experts have been able to capitalize and organize.

## EXTOLLING THE MAVERICK AS TRUSTWORTHY

The maverick's work takes place on the public stage, rather than within the confines of scientific communities. This complicates the sites of science-publics exchange, which are governed by external relations of trust (see chapter 5). Wakefield influences science discourse and progress in the public arena rather than in research laboratories, academic conferences, and peer-reviewed journals. This creates a familiar problem for democratic societies. While, broadly speaking, increased perspectives and alternative views can improve critical debate and decision-making (this is a standard justification for free speech), the worry with this crowding of public expertise is that the publics are not in a good position to judge the merits and faults of conflicting expert opinion and are therefore vulnerable to making bad and/or misinformed choices. This concern highlights yet another philosophical tension regarding the role of experts in democratic decision-making.

Political theorists, as well as philosophers and sociologists of science, have reflected on a paradox of democracy and expertise: does deferring to expert authority for scientifically informed public policy issues compromise democratic legitimacy (Anderson 2011; Turner 2001; Jasanoff 2003; Collins and Evans 2007; Kitcher 2011a; see the scholarly exchange between Lippman [1922; 1925] and Dewey [1922; 1925; 1927])? This concern is part of the broader complaint by critics of democracy that ordinary citizens are not competent to perform the epistemic tasks that democracy requires of them. That is, the lay populace is poorly equipped to properly inform themselves on the complex social and policy issues that majority vote determines in democratic political systems (Anderson 2006). Stephen Turner sees no problem with relying on experts to create the desired conditions of informed democratic choice. There is no inherent contradiction between expertise and democracy so long as a critical (but not cynical) stance is sustained. He explains that "to grant a role to expert knowledge does not require us to accept the immaculate conception of expertise" (Turner 2001, 146). Elizabeth Anderson similarly finds this criticism of democracy to be "doubtful as a general matter" but allows that the concern arguably has some force when applied to science-based public policy: "Responsible public policy making in a technological society relies on complex research. Lay citizens—those without scientific training—lack the knowledge needed to directly assess the merits of this research. Hence, there appears to be a tension between two demands— that public policies be empirically responsible and that they be democratically legitimate" (Anderson 2011). She concludes, optimistically, that the publics are quite capable of reasonably assessing scientific claims because its members *are* competent to make reliable second-order assessments of those claims, namely judgments of the trustworthiness of the scientist's character. This view that non-experts can judge expert claims via judgment of the testifier's character is held by numerous other philosophers and sociologists of expertise (see Lehrer 1977; Hardwig 1991; Fuller 1992; Goldman 2001; Selinger and Crease 2007; Whyte and Crease 2010; Selinger 2011; Grasswick 2010; Collins and Weinel 2011). Because the publics can effectively judge the trustworthiness of the expert speaker, Anderson holds, democracy is preserved. So are the decision-making capabilities of the nonexpert publics.

To make her case for reliable lay assessments of scientific claims, Anderson needs to demonstrate that the tools for doing so are widely available to the general publics. She sets out three-part criteria for assessing the trustworthiness of scientific experts that are available to anyone with a high-school education or equivalent and access to the internet:

(1)   an evaluation of the speaker's scientific expertise
(2)   assessment of the speakers' moral character (specifically their tendency to report honestly)
(3)   evaluation of the speaker's epistemic character (especially accountability to counterevidence and criticism).

**TABLE 6.1.** A hierarchy of expertise (in Anderson 2011)

| HIERARCHY OF EXPERTISE |
| --- |
| Scientists who are leaders in the field |
| Scientists whose research in the field is recognized and cited by peers |
| PhD scientists trained in the field |
| PhD scientists outside the field, but with collateral expertise (e.g., statistics in the relevant field) |
| PhD scientists outside the field of inquiry |
| People with a bachelor's or professional degree in an applied science specialty far removed from the field |
| Laypersons |

For (1), Anderson offers *criteria for judging scientific expertise* by outlining a hierarchy of expertise against which the speaker can be evaluated (see table 6.1).

The hierarchy of expertise places those influential thought leaders in the scientific field relevant to the policy or public debate in question on top, followed by those on the scientific periphery, and finally those with no expertise in the field. For (2), *criteria for assessing the honesty of the expert*, Anderson offers some red flags to look out for: financial conflicts of interest, for instance, bring that honesty into question, as does disciplinary action or inquiries into the expert's conduct. Finally, to assess (3), the expert's *epistemic responsibility*, the question must be asked whether they have submitted their work for peer review and responded to criticism and counterevidence.

Anderson then demonstrates the public accessibility of this second-order assessment of experts' credibility by applying the proposed criteria to the climate change debate. She uses a Wikipedia entry on the climate science debate and its links to relevant documents, like reports from the IPCC and the biographical details of the pundits on both sides, to establish quite convincingly that the majority opinion that anthropogenic climate change is a real and threatening phenomenon is more trustworthy than the opposing climate change agnostic and denialist positions. There was sufficient open-access material for Anderson to meaningfully assess all three criteria for second-order lay assessment of the scientific claims regarding global warming. For instance, the Wikipedia entry discussed and linked to a survey of the peer-reviewed literature on climate science (Oreskes 2004a), which found 75 percent of papers to endorse or presume the veracity of anthropogenic climate change. The remaining 25 percent dealt with methodology or paleoclimate and therefore took no position on recent climate change. Notably, no single peer-reviewed paper rejected the theory of anthropogenic climate change (Anderson 2011, 150–51).

This exercise of online research helpfully addresses two of Anderson's three criteria, showing that those with expertise in the field (i.e., those who publish in peer-reviewed scientific journals) overwhelmingly accept the theory of global warming. Furthermore, dissenters "have either been unwilling to submit their dissenting views to the judgment of their peers or have been unable to pass peer-review" (Anderson 2011, 151). Climate skeptics eagerly speak to the press and the publics but do *not* hold themselves accountable to the scientific community. This practice "impugns both their expertise and their epistemic responsibility." With the character of these experts in question, the force of their dissent presumably loses ground too. Because limits have been placed on "reasonable" dissent, as not all dissent is valuable for scientific inquiry, and because the contents of dissenting scientific claims are often beyond lay capacities for assessment, nonexperts rely on second-order assessments of the speakers to determine the extent to which they offer reasonable dissent.

Following these reasonable sounding three-part criteria, Wakefield, as a public face of vaccine hesitancy and dissent, scores low for trustworthiness. Yet Wakefield is still supported and trusted, a phenomenon that may appear as a strike in favor of the public ignorance thesis. Wakefield scores low on Anderson's hierarchy of expertise, having fallen from the top rung of recognized leader in the relevant field of research to the lower status of "PhD scientists trained in the field" (Anderson 2011, 146). His financial conflicts of interest discredit the honesty of his claims, and he has evaded accountability for his pronouncements on numerous occasions. But, in the eyes of his supporters, Wakefield's maverick status largely pardons him for these improprieties. All sanctions against him are interpreted by his supporters as the self-preserving actions taken by an establishment with something to hide. Wakefield's supporters have diligently pointed to the important function of dissenting views in scientific inquiry, thereby suggesting that it is the scientific establishment and not Wakefield who have acted in bad faith. Deer's damning investigative report was described on numerous occasions as a "witch hunt" (Nass 2011; Scott-Mumby n.d.; Taylor 2010).

Wakefield's persisting maverick status reveals a reversal of the hierarchy of expertise offered by Anderson (2011) (a similar hierarchy is offered in Selinger and Crease [2007] and Selinger [2011]). The perceived trustworthiness of the maverick lies in his *distance* from organized science; this contradicts Anderson's hierarchy, in which *near proximity* to the establishment's core ensures credibility. Similarly, Collins and Evans (2007) highlighted *interactional* expertise as uniquely credible, because the expert was imbedded *within* the research community. Both Anderson and Collins and Evans assume it uncontroversial to tie expertise to one's place within the research community, because that very community is thought to be the site of reliable knowledge. But the status of the maverick suggests that in-group membership does not induce public confidence so easily. The maverick upends that relationship by maintaining an image of unfettered and uncorrupted thought and action, thereby gaining credibility by being *outside* of the interpersonal and professional pressures and constraints of the research community. Wakefield's appeal is illustrative of the downgrading of expertise that worries Collins (2014) and Kitcher (2011), and the appeal of the outsider highlights that the trustworthiness of the group, and the home institutions, is questioned.

Where the problem of expertise (chapter 3) has focused only on the downgrading of expertise, this investigation into the ascent of the maverick helpfully assists in addressing the problem by highlighting weak points in conventional experts and expert bodies that can to be strengthened in order to improve public trust in experts. This analysis also frames the challenge of expertise *from the perspective of the publics* rather than privileging the perspectives of frustrated experts. The conventional framing of the problem of expertise assumes the problem largely lies in the misinformed publics; while commentators have acknowledged that experts make scientific mistakes (Nichols 2017, 10, 170–77; Collins 2014, 1–11) and sometimes abuse public trust (Nichols 2017, xiii, 179–88; Collins 2014, 1–11), those shortcomings have not been taken to be central to the problem. In the preface to *Death of Expertise* (2017), Nichols quickly shifts from past abuse of public trust (he cites US military strategists responsible for the Khe Sanh and Ia Drang losses during the Vietnam War) to the pressing contemporary overreaction by the publics, who have problematically gone beyond the necessary "healthy skepticism" in favor of unwarranted blanket skepticism of expertise (xiii). Again, in his view, the problem lies with the publics for misjudging the scale and scope of the problem, rather than with expert bodies for being inattentive to the sources of public mistrust in experts and expertise.

Yet where Nichols, Collins, and I agree is on the point that the publics are not benefitting maximally from expert knowledge. I characterized the optimal

relationship to be well-placed trust in expert sources (chapter 5). Just as Nichols
thinks the publics overreact in refusing expert opinion, I posit that Wakefield's
defenders trust him more than he deserves. But this is a reactive move, created by
persistent nonresponse by expert institutions to pressing sources of public mistrust. Wakefield listens to mothers and questions regimes of power and privilege
in expert bodies, two measures that expert institutions should be doing more of
to foster positive and trusting relationships with the publics. These measures
are so highly valued by members of the publics that Wakefield's supporters are
willing to overlook many of the maverick's questionable and concerning actions
and behaviors. This again should tell traditional experts that they are failing on
two important counts.

## THE BURDEN OF RISK

The puzzling discourse of distrust surrounding vaccine hesitancy has been
characterized by some social scientists as an illustrative feature of the *risk society*
(Leach and Fairhead [2007]; Hobson-West [2007]; Kaufman [2010]). I propose
that the ascendancy of the scientific maverick in light of a reversed hierarchy of
expertise offers an epistemic dimension to this sociological framework.

The "risk society" was first theorized by German sociologist Ulrich Beck[27]
(1992) in the wake of the Chernobyl nuclear disaster to denote the failures of
the "modern project." A risk society is defined by British sociologist Anthony
Giddens as "a society increasingly preoccupied with the future (and also with
safety), which generates the notion of risk" (Giddens and Pierson 1998, 209). Beck
defined the risk that preoccupies industrialized countries in late modernity as
"hazards and insecurities *induced and introduced by modernisation itself*" (Beck
1992, 21). Chernobyl was the defining case study. Human civilizations have always had to manage risk of, say, natural disasters, disease outbreaks, and enemy
conflict. Modernity uniquely introduced institutions like business, politics, and
science that fostered unprecedented rationality and security to everyday life.
These key institutions managed the "external risks" that threatened human life
and well-being, and in doing so, created new "manufactured risks" (Giddens
1999). Modernization involves much more than new technologies and changes in
work and organization: "the change in societal characteristics and normal biographies, changes in lifestyle and forms of love, change in the structures of power
and influence, in the forms of political repression and participation, in views
of reality and in the norms of knowledge" (Beck 1992, 50). New technologies

thereby reshape entire social structures. Chernobyl is an example of how the hazards produced by industrial practices—nuclear disaster, pollution, crime, and modern illnesses—are often not successfully managed by the very institutions that created them in the effort to manage external risks. That failure of modern institutions to manage risks and mitigate the harms they had created has led to public distrust of industry, government, experts, and all other facets of modern governance (Giddens 1999).

Vaccines, of course, are scientific marvels, regarded as one of the most significant accomplishments of modern medicine. Adverse events are manufactured risks that came out of this wondrous technological advancement. The public perception that the risk is not managed effectively indicates distrust in the scientific and government institutions that orchestrate current vaccination practices.

Childhood vaccination is an act of civic engagement. Vaccine requirements weigh personal rights against public health in their demand for collective participation. Public confidence in the scientific, political, and regulatory processes are necessary for acceptance of these requirements (Kaufman 2010). Parents vaccinate their children (and themselves) because they trust these systems of expertise and the modern institutions tasked with effectively managing public health threats while respecting democratic values. Some parents also value herd immunity, but the sociology literature suggests parents are motivated by individual responsibility for their own children (Reich 2016). Parents who do not vaccinate or are ambivalent about vaccines do not share that trust. Lowered public confidence is not created by poor scientific literacy, misinformation on the internet, or persuasive celebrity endorsements. Instead those confounding aspects of life influence understanding and behavior when social trust in the institutional apparatuses available for managing risk wanes (see chapter 5 on leaps of faith).

This claim is supported by research demonstrating that confidence in government plays a key role in the publics' willingness to vaccinate. Looking at public uptake of the 2009 H1N1 ("swine flu") vaccine in the United States, Mesch and Schwirian (2015) found that people who trusted the government's ability to deal with an epidemic were almost three times more likely to take the vaccine than those who did not. This finding might help explain why vaccine refusal is found both on the political left and right. It is not political affiliation that determines vaccine uptake, but rather confidence in governance.

With those perceived failures of institutions of government to control risk, the publics take on significant burdens of risk management. Beck-Gernsheim (2000) highlights how individual responsibility becomes a major preoccupation in the risk society; this emphasis recalls the characterization of the "public health citizen" (in chapter 1) and the pressure parents feel to "do the research" as a sign of good parenting (chapter 5). Specifically, "People think if you blindly follow experts, you're not taking personal responsibility" (Hobson-West 2007). The failure of experts and institutions to ground that trust leaves the publics searching for new sources to trust in order to manage risk. For some, Wakefield fulfills that need. In addition to flipping the hierarchy, Wakefield's maverick-as-hero status demonstrates the epistemic failings of biomedical and governmental institutions to foster social trust. Poor institutional trust permitted the narrative of biomedicine's intentional muzzling of Wakefield's dissent to gain traction among a questioning and skeptical publics.

As previously discussed in chapter 5, the quick dismissal by vaccine supporters of such public concerns as conspiratorial (and therefore unworthy of consideration) misses the distinction between trustworthiness and credibility. Since the two are separate, we do not need to agree on whether academic medicine's financial ties to industry in fact corrupt medical research and therefore make biomedical claims untrustworthy. This debate is controversial, because a researchers' motives are not always clear to outside observers or even to the conflicted party (Wilson 2016). However, it is *not* controversial to say that well-documented public discomfort over financial conflicts of interest in medical research and practice creates a credibility problem (regarding vaccines, see Navin and Largent [2017]). Anderson's insight that the lay publics perform second-order assessments of scientific claims explains how and why poor credibility is a problem for scientific institutions. Modern institutions like public health are tasked with managing risk, and risk management in democratically accountable political frameworks crucially relies on high public confidence and support. The financial conflicts of interest (regardless of whether the research is actually corrupted) are perceived as threatening by the vulnerable publics. Indeed, the maverick becomes hero, and the outsider the new scientific expert, when institutional credibility lowers. The solution lies in institutional efforts to regain the publics' trust and thereby upend the appeal of the maverick.

## THE MAVERICK AND PUBLIC TRUST IN SCIENCE

Extolling the maverick only sounds outrageous if pitted against "science" as an unquestionably open and trustworthy institution. Our scientific institutions do not enjoy such good public relations, which invites, even encourages, those outliers who soothe as much as they stoke public fear. Experts and expert institutions would do well to think beyond the maverick as a nuisance getting in the way of their good practices and confusing the publics. Rather, the ascendancy of the maverick is a signal for them to reflect on their own shortcomings in earning the publics' trust. Public mistrust of science has reconfigured the scientific expert, flipping the traditional hierarchy of expertise and elevating the maverick while undermining the credibility of the (institutionally sanctioned) hero-expert. The concluding chapter of this book proposes strategies for rebuilding trust, by diffusing the sources of distrust and improving communications between stakeholders.

# CONCLUSION

## REBUILDING TRUST

This book has presented two alternative frameworks for understanding and addressing vaccine hesitancy and refusal. The dominant framework that currently shapes scholarly and popular discourses on the problem of vaccine hesitancy employs a war metaphor to capture the intractability of the problem. The war metaphor also entrenches an "us" (science) versus "them" (publics) division that is not conducive to engagement and resolution. The "war on science" metaphor described a scientized politics (chapter 4) captured in three popular explanations for vaccine hesitancy: public misunderstanding of science (chapter 1), the influence of cognitive biases on the publics' reasoning about vaccines (chapter 2), and antiexpertise and science denialism among the publics (chapter 3). All three narratives point to the publics as the problem (and even the enemy), with little attention to "us," the courageous defenders of science. Yet, as I have shown, the scientizing force of "evidence-based everything" and the linear model of science-to-policy contribute to antagonizing science-publics relations (chapter 4).

I have presented an alternative framework for understanding vaccine hesitancy and refusal, namely a "crisis of trust." The link between trust and vaccines has been undertheorized, a gap that this book has worked to address. There is some recognition of a crisis of trust in healthcare (for example, Shore 2007; Lee,

McGlynn, and Safran 2019), resulting in fractured care, both undertreatment and overtreatment (Brownlee 2010), and patient dissatisfaction (Norris 2007). For marginalized populations, that mistrust is not new; nor is it driven by technology. Vaccine hesitancy, however, is still curiously framed as a war on science.

The alternative framework's emphasis on trust better captures the problem of vaccine hesitancy and offers a more enabling edifice for addressing it. It calls on scientific experts to be part of an active bridging response rather than lament the end of expertise in defeat. To counter falling public trust in scientific institutions, public health agencies and experts must move their ideas and communications beyond false ideals of scientism and work to address vaccine hesitancy by responding to discrimination within their institutions, reforming their susceptibility to industry influence, and appealing to shared values and priorities with public stakeholders. Outreach efforts must not re-entrench the idea of a war.

The analysis of the sources of mistrust developed in chapter 5, with further elaboration in chapter 6 vis-à-vis "the maverick," suggests that broad challenges to scientific governance have farther reach than vaccine hesitancy. The kind of trust-building redress that I will now propose could potentially positively impact public uptake of communications regarding other contested areas of science, like anthropogenic climate change, genetically modified organisms, and viral pandemic response. I hope this book motivates further research into public trust in these and other science-publics flashpoints.

Because much of what members of the publics know about vaccines pivots on epistemic trust, the security of relations between scientific institutions and the publics is a key determinant of vaccine confidence and uptake. The scientific consensus is designed to direct public opinion and action; yet, tied into the consensus is a claim to the epistemic and moral legitimacy of its authors and their institutions. While most of the publics accept the legitimacy of scientific pronouncements, vaccine hesitators and more strident vaccine refusers reject those claims of legitimacy. They do not trust the source.

This investigation into trust and science resulted in a more charitable reading of the much-maligned vaccine hesitator and refuser, not because of the contents of vaccine-skeptical claims but because of the challenges inherent in trusting. I have argued that it is a mistake that scientific institutions take little interest and responsibility for the well-documented public trust deficit. Public-health and vaccine advocates are aware of poor public trust in vaccines but see this as a problem with the publics rather than signalling one in scientific governance. Vaccine pundits often contribute to public shaming and disparaging of vaccine hesitators and refusers rather than trying to build bridges. This lack of priority must be rethought, given that public health is so dependent on public trust for achieving its community health goals.

Vaccine-critical sources are quite attuned to the moral and epistemic difficulty of trusting and employ this to hone a persuasive message of informed decision-making. An analysis of vaccine-critical websites (Hobson-West 2007) found a persistent framing of trust in negative terms, in which following recommended vaccine guidelines was presented as an "easy option" for parents who did not give the issue sufficient study and attention. These groups wisely do not try to place themselves in positions of new authority. Instead they overstate the uncertainty regarding vaccine safety, which, they argue, should compel all parents to study the issue carefully and consider what is best for their own children. Vaccine questioners, regardless of the final choice made, are empowered by their critical questioning and study. The vaccine-skeptical website vaccination.co.uk explains that

> good parents are not necessarily by definition those who vaccinate their children And bad parents those who don't or vice versa . . . Making informed vaccine/vaccination decisions and taking responsibility for them is not an easy thing to do. It may seem a lot easier to simply go along with whatever the prevailing wind tells us to do. *But remaining ignorant and trusting blindly can be the biggest risk of all.* Only you really know what is the best decision for your child and hence the importance of learning enough to give you the ability to make that decision. (vaccination.co.uk, emphasis added in Hobson-West 2007)

This language of informed consent, critical thinking, and parents as experts on their own children is the antithesis of blind trust.[1] But skepticism and critical thinking does not replace trust in expert sources. In knowledge pursuits, trust is inescapable (see chapter 5). The lesson here is that public trust is hard won. Biomedical and scientific institutions cannot take it as a given that they should be trusted; instead, trust must be earned and maintained. This argument should motivate experts to disown the doomsday reading that expertise is dead. Instead, experts can re-center themselves in public conversations about vaccines and public health.

To confront public resistance to scientific claims, focus should be placed on building and maintaining that trust. Misinformation should still be corrected but should be understood to be a "downstream" symptom of poor public relations.[2] Public health practitioners should look upstream to see what is causing this misinformation to take hold. Doing this does not discount that public health agencies have good scientific backing for their claims. It *does* mean that having good science is not enough. This is a different picture of science in relation to the publics than science anchoring democratic decision-making. Science should still be understood to hold firm ground, but evidence does not replace values in policy action (chapter 4). All evidence is subject to interpretation, and political and policy decision-making requires numerous nonscientific considerations. Scientific evidence operates within a constellation of social influences that guide personal decision-making and policy formation. Good public relations ensure that science stands prominently within social frameworks. Defending public health by waging war on the publics is not a good strategy. Public health, a collective good that requires community, depends on public trust.

## HOW TO ADDRESS VACCINE HESITANCY AND REFUSAL

Since blaming, shaming, and punishing the wayward publics hardens anti-vaccine views and entrenches polarities rather than encouraging community, a different strategy is needed. What can vaccine advocates and experts do to build public trust in vaccines? Trust is built and maintained in relationships that are respectful, open, and honest (Peters, Covello, and McCallum 1997). The critical relationships enabling successful vaccination programs are at the individual level, between patient and provider, and the institutional level, between the publics and the scientific and government agencies that enact vaccine programs as a public health measure. These relationships can be optimized, and the following recommendations are general measures for countering sources of mistrust and promoting more trust. These suggestions are not, and cannot be, ready for use. Instead, they serve to direct the development of context-sensitive practical interventions, all of which must be subject to testing.[3] I highlight five areas where public trust in vaccines can be encouraged or discouraged: (1) healthcare provider-patient encounters; (2) public health messaging; (3) vaccine mandates; (4) diversity, inclusion, and representation in health sectors; and (5) industry influence on healthcare. All the recommendations below work toward building cultures of public trust.

### Healthcare Provider-Patient Encounters

A great boon for vaccination programs is that, despite many misgivings at the institutional level (especially government institutions, see Clifton 2019), the publics still trust their healthcare providers for vaccination information and healthcare in general (Wellcome Global Monitor 2019). The 2018 Wellcome Global Monitor, a global study of public attitudes about health and science,[4] found more than eight in ten people trust medical workers for health advice and that the most trusted source of health advice is a physician or a nurse (Wellcome Global Monitor 2019).[5] Vaccine-hesitant and -refusing parents often describe their skepticism as arising from having their vaccine-related concerns dismissed and feeling disrespected by their primary care providers (Kirby 2006; Navin 2015). This suggests a breakdown of prior trust after the patient's expectations were not met. Thus, the patient-provider interaction is critical. Primary care providers need the time (and billing codes[6]) to respond patiently and nonjudgmentally to parents' questions and to build on shared goals like ensuring children's health and safety. Listening to parents' concerns will lead to more effective responses. For instance, the many parents who think vaccines are generally safe but may not be safe for their *own* child (see chapter 1) will not have their fears allayed when well-meaning healthcare providers point to the latest epidemiological study demonstrating vaccines to be safe at the population level. Patients also want honest information, which may require admitting to gaps in the research, for instance, regarding what conditions precipitate serious adverse events. Admitting to uncertainty does not undermine trust, as patients look for providers who have their interests at heart and communicate honestly more than they look for unequivocal scientific pronouncements (Larson et al. 2011).

Any criticism that providing healthcare professionals with remuneration for this kind of time requirement is too expensive and a drain on limited resources may be correct given current arrangements of taxation and healthcare spending. That said, when serious public health crises emerge, prior investment in establishing relationships of trust pays off. The cost of containing infectious disease epidemics is very high. The cost of poor public trust in public health and government messaging during a pandemic is even higher, as may be seen in the United States' floundering response to COVID-19.

## Public Health Messaging

Seeing that there is some evidence for the effectiveness of indirect means of communication targeting the values instead of the scientific facts (see chapter 2), it is a good time to consider what values public health is promoting in its messaging. There are some instances of contrasting values being promoted, thereby giving the impression of contradictory advice to parents. Public health messaging must address those seeming contradictions. Additionally, renewed emphasis on the *public* in public health serves to benefit vaccine programs more than current consumerist messaging emphasizing individual choice and parental responsibility for one's own children.

Running alongside vaccine messaging are communications about *personalized* medicine. With the advancement of precision medicine comes the promise of no more "one size fits all" medicine in treatment and prevention (Health 2.0 2018). Parents see it as justified to ask why this isn't the same for vaccines. Vaccine communications also run into difficulties due to public health messaging about the naturalness of breastfeeding. Public health agencies promote breastfeeding as a preferred choice for responsible mothers,[7] using communications that valorize the "natural" and convey the message that immunity is conferred to the child through breast milk (Martucci and Barnhill 2016). It is hardly surprising to hear parents disparaging vaccines as "unnatural" as well as unnecessary when coupled with prolonged breastfeeding strategies (Reich 2016; Dubé et al. 2015).

In trying to appeal to maternal responsibility as a reason to vaccinate, public health messaging and vaccine advertising have contributed to the cultural image of vaccines as a personal choice and an individual good, thus losing the important message of community benefit. The problem with this strategy of emphasizing self-interest (i.e., a good mother is responsible for protecting her own children) is that vaccine refusal is, in fact, a logical conclusion for parents who see vaccination as one choice to make as part of the overall health strategy they put in place for (only) their children's benefit (Reich 2016). Colgrove (2006) details how early nineteenth-century advertising for the diphtheria vaccine in America shifted attention to responsible mothering practices for protecting one's own child. This contrasted with prior messaging about the smallpox vaccine as a community good. Individual decisions to vaccinate do, of course, lead to community protection, but at the cost of shifting focus from the greatest power of vaccines, namely, their ability to lower the risk of infection for everybody.

Current vaccine campaigns still work to persuade women to be responsible mothers by vaccinating their children. For example, the American national nonprofit organization Vaccinate Your Family: The Next Generation of Every Child by Two (formerly Every Child by Two) appeals to the healthcare decision maker in the family (usually a mother) by encouraging its website visitors to learn more about how "vaccinations can protect every member of your family" (Vaccinate Your Family 2019). The Public Health Agency of Canada's widely distributed booklet, *A Parent's Guide to Vaccination* (2018), begins with the statement, "Vaccination is the best way to protect your child's health" and further explains, "Parents are responsible for the well-being of their children, including protecting them from illness caused by diseases that are vaccine-preventable. Learn about vaccination and why it is important to your child's health. Parents agree that feeding and sleeping schedules are important to help keep children healthy. The same goes for childhood vaccinations. Vaccinating your children is the best way to keep them safe from many serious and potentially deadly diseases. You can help protect your children by getting them vaccinated on time and keeping their shots up to date" (2). Vaccination is therefore likened to other health and wellness choices that parents make for their own children. To explain how vaccine protection works, vaccines are compared to seatbelts: "It's just like . . . seatbelts are not 100% effective at protecting you while driving, but they significantly reduce your risk of being injured" (Public Health Agency of Canada 2018, 4). The analogy to seatbelts works with respect to reducing the risk of personal injury, but seatbelts have no collective protective effects.

The benefits of herd immunity only get mentioned in an oddly placed statement about "What if my child can't be vaccinated?" To this question, the information booklet responds, "You can help protect your children by encouraging those around your child to be up to date with their vaccination. Diseases that may not seem serious to adults can be very harmful to vulnerable children" (Public Health Agency of Canada 2018, 5). While it is surely reasonable to coach a new parent on the difficult task of raising their own child, losing the message of public benefits of vaccines instantiates the idea that individuals are primarily responsible for their immediate interests and community obligations fall to second place. Vaccine-refusing mothers in Reich's study (2016) exemplified that attitude; they understood the risk that their own unvaccinated children presented to other children but did not perceive themselves to have responsibilities to protect other children, only their own. This hyperindividualistic messaging does not come from public health alone; the pressures put on mothers to make the right choices for their children and thereby carry almost singular responsibility for their children's success are seen most noxiously in the "mother blaming"[8] that takes place when children fail. Furthermore, it may be hard to make good choices when one is put under this kind of scrutiny and pressure. A more compassionate response to mothers, with less blame and more support, would be a progressive move.[9]

Important for public health is the knowledge that our best public health interventions and social programs result from collective action. We can accomplish more together than we can alone. The collective funding and support of public education, libraries, sanitation, public parks, and more, benefits everyone, even if each person does not benefit from these programs equally. Vaccines should be similarly understood, but instead healthcare consumers are encouraged to do individual costing of vaccines (i.e., "the best way to protect yourself and your children") with the expectation that the individual calculus will land squarely in favor of vaccines. The science, after all, supports that hypothetical cost-benefit calculation. Yet people bring other considerations into their healthcare choices. Throughout, vaccines are conceptualized as a consumer product rather than a public good, so that like with all consumer products, it's up to you to decide if you need it, want it, and benefit from it. We do it for our own children, not everyone's children.

As a whole, these recommendations targeting clinical interactions and public health messaging amount to a call for better and more effective communications regarding vaccines, and I make these suggestions despite vaccine communications' poor record of efficacy. Health behavior research into vaccine uptake and refusal shows poor outcomes from interventions focused on communications and shared decision-making models. A 2017 systematic review (Brewer et al. 2017) concluded that no intervention targeting vaccine attitudes has been demonstrated to significantly improve vaccine attitudes or to increase vaccine uptake. The only programs that have successfully increased vaccination uptake have been those that nudge people with positive intention to vaccinate into action, through prompts, reminders, and incentives.

This finding, that very little is known about which interventions work, and that attempts to change attitudes have had little success in changing beliefs or behaviors, should not discourage efforts to address vaccine hesitancy. Addressing the underlying attitudes remains critical for the very same reason that vaccine hesitancy became a research priority for public health in the first place (see introduction). Specifically, vaccination programs and public health efforts are impacted by attitudes, not just behavior. Focusing on behavior misses the context in which vaccine hesitancy arises and can miss the predictive determinants of vaccine refusal. The poor outcomes for vaccine communication interventions should inspire researchers and frontline workers to try different tactics. My research asks behaviorists and healthcare workers to step back and consider the assumptions built into the very framework in which communication and persuasion efforts have taken place and failed. Reframing the issue, and redirecting efforts to address trust rather than information and misinformation alone, can and should motivate the development of new ethical persuasion interventions.

## Vaccine Mandates

Even with effective communications, vaccination programs cannot succeed through word of mouth and goodwill alone. Effective policy is crucial. It is difficult to assure coverage as high as 95 percent (for collective protection against measles outbreaks) without some sort of governance mechanism (i.e., penalty or reward, whether legislative or financial). Vaccine mandates have been shown to be effective for, even essential to, maintaining high levels of immunization coverage and low rates of vaccine-preventable diseases in high-income countries.[10] There is limited evidence of the impact of such requirements in low- or middle-income countries (Omer, Betsch, and Leask 2019).

Can mandates be reconciled with improving public trust? Vaccine mandates, an exercise of state authority, are generally contrasted with positive political values like liberty and free choice.[11] But laws also function to enable the public good by encouraging collective action, and they do so when they are created using democratic processes to ensure legitimacy and fairness. Not everyone will like the outcome, but fair procedure is valued and conducive to public trust.

Vaccine mandates are valuable public health tools that require careful use. They can convey the importance of the intervention in question and offer minimal individual burden for collective maximal benefit when they target disease spread effectively (e.g., influenza vaccines for healthcare workers). They must also distribute the burden of constrained choice equitably throughout the population (i.e., vaccine exemptions should not be easier for affluent people to access than they are for poor people). These efforts aim to minimize public pushback as much as possible, but this is a delicate balancing act between the force of the mandate (which favors minimal exceptions) and the force of the backlash (which can create many unintended harms like galvanizing anti-vaccine politics).

The most commonly used vaccine mandates are school-entry mandates that make access to schools and daycares conditional on vaccination. France responded to its globally high rates of vaccine hesitancy and increases in measles outbreaks in January 2018 by strengthening the school entry mandates, from a previous three vaccines (diphtheria, tetanus, and polio) to eleven vaccines, including the measles vaccine. Health officials had noticed good coverage for the mandated vaccines (95 percent or higher), while the latter "recommended" vaccines were dangerously low. Changing the directive from "recommended" to "required" seemed to convey the message that the latter vaccines, including measles, were important measures for public health. Physicians soon reported less questions from their patients regarding the newly mandated vaccines than before, and coverage increased (Whiting 2019). School-entry vaccine requirements have a huge public health impact because they focus on children, who are vulnerable to infectious disease due to their young age and high levels of sociality. Most children are impacted by a population-wide school-entry vaccine mandate, with only homeschooled children falling outside of the mandate's purview. But the details of the mandate matter too.

Mandates must be sensitive to the needs and interests of the community they serve. This involves careful analysis and justification for which vaccines should be required, how mandates should be enforced, if exemptions should be allowed, and what incentives and deterrents should be in place to encourage compliance with the mandates.[12] The many different mandates available throughout the industrialized North tells us that public health officials recognize the practicality of context-sensitive mandates (see Attwell et al. [2018] for a comparative review).[13]

Bolstered by penalty or reward, vaccine mandates shift the choice set of parents, but the shift is not distributed equally. The extra time required to gain a nonmedical exemption for vaccines lessens use of this administrative option, but the cost is far greater for people with lower socioeconomic advantage. Financial penalties or loss of welfare payment further impacts some families disproportionally. Vaccine mandates are justified insofar as they can minimize vaccine exemptions and thereby protect the populations, but the unequal impact of vaccine exemptions being more at the disposal of wealthy citizens reproduces inequalities. Public health agencies need to be accountable to inequality produced and/or entrenched by vaccine mandates and must locally grapple with equity-responsive measures alongside these directives.

Because successful mandates require public buy-in, transparency is crucial regarding the justification for their specifications. The Colorado-based vaccine-hesitant parents interviewed by Reich (2016) had little understanding of their state's vaccine requirements, which spurred mistrust and resentment. Why, for example, must infants be vaccinated against rubella, which is experienced as a fairly mild disease? Here, the emphasis on public good again offers clarity. Children are vaccinated to protect pregnant women from rubella, because exposure during pregnancy commonly leads to birth defects. A public relations campaign emphasizing this little-known fact may go far to convince otherwise-reluctant parents.

Vaccine mandates are also more recognizable as a reasonable public health measure when they are introduced during moments of political calm. Mandates will be less polarizing if they are introduced as health-promoting behavior rather than punishment for vaccine-skeptical families. The current tendency to use mandates as political muscle during outbreaks (as seen, for example, in response to outbreaks in California in 2016[14] and New York in 2019[15]) takes attention away from the community benefit that a well-designed, transparent, and equitable vaccine mandate can provide.

Despite the stringent sound of the term "mandate," there is great variety in how strictly those requirements are enforced and the extent to which parents can refuse school-entry vaccination. Medical exemptions for those with weak immune systems are not controversial; if anything, the vulnerability of immunocompromised individuals to vaccine-preventable diseases is good reason to insist on others getting vaccinated. The controversy surrounds the availability and accessibility of nonmedical exemptions, whether on grounds of religious or personal belief.[16] Many jurisdictions are making these exemptions more difficult to acquire by adding bureaucratic burdens like requiring education or counselling sessions, and signatures from medical personnel and notaries. Introducing such burdens has been shown to successfully reduce the number of requests for nonmedical exemptions (Blank et al. 2013; Omer et al. 2006). Some US states, Australia,[17] and several European countries[18] have more boldly eliminated nonmedical exemptions by attaching vaccine refusal to financial penalty, the possibility of jail time, and lost child benefit payments. These methods tend to increase vaccination rates by motivating the "fence sitters" to vaccinate their children in response to the increasing burden of nonvaccination. Yet, when restrictions are placed on family autonomy, there is the risk of hardening anti-vaccine views, notably among those who may support vaccines as a health measure but bristle at government compulsion. Mandates need to be approached with care (see Omer, Betsch, and Leask 2019), and with attention to the local context. Each jurisdiction will have unique considerations: How accessible are vaccines? What (if any) are the sources of undervaccination and nonvaccination of local children? How much legislative interference will the publics tolerate? A recent global study of vaccine mandates showed that there is no straightforward relationship between the forcefulness of a policy and its impact on the rate of vaccination (Omer, Betsch, and Leask 2019). What works in one jurisdiction may backfire in others by stoking resentment due to entrenched inequality (e.g., lesser-resourced families will feel the burden of lost benefits or lost access to public schools more dramatically) and by fueling anti-vaccine sentiments and activism.

## Diversity, Inclusion, and Representation in Health Sciences, Healthcare, and Public Health

Public trust in scientific institutions will remain on shaky ground without redress of historic and current injustices against marginalized communities by scientists and health practitioners. Prioritizing public trust must include strong efforts to increase diversity and representation within health research and practice. This includes (1) diversifying the workforce of health science and healthcare researchers and practitioners and (2) increasing community participation in public health research and practice. There are good reasons to promote diversity within any workplace—increasing perspectives and incorporating a broader range of ideas allows for innovation and improvement (Altman 2017). This is the case for scientific research institutions too.

Diversity in science achieves both social ends, like justice and equity, and epistemic ends, by improving the quality of scientific research. When scientific training is accessible and inclusive for traditionally underrepresented groups, the most talented workforce can be generated. Current barriers that exclude people who cannot afford years devoted to higher education, who cannot balance the demands of childcare, or who cannot tolerate training and workplace discrimination, limits the talent pool. An additional epistemic benefit of increasing participation of underrepresented groups is increased scientific objectivity[19] and minimizing the negative influences of bias in scientific reasoning (Nelson 1990; Harding 1991; Code 1991; Kitcher 2001; Longino 1990, 2002; Solomon 2001, 2006; Wylie and Nelson 2007). Philosophers of science—especially feminist philosophers—have used case studies from the history of science to demonstrate how even conscientious and well-intentioned scientists can make problematic assumptions, adopt racial and gender stereotypes, or reason in ways that reflect and project their own experiences, values, and interests (Fausto-Sterling 1985; Gould 1996; Longino 1990; Martin 1996; Solomon 2001; Intemann 2009). It is difficult to see one's own biases, or the biases shared by one's social group, and so diversity within scientific communities becomes a critical component of values testing. Since science is not value-free, those values must be rigorously examined to determine which ones are present in any scientific investigation and whether they should be. Diverse communities of researchers bring in a broader range of perspectives for critically engaging the working assumptions, values, and interests operating within any research domain. By bringing different points of view into critical tension with each other, and structuring scientific communities in ways that criticism is taken seriously (Longino 2002, 51), diverse epistemic communities can produce more informed views on what values and assumptions ought to inform the research than would a homogenous group of scientists (Harding 1991; Nelson 1990; Longino 1990, 2002; Intemann 2009). This critical scrutiny can be taken further by permitting community or public input on research priorities and projects.

The Sullivan Commission on Diversity in the Healthcare Workforce (USA) prefaced its influential 2004 report on the representation of minorities among American healthcare professionals with the statement: "Today's physicians, nurses and dentists have too little resemblance to the diverse populations they serve, leaving many Americans feeling excluded by a system that seems distant and uncaring" (Sullivan Commission 2004, iii). The Sullivan commission regards the failure of the nation's health professions to keep pace with changing demographics as possibly "an even greater cause of disparities in health access and outcomes than the persistent lack of health insurance of millions of Americans" (iii). Numerous studies show that representation matters to patients, who associate racial and gender concordance between patient and physician with better healthcare (Street et al. 2008). Lack of diversity and representation in the healthcare workforce impacts health disparities in underrepresented patient populations (Institute of Medicine 2003). Street et al. explain that "the physician-patient relationship is strengthened, when patients see themselves as similar to their physicians in personal beliefs, values, and communication. Perceived personal similarity is associated with higher ratings of trust, satisfaction, and intention to adhere" (Street et al. 2008). In short, building public trust and building both diverse scientific research communities and a diverse healthcare workforce go together.

Public health must similarly prioritize diversity in its workforce as part of the social justice and equity commitments that guide public health practice (see, for example, Office of Disease Prevention and Health Promotion 2020) and as a means for improving public trust. Because sociocultural competencies are so necessary for working with diverse individuals, groups, and communities, the Public Health Agency of Canada lists "diversity and inclusion" as one of its seven public health competencies.[20] Diversity and inclusion are therefore recognized to be among "the essential knowledge, skills and attitudes necessary for the practice of public health" (Public Health Agency of Canada 2007) and for building an effective public health workforce (Joint Task Group on Public

Health Human Resources 2005). A public health practitioner must be able to: "Recognize how the determinants of health (biological, social, cultural, economic and physical) influence the health and well-being of specific population groups; Address population diversity when planning, implementing, adapting and evaluating public health programs and policies; Apply culturally-relevant and appropriate approaches with people from diverse cultural, socioeconomic and educational backgrounds, and persons of all ages, genders, health status, sexual orientations and abilities" (Public Health Agency of Canada 2007). The "diversity and inclusion" slogan thereby captures a host of culturally inclusive and anti-oppressive[21] skills, attitudes, and practices necessary for effective communications with diverse publics, and for creating inclusive practices, programs, and policies. The Core Competencies document does not speak directly to representation within the public health workforce, but workforce diversity should be understood to be important for promoting an inclusive and equitable public health approach. A diverse public health workforce is vital for defining sociocultural competencies and developing adequate training, for challenging entrenched attitudes and practices within public health units, for developing effective relationships with marginalized communities, and for improving public health for everyone. Diversity and inclusion must be prioritized in faculty hiring and student admissions in research units and schools of medicine and public health; it should also be reflected in all levels of administration in public health units. Without diversity and representation, public health efforts will struggle to grasp culturally sensitive structural barriers to health, to examine patterns of health and disease, and to narrow health gaps. Shahi, Karachiwalla, and Grewal (2019) have recently called on the Canadian public health sector to "walk the walk" by promoting equity, diversity, and inclusion within public health units.

When it comes to explicit commitments to social justice, public health science and practice needs community participation. Insofar as public health science works in the public interest and relies on public trust to achieve public health, broad public consultation is needed. Community organizers should have a seat at the table when setting research priorities for community-based interventions to make sure that they are culturally appropriate, and that public health interests and community interests are in line. Participatory research, where scientists and nonscientists work together, would further health equity goals not only by crafting and honing effective interventions but also by empowering members of underrepresented communities (Wallerstein and Duran 2010).

## INDUSTRY INFLUENCE ON HEALTHCARE

Healthcare operations face an additional challenge in the urgent need to recon-
figure industry ties to healthcare practice. Empirical research shows lower public
trust in scientists and physicians perceived to suffer from financial conflicts of
interests or loss of independence (Hargreaves, Lewis, and Spears 2003). Industry influence can bias research outcomes and study design (Bekelman, Li, and
Gross 2003; Lexchin et al. 2003), weaken regulatory agencies' necessary "arm's
length" scrutiny of industry-funded research (see, for example, concern about
the "revolving door" problem for the FDA [Piller 2018; Z. Brennan 2018], and
Health Canada [Lexchin 2019; Lexchin 2016; Grundy 2018]), and create conflicts
of interest in clinical guidelines development (see Moynihan et al. 2018; Neuman et al. 2011). Physicians' prescribing patterns are also influenced by direct
meetings with pharmaceutical sales representatives and by attending sponsored
seminars (often held in fancy restaurants and sunbelt locations) (Gray, Hofmann,
and Mansfield 2010). Numerous observational studies have found association
between prescriber interactions with sales representatives and more frequent
or lower quality prescribing (e.g., De Bakker et al. 2007; Steinman et al. 2007).

These issues were addressed in chapter 5, along with acknowledgment of
the counterargument that the pharmaceutical industry has done a lot of good in
terms of creating helpful pharmaceuticals. Indeed, it has. But this industry has
earned a poor reputation among the publics due to shocking scandals that have
harmed and killed patients (Lenzer 2004), as well as use of its financial clout to
lobby politicians and university administrators into weakening the necessary
checks on pharmaceutical products by way of independent clinical trials (Schafer
2004; Godlee 2006), unbiased medical education (Persaud 2013), and independent regulatory review (Ray and Stein 2006; Lexchin 2017). Defenders will insist
that market forces and deregulation encourage innovation, but patients are the
victims when speed compromises quality and when markets do not distribute
health resources equitably (e.g., price gouging and neglected diseases [see Light
2020]). Health professionals and publicly accountable institutional bodies suffer as well in strained relationships with the publics. Professional groups and
scientific bodies have the choice to define the limits of their associations with
private industry. Current efforts to manage financial conflicts of interest in the
health professions are weak. Disclosure statements and sunshine lists are not
enough to ensure the levels of public confidence needed to stave off persistent
vaccine hesitancy.

## IN CLOSING

As I write this concluding paragraph, we are in the fifth month of a global pandemic that may be effectively contained or eradicated through the invention and uptake of a vaccine. An unprecedented global effort is underway to develop a COVID-19 vaccine within twelve to eighteen months (rather than the usual five to ten years) (Steenhuysen et al. 2020). Many world leaders accept that fully reopening society after the period of "physical distancing"[22] and varying degrees of lockdown requires a vaccine (Britneff 2020). The return to "normal" will involve impressive technological and manufacturing capability, massive public health immunization drives, and wide public acceptance of the new vaccine once it is ready. So much of what has been considered in this book has vital relevancy for pandemic response both in the short and long term. Without question, trust as explained here is at the center of effective response. Those who think that the measures suggested in this final chapter can be minimized, put off, or ignored altogether must consider the alternative burden of vaccine hesitancy and refusal in response to this and future epidemics and pandemics. Enacting change is difficult, but the status quo is a plague.

# NOTES

**Introduction: Vaccine Hesitancy in the Industrialized North**

1. WHO's "Ten Threats to Global Health in 2019" were listed as: air pollution and climate change; noncommunicable diseases; global influenza pandemic; fragile and vulnerable settings; antimicrobial resistance; Ebola and other high-threat pathogens; weak primary healthcare; vaccine hesitancy; dengue; and HIV.

2. Philosopher of population health Sean Valles (2018; esp. chapter 2) traces the population health roots of the WHO, seen especially in the WHO definition of health. Adopted in 1946 and still found today, unamended, in the Preamble to the Constitution of WHO, health is defined as "a state of complete physical, mental and social well-being and not merely the absence of disease or infirmity."

3. The meeting notes specifically highlighted challenges with polio vaccine drives in India and Nigeria.

4. Industrialized countries are countries with developed economies and advanced technological infrastructure relative to less industrialized nations. The criteria for evaluating the degree of economic development in a country are gross domestic product (GDP), gross national product (GNP), average per capita income, level of industrialization, amount of widespread infrastructure, and general standard of living. Some development measures also use noneconomic factors like the human development index (HDI), which quantifies a country's levels of education, literacy, and health into a single figure.

5. The terms "Global North" and "Global South"(or "North" and "South") divide nations into two categories, the former capturing those that are wealthiest and most powerful and the latter including a disproportionate number of nations that rank at or near the bottom in terms of global wealth and power (Ritzer 2013, 312). The North houses one-quarter of the world population and controls four-fifth of global wealth, while the South has three-quarters of the world population and accesses one-fifth of global wealth (Mimiko 2012). "North" and "South" also refer to rough geographical location, specifically location north or south of the thirtieth parallel north circle of latitude. Most wealthy nations are located north of the circle of latitude that is thirty degrees north of the Earth's equatorial plane, while most of the lesser developed countries are south of the thirtieth parallel north (Ritzer 2013). The geographic designation has exceptions, such as Australia and New Zealand, located in the South but designated as North due to their robust economies and infrastructure. "North" and "South" are often used as short hands for "developed" and "developing," and to a lesser extent, "industrialized" and "nonindustrialized," although there are disagreements among development theorists about the precise definitions as well as the membership of some countries. China, for example, carry some features of North (industrial power), and other features of South (extreme poverty among a good portion of its population) (Jackson et al. 2016).

6. Opel et al. (2011) measure 20–30 percent of American parents to be vaccine hesitant, while Largent (2012) cites literature estimating 40 percent of American parents.

7. The first vaccine was administered two years before Jenner's experiment by Benjamin Jesty, a

Dorset farmer, but not in an experimental context. Jesty vaccinated his family during a local small-pox epidemic (Pead 2003).

8. To clarify the terminology, *inoculation* refers to any method of inducing immunity against infectious disease other than acquiring the disease. Prior to Jenner, smallpox inoculation involved inserting pus from a smallpox below the skin in order to create an immune response. This form of inoculation was called *variolation* because it used the smallpox virus (variola) to build immunity. While effective, it was dangerous and at times lethal to be exposed to even small amounts of the deadly smallpox virus. Jesty, and then Jenner, were able to create the same immune response to smallpox without the risk by subcutaneous exposure to cowpox, a bovine disease that was closely related to smallpox but presented no risk to human health. Jenner observed that Dutch milk maids did not contract smallpox during local outbreaks and reasoned that the *vaccinia* (cowpox) virus was the source. The term "vaccine" came from the use of the vaccinia virus as a mode of inoculation.

9. Wealth and education encourage better health by increasing effective agency, a sense of personal control that encourages healthy living, as well as providing the material and social resources for enabling good health. Wealth and education are "fundamental causes" of health (Link and Phelan 1995), that is, social buffers against health harms caused by unsafe neighborhoods, poor access to quality healthcare, chronic stress, occupational hazards, and more. For a review of public health research into education and population health outcomes, see Hahn and Truman (2015).

10. The association of vaccine refusal and affluence has triggered class tensions in some instances. During a 2014 pertussis outbreak in Los Angeles, *The Hollywood Reporter* published a cover story titled "Hollywood's Vaccine Wars: L.A.'s 'Entitled' Westsiders behind City's Epidemic" (Baum and Gall 2014). The story was reposted on the *Data Lounge* blog with the more colorful title, "Entitled Rich Hollywood Assholes Are to Blame for Recent Whooping Cough Epidemic" (Anonymous 2014).

11. There is more discussion on Paul Offit's work in chapter 1, including criticisms of his divisive and sometimes disparaging language when characterizing vaccine hesitators and refusers.

12. Gavi, the Vaccine Alliance, is a public-private global health partnership committed to increasing access to immunization in under-resourced countries. Based in Geneva, Switzerland, the alliance was founded by and is supported by the Bill and Melinda Gates Foundation.

13. Orr and Beck (2017) found that the Parent Attitudes about Childhood Vaccines (PACV) survey tool successfully identified influenza vaccine-hesitant caregivers in a primary care center that serves a largely urban, low-income, and racialized patient population in Cincinnati, Ohio.

14. Convenience sampling is a type of nonprobability sampling that involves drawing study participants from a population that is easy to access. For example, vaccine hesitancy research might seek participants among patients at a particular healthcare clinic.

15. Self-selection and nonresponse biases are common problems in survey research because participants decide whether they want to participate in the survey. These individual choices can result in nonrepresentative study populations.

16. The two studies thereby offered a mixed methods approach, combining qualitative and quantitative methods.

17. *Affluenza*, a portmanteau of *affluence* and *influenza*, is a term used by critics of consumerism to describe a psychological malaise affecting wealthy young people. It is not a medically recognized disease, but it does carry cultural cachet. The term was coined in the mid-twentieth century and popularized in a 1997 PBS documentary by the same name and follow-up book (de Graff et al. 2001). Affluenza is defined as "a painful, contagious, socially transmitted condition of overload, debt, anxiety, and waste resulting from the dogged pursuit of more" (de Graff et al. 2001). The 2005 book *Affluenza: When Too Much is Never Enough* (Hamilton and Denniss 2001) posed the question, "If the economy has been doing so well, why are we not becoming happier?" (viii). The answer that is

offered is that consumer culture invites overconsumption, consumer debt, environmental destruction, and mental illness due to alienation and distress (179–80). "Affluenza" resurged in popular
usage in 2013 with the trial of Ethan Couch, a teenager in Texas arrested for killing and injuring
pedestrians while driving under the influence of alcohol. In court, a psychologist argued for affluenza in Couch's defense, specifically that the accused was unable to understand the consequences of
his actions because of financial privilege. This argument sparked a media frenzy about the term; see
especially the response by de Graff (2014).

18. The war on science terminology does not appear to extend into non-English language media,
with the exception of some usage in French Canadian media. See for example, "Guerre à la science:
Le temps de la contre-attaque" (Agence Science-Presse 2016), describing political assault on science
in Canada and the USA. Outside of the French Canadian press, the "war on science" only appears
as translation of or commentary on English-language content. For example, see Italian coverage of
*National Geographic*'s March 2015 issue, "Guerra alla scienza" (Pennetta 2015).

19. The cover page image can be viewed online, including here: http://coolsciencedad.blogspot.
com/2015/03/the-war-on-science-national-geographic.html. The bold text appears in all caps
against black background and the image of a worker adjusting an exhibit of the moon landing at
NASA's Kennedy Space Center in Florida.

20. While the origins of the term are unknown to me, its current usage traces back to American political journalist Katerina vanden Heuvel's (2004) article in the *Nation* about then-president George
W. Bush's antiscience policies, and science journalist Chris Mooney's (2005) book *The Republican
War on Science*. The book traces a longer history of political interference with science by conserva-
tive politicians, a narrative that escalated during the Reagan years (as seen in that administration's
apathy toward the science of evolution, HIV/AIDS, and acid rain) and came to a head during George
W. Bush's administration. Bush gained notoriety as "the antiscience president" (Mooney 2005, 223;
Duncan 2007) when the Union of Concerned Scientists published a report in 2004 detailing the
Bush administration's unprecedented scientific interference. The document was signed by over sixty
leading scientists and Nobel laureates (Union of Concerned Scientists, 2004). According to Mooney,
this highly publicized report "finally jolted" public attention to the decades-long conservative war
on science, prompted Mooney's journalistic endeavor, and made "war on science" a common phrase
for denoting politicized science and the belief that science was under political attack. Canadian and
Australian media have used the term to refer to their respective national governments' interference
in scientific research (Turner 2013; Dupuis 2013; Eyb 2014); in the UK, the BBC produced the 2006
documentary *A War on Science*, on intelligent design challenges to the theory of evolution.

21. American writers extend the term to describe antiscience events in other countries too. Otto
(2016) applies the charge to Canadian suppression of environmental science by its federal government,
anti-GMO activism in Europe and China, and antifluoridation and anti-windfarm politics in Australia.

22. There are some exceptions, of course, to caricatures of vaccine refusers. See, for example,
health journalist Tara Haelle's "15 Myths about Anti-Vaxxers, Debunked" (2015a; 2015b; 2015c).

23. Chemophobia is an irrational fear of chemicals. Despite containing the suffix -*phobia*, it is
not a phobia by standard medical definition. Most of the writing on chemophobia treats it as a
prejudice. Michelle Frankl, an American chemist, has written that "we are a chemophobic culture.
*Chemical* has become a synonym for something artificial, adulterated, hazardous, or toxic. . . . [but]
absolutely everything is made of atoms and molecules. It's all chemistry" (Frankl 2013). This bifurcation of natural and unnatural, organic and chemical, is thought to drive the unfounded view that
alternative medicine is safe.

24. Some of the works that have inspired this area of study are philosopher of science John Hardwig's (1985; 1991; 1994) papers on epistemic dependence in science, and the scholarship of historian

and sociologist of science Steven Shapin and historian Simon Schaffer, notably their coauthored book, *Leviathan and the Air Pump* (Shapin and Schaffer 1985).

25. This book will refrain from using the disparaging terminology of *anti-vaxxer* unless used in quotation marks to denote use of the term as relevant to the arguments put forth by others.

26. Biomedical science has a fraught history of research on vulnerable people and populations. Some unforgettable cases include: The Tuskegee Syphilis Study (where Black men with untreated syphilis were unknowingly observed for years and denied treatment in order to study disease progression [see Jones 1981]); Henrietta Lax (whose cancerous cells were obtained without permission and who never received dividends for the creation of the HeLa cell line that is still used widely in medical research [see Skloot 2011]); the Willowbrook hepatitis experiments (which involved infecting institutionalized children at the Willowbrook State School with hepatitis in order to observe disease progression [see Rothman and Rothman 2009]). Dangerous covert nutritional experiments were performed on Aboriginal children in Canadian residential schools (Mosby 2013). See also Schroeder et al.'s (2018) case studies on exploitative research in North-South research collaborations.

27. The rates of vaccination coverage needed within a population to curb the spread of infectious diseases ("herd immunity thresholds") will vary based on how contagious the disease is, how effective the vaccine is, how long immunity lasts for vaccinated and previously infected people, and how vulnerable the specific population is to infection. Measles, the most infectious of vaccine-preventable diseases, requires population coverage as high as 95 percent (and arguably higher in some highly social communities) to curb the spread of measles. Polio, a comparatively less contagious disease, can be contained with vaccination coverage ranging from 80 to 86 percent (depending on specific features of the population) (Helft and Willingham 2014).

28. Science and Communications Studies prefer use of the term "the publics" instead of "the public" or "public sphere" to highlight the diversity of people represented under the phrase and the plurality of nonexpert ways of engaging with science.

29. The rising tide of mistrust only captures the experiences of some members of the publics. Other publics, especially members of marginalized communities, have never felt equality in terms of their relationships to government and the benefits of science.

30. It warrants mention that science has historically served state-sanctioned injustices. See, for example, Saini's (2019) *Superior: On the Return of Race Science*, which documents the disturbing resilience of scientific racism. I discuss this further in chapter 5.

31. Largent saw the autism–vaccine controversy as a proxy debate that obscures a constellation of concerns held by many parents about the number of vaccines required (some for diseases that the children are unlikely to ever encounter); the desire for more flexibility and choice regarding the vaccine schedule; and fear of known side effects that, while rare, can be serious and even life-threatening. These, he explains, are "essential problems with our vaccine regime" (Largent 2012, 158). Navin offers a broader social accounting of vaccine refusal as "a symptom of changes in the educated public's relationship with both health care and the political community" (Navin 2015, 1). Hausman (2019) characterizes vaccine controversy as a social problem, rather than a scientific one, and which includes critiques of medicalization and concerns about the dangers of modern medicine.

### Chapter 1. The "Ignorant Public"
*Epigraph:* Fischer 2019.

1. The London Royal Society's (1985) report lead to the development of a now-thriving area of science communications studies by the same name, although "public understanding of science" is now interpreted very differently than the account offered in the report.

2. This book focuses on what historian Mark Largent (2012) referred to as the "current" anti-vac-

cine movement that started with the Wakefield scandal and continues today. While there were previous anti-vaccine movements, Largent claims that there are very few historical links between previous movements and the current situation. For some history on anti-vaccine movements in the USA, see Kaufman (1967), Colgrove (2006), Conis (2015b). For a history of anti-vaccination in the UK, see Durbach (2000; 2002; 2004), and for Canada, see MacDougall and Monnais (2017).

3. Some commentators still acknowledge that there were precipitating factors leading up to the explosive reaction to Wakefield et al.'s 1998 study. Fitzpatrick, for instance, notes that a few years prior to Wakefield and colleagues' first suggestion of an MMR-autism link, "there were already signs that MMR was in trouble" (2004a, 11). The UK had experienced its first decline in MMR vaccine uptake (from a 92 percent average to roughly 91 percent) in 1997 following bad press over the 1994 "Operation Safeguard" school immunization program that offered a combined measles-rubella vaccine. There had also been publicity in 1995 for Wakefield and colleagues' earlier work suggesting a link between measles or the measles vaccine and inflammatory bowel disease (Fitzpatrick 2004a, 11–12).

4. The recommendation is for the first dose of the MMR vaccine to be administered at twelve to fifteen months of age in the USA (Center for Disease Control and Prevention ND), at twelve months in all Canadian provinces (Public Health Agency of Canada 2011), and twelve to thirteen months in the UK (patient.co.uk ND)

5. *Lancet* editor Richard Horton was strongly criticized for his decision to publish the paper. See, for example, Greenhalgh (2004).

6. In 1982 an American TV documentary titled *DPT: Vaccine Roulette* aired on NBC local stations; it emphasized the risks of the diphtheria, pertussis, and tetanus (DPT) vaccine while ignoring the dangers of the diseases themselves, prompting wide public concern and harsh rebuke from the American Academy of Pediatrics and the Center for Disease Control and Prevention. Despite decades of use—the DPT vaccine was first licenced in the USA in 1949—the documentary galvanized public concern and prompted grassroots organizing by parents who believed their children had been injured by the DPT vaccine.

7. For an analysis of the influence of Jenny McCarthy, the former celebrity face of the "anti-vaxx" movement, on vaccine hesitancy, see Largent (2012, 138–48). See also Patrick Coleman's (2019) "Reminder Jenny McCarthy Helped Cause the Anti-Vaxxer Measles Outbreak" in the February 2019 issue of *Fatherly*. Also, TV producer Derek Batholomous's website, jennymccarthybodycount.com, started in 2009. When the count ended six years later, the website listed 152,763 illnesses and 9,028 preventable deaths.

8. This thesis permits the increasingly popular option among parents of a modified or "alternative" vaccine schedule rather than indiscriminate rejection of all vaccines. Some vaccines could be eliminated, combined vaccines could be unbundled, and vaccines could be introduced more slowly. See for instance, "Dr. Bob's Alternative Vaccine Schedule" promoted by best-selling author and physician Dr. Robert Sears (Sears 2007).

9. Those estimates and the detailed calculations are reviewed in Offit et al. (2002).

10. Offit made the now infamous "hundred thousand vaccines" argument in response to Dr. Sears's claim that the combination MMR booster should be withheld until age five when the immune system is more mature. Offit hoped to prove, to the contrary, that vaccines given in the first year of life induce an excellent immune response. Instead the "hundred thousand" comment raised the ire of many vaccine hesitators and deniers, who perceived Offit as being insensitive and uncaring toward vulnerable children. See Huff (2012).

11. Gerber and Offit (2009) describe the three popular vaccine danger theses as "shifting" because, by their account, the anti-vaccine movement has shifted public fear and attention from one theory to another as evidence mounted against any one of them and threatened to undermine it.

12. This theory of public misunderstanding of the science has been stated explicitly in some instances. For example, see the 2008 *New York Times* headline "Measles Cases Grow in Number, and Officials Blame Parents' Fear of Autism" (Harris 2008).

13. A 2019 study examining the Danish national registry records of over 650,000 people (the largest study to date) showed no autism-vaccine connection (Hviid et al. 2019).

14. An ESRC commissioned report on science, the publics, and the media, which comprehensively reviewed media coverage of the MMR-autism debate in 2,214 newspaper, radio, and television reports from January to September 2002 and surveyed over 1,000 British residents, came to the same conclusion. See Hargreaves et al. (2003).

15. Offit explained to a reporter for *Baby Talk* magazine that vaccines are "under fire" due to their success. He explained that "it's the natural evolution of a vaccine program" (in Howard 2005).

16. This kind of vaccine messaging still accomplishes maintenance of positive attitudes toward vaccines and vaccine compliance by most publics. The difficulty is in changing the attitudes and behaviors of vaccine-hesitant and vaccine-refusing people.

17. See chapter 6 for more on Andrew Wakefield as maverick.

18. Historian of science Naomi Oreskes entertained this option in editorials on public resistance toward the overwhelmingly strong climate change consensus offered by the Intergovernmental Panel on Climate Change, National Academy of Sciences, American Meteorological Society, the American Geophysical Union, and the American Association for the Advancement of Science. In these writings, she attempted to clarify what the consensus represents (a justified majority opinion rather than unanimous agreement), the rigorous analysis with which the climate change conclusion was reached, and why the publics should not be concerned by a few outlier scientists who challenge the consensus (Oreskes 2004a; 2004b).

19. Hobson-West (2007) found this language of individualized needs of the child being heavily used by British "vaccine-critical" groups (including JABS) in her interviews with the leaders of ten such groups. This suggests that the anti-vaccine rhetoric is more in tune with parental thinking and attitudes (whether influencing or being influenced by those parents) than the population-level language of risk employed by pro-vaccine sources.

20. This network was founded by Del Bigtree, TV producer of the *Dr. Phil Show* and *The Doctors*, a medical talk show. As a prominent voice among vaccine skeptics, he hosts a radio talk show and was a producer of *Vaxxed*, the 2016 Andrew Wakefield film project.

21. https://www.informedparent.co.uk/.

22. ICD-10 refers to the tenth revision of the *International Statistical Classification of Diseases and Related Health Problems* (ICD), a medical classification list compiled by the World Health Organization (World Health Organization 2016). Medical classification transforms descriptions of medical diagnoses and procedures into standardized statistical codes. The ICD-10 includes codes for diseases, signs and symptoms, abnormal findings, complaints, social circumstances, and external causes of injury or disease (World Health Organization 2020). The codes are widely used for billing purposes by health professionals. Work on ICD-10 began in 1983 and was endorsed by the Forty-Third World Health Assembly in 1990 (World Health Organization 2016, 1–3). Member states will use the ICD-10 until January 1, 2022, when it will be replaced by ICD-11. The ICD-10 description of Childhood Autism is available on pages 147–49 of the list (World Health Organization 1993).

23. The link for "MMR and Acquired Autism (Autistic Enterocolitis)—A Briefing Note" (Trowther 2003) was still live in May 2020.

24. From 1932 to 1972, the United States Public Health Service conducted a nontherapeutic experiment involving over four hundred black male sharecroppers infected with syphilis. The study traced disease progression in the subjects until death. The men were not told they had syphilis and

were not given treatment when penicillin became publicly available. Health officials deceived the men into believing they were patients in a government study of "bad blood," a catch-all phrase Black sharecroppers used to describe a host of illnesses (Jones 1993). The study was discontinued when the *Washington Evening Star* broke the story in 1972, following leaked information from Peter Buxton, a US Public Health Service employee. At the end of this forty- year study, more than one hundred men had died from syphilis or related complications, forty wives of Tuskegee participants had been infected, and nineteen children were born with congenital syphilis.

25. The ethical violations against Tuskegee subjects far exceeded knowledge suppression. The subjects were deliberately deceived about their health conditions and the nature of the treatment they were receiving, and they were denied the standard of care (see Brandt 1978).

26. Thomas and Quinn argued in 1991 that "almost sixty years after the [Tuskegee] study began, there remains a trail of distrust and suspicion that hampers HIV education efforts in Black communities" (Thomas and Quinn 1991; see also Jones 1993, chapter 14).

27. Those values are buried, however, as the value-free ideal strongly persists in policy circles (Douglas 2009).

28. Brossard and Lewenstein (2009) further divide Miller's (2001) second model of public understanding of science, the contextualist foil to the deficit model, into three: contextualist, lay expert, and finally, public engagement models. The latter is the most desirable model by their account.

29. The House of Lords claims to have shifted its focus from public misunderstanding, articulated in the Bodmer report, to a communicative approach. A 2004 publication reads, "While the themes the Bodmer report deals with are still of crucial importance today—not least to encourage young people to study and develop an interest in science—things have moved on since this time. The public understanding of science approach has been questioned as a deficit model of understanding. The implied relationship that support for science can be achieved through better communication overlooks the fact that different groups may frame scientific issues differently" (House of Lords 2004, 11).

## Chapter 2. The "Stubborn Mind"

1. Critical for gaining solid empirical support and understanding of motivated reasoning is identifying these more empirically established mechanisms and giving a plausible account of how they work in goal-directed reasoning. Otherwise, as Kahan (2011) points out, "assertions of 'motivated cognition' become circular—'x believes that [y] because it was useful; the evidence is that it was useful for x to believe that [y].'"

2. Hume's quote comes from his writing on moral psychology, the study of how we are motivated to act morally, in *Treatise of Human Nature*, book 2, section 3, part 3.

3. The "group-grid" has animated two decades' worth of empirical research aimed at testing the cultural theory of risk (of which cultural cognition is just one operational framework). See Kahan (2012).

4. Health and science journalists seemed to demonstrate their own confirmation bias with regards to thinking about vaccine hesitancy. I thank Ben Chin-Yee for pointing this out to me.

5. On the facticity of values, see Anderson (2004; 2010); Clough (2003a; 2003b; 2014); Goldenberg (2015; 2014). See also Brown (2020) on the reliability of value judgments.

6. The "I Immunise" campaign is described by its organizers as "leading with facts instead of values" (Fisher et al. 2014), language that I have flagged as probably unwittingly invoking an untenable fact-value distinction. While the campaign does focus on identity rather than the facts about vaccine safety and efficacy ("indirect means" in table 2.2), I read the campaign work done here as an interrogation of values, especially how they relate to vaccination.

7. When the campaign was launched in early 2014, Fremantle and surrounding suburbs' rates of immunization were roughly 5 percent lower than the rest of the country. Vaccination rates of 93 per-

cent among one-year olds, and 82 percent for five-year olds made the city vulnerable to infectious disease outbreaks. Herd immunity for measles is only reached when 95 percent of the population are vaccinated. Two years later, Australia gained international attention for its strong legislative action to confront vaccine refusal. The "No Jab, No Pay" policy withholds three state payments (Child Care Benefits, Child Care Rebate, Family Tax Benefit Part A end of year supplement) and imposes fines on childcare centers that admit unvaccinated children. Since the policy's introduction, vaccination rates have increased minimally in Western Australia (Satti 2018).

8. The designation of the Freo parents who appeared on the ads as "local experts" challenges the concept of expert beyond its usual bounds. Experts are understood to have specialized knowledge about the issue in question, yet there is debate over whose expertise is recognized and what expert knowledge is relevant to the issue at hand. Science studies researchers have enlarged expertise beyond academic credentialed knowledge to include lay expertise (Wynne 1996), or experience-based expertise (Collins and Evans 2002), based on experience acquired in everyday life. Health research now recognizes "expert patients," people whose experience living with long-term chronic illness affords them unique and valuable insight into their condition and their care needs that is distinct from the expertise of physicians and medical researchers and relevant to successful health management (for example, Lindsay and Vrijhoef 2009). But there is still disagreement about when lay expertise is relevant to the debate. Is vaccine controversy settled by expert knowledge on vaccine safety and efficacy, or do other stakeholders like parents bring in relevant knowledge, even expert knowledge? Experts and expertise are examined in chapters 3 and 6 of this book.

9. Importantly, this isn't a replacement of facts with values in vaccine debates. Instead the facts surrounding identity-constituting value preferences are foregrounded in order to demonstrate their fit with vaccination practices. This campaign can be understood to expand the rhetorical strategy of vaccine outreach beyond the facts about vaccine safety and efficacy to include facts that inform social and cultural identities. I thank Sharyn Clough for making this important point to me in private correspondence and refer readers to her work on the factual basis of value judgments (2003a; 2003b; 2014).

10. The webpage http://immunise.org.au/renee/ is no longer available.

11. For an analysis of vaccine mandates, see Attwell and Navin (2019).

12. Behavior-augmenting incentives include: fear of penalty (hierarchy), financial gain (markets), and peer-acceptance (networks) (Mols et al. 2015).

13. Nudges are limited to "easy and cheap" changes to the choice architecture (Thaler and Sunstein 2008). Thus financial incentives fall out of the purview of nudges.

14. For an ethical analysis of vaccine mandates, see Navin and Largent (2017).

15. Also, Navin and Attwell (2019) argue for diversity of values regarding the ethical justification of any communities' vaccine-mandate policies.

### Chapter 3. The "Death of Expertise"
*Epigraph:* Nichols 2014.

1. For analysis of populist epistemologies and their reverence for the "common sense" of the people over expert wisdom and knowledge, see Ylä-Anttila (2018).

2. Whereas Fischer is a professor of business and management, Nichols is a political scientist who presumably would be aware of this area of political science scholarship. Yet Nichols (2017a) limits his discussion of populism to a characterization of uninformed popular opinion as "populist."

3. Anti-intellectualism is hostility toward or mistrust of intellectuals and intellectualism and is commonly expressed in depreciation of art, literature, and science as contemptible human pursuits. This supposed championing of the "common folk" vilifies educated people, such as academics and other professional experts, as detached from and dismissive of the concerns of ordinary people.

4. The contact point between death of expertise and anti-intellectualism lies in the rejection of elites. American commentators root the tendency toward anti-intellectualism in a distinctly American affection for social egalitarianism that came with the nation's historical rejection of European hierarchy based on birth and class (see Bruinius 2018; Nichols in Buck [2017]). But this anti-elitist tendency is seen in non-American contexts as well. Totalitarian governments have long manipulated and applied anti-intellectualism to repress political dissent. In political situations as diverse as the Spanish Civil war and the Khmer Rouge regime, the intelligentsia were targeted and killed.

5. The Dunning-Kruger effect refers to social psychology research by David Dunning and Justin Kruger into metacognition, the capacity to self-assess how much we know. Kruger and Dunning (1999) found that people with the lowest knowledge or skills tended to overestimate their knowledge and ability as superior. These subjects were "unskilled and unaware of it," that is, they lacked the self-awareness to recognize their own limits and to appreciate the actually superior knowledge, skills, and abilities of other individuals compared to themselves.

6. See the PBS NewsHour interview with Nichols, "The Problem with Thinking You Know More than Experts" (PBS NewsHour 2017).

7. Institutional governance refers to the configuration of state and private organizations that shape national, economic, and social outcomes (Griffiths and Zammuto 2005).

8. Kitcher's work admittedly does not fit some characterizations of science studies, and so there may be disagreement with my description of him as a science studies scholar. If science studies is understood as the scholarly effort to challenge scientific authority, then Kitcher is out of place within this category. I use the term "science studies" to mean the social, philosophical, and historical study of science, a characterization of the field that easily includes Kitcher.

9. By some accounts he was more than just a veteran, but rather the catalyst of the Science Wars, the 1990s intellectual skirmish between scientists and so-called postmodern science studies scholars.

10. In the next chapter, the same phenomenon of distinguishing good and bad science by absence versus presence of values will be demonstrated to invite the manipulation of science for political ends.

11. See also Sokal and Bricmont (1999), *Fashionable Nonsense: Postmodern Intellectuals' Abuse of Science*, which dedicates a chapter to the work of Latour. One of the authors, Alan Sokal, is the instigator of the notorious "Sokal Hoax," a scholarly publishing sting that he, a physics professor, perpetrated to expose what he saw as lack of intellectual rigour in postmodern cultural studies. In 1996, Sokal submitted a nonsense article to the journal *Social Text* "to investigate whether a leading North American journal of cultural studies—whose editorial collective includes such luminaries as Frederic Jameson and Andrew Ross—[would] publish an article liberally salted with nonsense if (a) it sounded good and (b) it flattered the editors' ideological preconceptions" (Sokal 1996). Sokal's manuscript, "Transgressing the Boundaries: Towards a Transformative Hermeneutics of Quantum Gravity," was published in the *Social Text* spring/summer 1996 "Science Wars" issue. It proposed that quantum gravity is a social and linguistic construct. At that time, the journal did not practice academic peer review and it did not submit the article for outside expert review by a physicist (Robbins and Ross 1996). The hoax sparked debate about the scholarly merit of commentary on the physical sciences by humanities researchers, the status of postmodern philosophy, and the ethics of orchestrating such a hoax.

12. Sheila Jasanoff has similarly argued for science and technology studies (STS) research as the solution to, rather than the cause of, the problem of post-truth (Jasanoff and Simmett 2017). STS scholarship shows that moral panics about the status of knowledge in the public sphere are as old as knowledge itself. Also, against current laments about post-truth politics, there was no previous time when truth reigned uncontested and unfettered: "The road to knowledge was never so straight nor straightforward" (Jasanoff and Simmett 2017, 755).

13. The worry about excesses of second wave science studies appears similar to the criticisms its practitioners faced in real time by conservative critics of their supposed scientific relativism during the Science Wars. It seems curious that science studies survived the Science Wars of the 1990s, only to now waver in confidence. Yet Douglas (2009, see ch. 1) argues that the Science Wars were different from the current struggle, in part because the former was an academic debate while the present downgrading of experts comes from outside of the academy.

14. They key point is that communities shape and bound expertise. Collins uses the example of the fictitious community of Nobelskigrad, where all of its members have Nobel-winning levels of scientific training and knowledge. In Nobeslkigrad, high levels of scientific knowledge is ubiquitous knowledge because everyone has it, rather than specialist knowledge. Specialist expertise is special because not everyone has it.

15. Collins and Evans describe a tension between legitimation and extension. Democracy is supported by widening who gets a say, but this creates the "problem of extension," wherein expertise is broadened beyond the intellectual bounds that make expert knowledge useful (Collins and Evans 2002).

16. See https://www.facebook.com/pg/MalaysiaVaccine/photos/?tab=album&album_id=644 462025684284 (accessed April 18, 2019).

17. The letter was emailed to me and published on the group's website (see Kuntz 2017).

18. This is the same group responsible for the vaccine-skeptical billboards that appeared in downtown Toronto and were then promptly removed due to public pressure (Weeks 2019).

19. Navin (2015, ch. 1) presents further analysis of the epistemic cultures of vaccine skeptics.

20. Kitcher (1993) and other historians and philosophers of science also speak of the 1940s and 1950s as a time of high public optimism and confidence about science.

### Chapter 4. Politicized Science and Scientized Politics

1. Sam Harris (2011), for instance, argues that ethics should be fully supplanted by evolutionary theory and neuroscience. Defenders of the humanities disagree, claiming that the philosophical questions that vex us will not be answered by science. Neurohumanities (Quart 2013), for instance, the supposed savior of the liberal arts on college campuses, leads to a "shrinking world of ideas" (Krystal 2014). Krystal laments that assimilating humanities into neuroscience shifts "our focus from the meaning of ideas to the means by which they're produced." As a result, "the same questions that always intrigued us—What is justice? What is the good life? What is morally valid? What is free will?—take a back seat to the biases embedded in our neural circuitry. Instead of grappling with the gods, we seem to be more interested in the topography of Mount Olympus" (Krystal 2014; see also Roger Scruton's [2013] criticism of neuroaesthetics).

2. Hicks (2017) described science controversies as "proxy politics."

3. For social histories of evidence-based medicine, see Daly (2005) and Timmermans and Berg (2003).

4. The social constructedness of science need not be read in the strong sense (e.g., Bloor 2007). There are milder interpretations, like Barad's (2007) account of material-discursive practices, or the forms of plural realism mentioned in chapter 3.

5. I say "supposedly" because positivism framed moral and other value claims as empirically unfalsifiable, but philosophers of science have recently argued that value claims have empirical content and are therefore open to empirical assessment. See chapter 2, note 5.

6. "Junk science" refers to scientific data, research, or analysis considered to be inaccurate or fraudulent. It is contrasted with "sound science." The term also points to research driven by ideological motives. See Brandt (2007) on industry-influenced "junk science" regarding the health impacts of cigarettes, and Oreskes and Conway (2010) on cigarette and climate change junk science. Charges of "junk science" are often made in political and legal contexts where facts and scientific results have a

great amount of weight in the making of a determination. For historical use of the terms "junk" and "sound" science in American political and legal contexts, see chapter 6 of Mooney (2005). For a philosopher's analysis of contemporary sound vs. junk science rhetoric, see chapter 1 of Douglas (2009).

7. Among philosophers of science, realists think science offers not truth but the best approximations of truth. Philosophers of science since Duhem (1906/1962) have considered good science to offer approximations of truth and yet insist that it remain open to further inquiry and revision of prior views (i.e., Hempel, Popper).

8. Verificationism dismisses broad swaths of philosophical and theological investigation by arguing that statements regarding metaphysics, theology, ethics, and aesthetics are cognitively meaningless. Such statements may be meaningful in influencing emotions or behaviors, but not in terms of truth-value, information, or factual content.

9. My comments echo a large body of research in the philosophy of science on the relationship between science and values. Building on classic arguments by Rudner (1953) and Bahm (1971) and elements of pragmatist philosophy (e.g., the work of WVO Quine), contemporary research has variously demonstrated why the value-free ideal of science is implausible, which values enter scientific reasoning and where, which values benefit and which ones harm scientific inquiry, and how competing values should be adjudicated. Feminist philosophers of science have been particularly strong in this area of research (e.g.., Longino 1990; 2002; Kourany 2010; Solomon 2001; Wylie and Nelson 2007). For a good overview, see Douglas's (2016) "Values in Science" entry in the *Oxford Handbook of Philosophy of Science*.

10. This is what Jasanoff (2004) calls the "coproduction" of science and values or social norms.

11. For example, "Emergence of a Post Fact World" (Fukayama 2017) and *After the Fact* (Bomey 2018).

12. As I write this in May 2020, the COVID-19 outbreak is in its fifth month. Within weeks of the first observations of unusual cases of pneumonia in Wuhan, China, the causal link between the novel coronavirus and the emergence of a new strain of potentially acute respiratory illness was firmly established. Also well-established is the exponential increase in both disease incidence and mortality resulting from the illness. There remains uncertainty regarding ease of transmission, rates of misdiagnosis, and the numbers of asymptomatic cases, but the chain of causation is clear. The virus is identified, people are becoming ill from that virus, hospitals are filling up in disease "hot spots," patients are dying, and the number of deaths can be counted and communicated unequivocally. The proper response, however, is globally divisive: quarantine and the closing of schools and nonessential businesses are politically controversial. Those public health measures have social and economic costs that some argue outweigh the magnitude of the illness (Harel 2020; for the opposing view, see Crowe 2020). There is also a minority view that the virus ought to spread in order to generate widespread herd immunity (Straus 2020). The herd immunity approach was briefly touted by British prime minister Boris Johnson (Yong 2020; Mueller 2020).

## Chapter 5. Trust and Credibility in Science

*Epigraph:* American Academy of Arts and Sciences 2014b, 1; my emphasis.

1. There are small research bases investigating behavioral modifications and patient-provider communications in order to encourage vaccine uptake.

2. The press surrounding the report's release curiously made no mention of trust (see AAAS 2014a; Bloom et al. 2014). Why this oversight? Because despite motivating the investigation, trust was not reflected in the key findings. For example, the report's co-chairs summarized the report's conclusions without any mention of trust (in Bloom, Marcuse, and Mnookin [2014]). I argue that this shortcoming follows from building a research agenda on a weak theoretical foundation.

3. The desire to hide in the herd is the one exception, as it does not clearly follow from a challenging of scientific expert opinion. Instead it is a risk-reducing calculation based on the known presence of serious but rare adverse events following vaccination.

4. The scientific expert will be trusted to generate reliable knowledge rather than true knowledge, given the fallibility of science.

5. McLeod (2002) points out that sometimes the presumption of moral integrity of the trustee will suffice; proper motivation is not always expected or necessary.

6. Unlike mere reliance, which can only be disappointed, trust can be betrayed and give rise to reactive attitudes like resentment and anger (Holton 1994, 66–67).

7. This terminology can be traced back to the classic contributions by nineteenth-century German sociologist Georg Simmel (1900/1978), whose *lebensphilosophie* was inspired in part by philosopher Soren Kierkegaard's critiques of rationalism. Kierkegaard discussed the qualitative leap in the context of ethics and religious faith in his analysis of Abraham's would-be sacrifice of his son Isaac, in *Fear and Trembling* (Kierkegaard 1843/1985). See also Kierkegaard's analysis of Lessing's third thesis, in *Concluding Unscientific Postscript to Philosophical Fragments* (Kierkegaard 1846/1992). For discussion of Simmel's leap of faith and theory of trust, see Mollering (2001).

8. The individualist language is a break from the premodern emphasis on hierarchically powerful social bodies as knowledge authorities.

9. Philip Kitcher similarly addressed the epistemic role of trust in science, arguing specifically for its place as part of the optimal division of cognitive labor in science (Kitcher 1990, 1993).

10. The published manuscript includes 9 pages of text and 24 pages listing the names of all 5,154 authors. The article was a joint collaboration of two huge teams that operated two particle detectors at the Large Hadron Collider at CERN, the European particle physics lab near Geneva, Switzerland. The two research teams pooled their data to obtain the most precise estimate yet of the mass of the Higgs boson particle.

11. I am using the term "objectivity" in the pragmatic sense of intersubjective agreement, rather than the classical realist sense of "non-subjectivity." Feminist philosophers have strengthened the rigor of the intersubjective agreement by increasing the inclusivity of the communities of knowers striving for intersubjective criticism. See Harding (1993) on "strong objectivity" and Longino's (2002) transformative criticism as the standards that make a community of inquirers objective.

12. The exclusion of aristocratic and gentry women from the Royal Society fellowship, however, suggests class to be a necessary but not sufficient criterion for trustworthiness. The Royal Society did not admit women fellows until 1945, with only one exception: Queen Victoria (Murdoch 2014, 167).

13. For a review of the complex and multiple meanings of the term "objectivity," see Daston and Galison (2010) and Douglas (2004).

14. Hardwig recognizes that competence is not a character trait per se but allows it as part of the epistemic qualities required for trustworthiness, because competence depends largely on epistemic character. He explains that "becoming knowledgeable and then remaining current almost always requires habits of self-discipline, focus, and persistence" (1991, 700).

15. Luhmann (1979) explains that we benefit from well-placed trust more over time, as positive interactions result in less vigilance being required.

16. Climate experts are defined as "scientists who have published climate-related scientific research" (Cook et al. 2018, 3).

17. Almassi (2012) has made the same argument, that most of what we know about climate change rests on epistemic trust.

18. Once a central celebrity figure among vaccine skeptics, actress and comedian Jenny McCarthy famously dismissed the consensus view on vaccines and autism during a 2007 TV appearance

on *Oprah*; she defended her own expertise as a parent researcher and advocate for her son by claiming, "University of Google is where I got my degree from" (see vanden Heuvel 2013). For more on McCarthy's influence, see Largent (2012; 2013).

19. The links between medical racism and mistrust of healthcare personnel and institutions are found among other marginalized groups. For example, in Canada, Indigenous people's distrust and avoidance of contact with the medical system is tied to past and current abuse, coercion, and forced separation of Indigenous families in which health professionals and systems are implicated (Narine 2013; Vogel 2015; Goodman et al. 2017).

20. Eugenics programs aimed at "race betterment" were closely tied to public health and hygiene concerns in the early twentieth century. In the United States, the Race Betterment Foundation was founded by John Harvey Kellog to respond to supposed "race degeneracy." The foundation supported hygiene and eugenics programs, incorporating what are now seen as responsible public health efforts (physical fitness, nutrition, safe housing). However, they also espoused nefarious claims about heredity that were taken to justify eugenics registries and the sterilization of individuals deemed unfit or degenerate.

21. Bacher (1993, 45–49) chronicled the early twentieth-century public health response to Toronto's "slum" Ward District amid anti-immigrant sentiment. Bacher explains that interest in the housing conditions of the urban poor began to mount in Canadian cities as sensational accounts of immigrant life aroused fears for middle-class health and safety. Toronto public health officer Charles Hastings, author of the influential 1911 Toronto housing survey, blamed "the foreign element" for the "exorbitant rents" they endured. He warned the city against immigrants whose "ideas of sanitation are not ours." His 1914 *Report of the Medical Health Officer* led to the displacement of many vulnerable individuals and families from the Ward District. Other public health officials similarly endorsed anti-immigrant views regarding hygiene and health. Dr Charles Hodgetts, head of the Commission of Conservation's public health committee, viewed immigrants as "willing to live like swine," while Hamilton, Ontario's, public health officer James Roberts wrote that only the "drunken, lazy, and improvident" poor experienced housing problems (Bacher 1993, 46).

22. Swope (2018) examines public health's "problematic role" in urban renewal in Washington, DC, since the passing of the 1949 Housing Act. Public health officials worked with urban planners, offering "healthy housing standards" to assist in urban renewal programs across the USA. Yet research shows that urban renewal resulted in far more housing units destroyed than created, and that the majority of both relocated and displaced families were Black low-income residents (Swope 2018).

23. The connection between US and Nazi eugenicists is discussed in Kuhl (1994).

24. Pharmascolds are defined as "prominent critics . . . who routinely vilify the medical products industry and portray academics working with it as traitors and sellouts" (Shaywitz and Stossell 2009).

25. The so-called "pharmascolds" have embraced the moniker and dubbed their adversaries "pharmapologists."

26. When a vaccine is widely recommended and licensing is restricted to a few manufacturers, it can be extremely profitable. For example, Merck Pharmaceuticals, the only company licensed to offer the measles vaccine in the USA, reported 2014 earnings of $1.4 billion in sales for ProdQuad (a vaccine for measles, mumps, rubella, and varicella). MMR II (for measles, mumps, rubella), and Varivax (a chicken pox vaccine) together came in at $1.4 billion. Their top selling vaccine, Gardasil, an HPV vaccine, brought in $1.7 billion in sales (Lam 2015).

27. Additional qualitative research on vaccine-hesitant parents have supported Kaufman's account of bricolage. See Ward et al. (2017) and Sobo et al.'s (2016) similar term, "curated assemblages," which are self-curated collections of stories, memories, and practices.

28. This is not a relativist position on scientific evidence.

## Chapter 6. The Scientific Expert as Hero and Maverick

1. Defenders of expertise like Collins (2014) hark back to the scientific optimism of post–World War II. This is not to suggest that there was no contestation of scientific expertise prior to, or during, this time.

2. Only a minority of orthodox scientific experts discuss problems of power and privilege within their domains, for example, the biomedical science researchers and academic physicians calling attention to the harms of financial conflicts in biomedical science research (see chapter 5). There are also some healthcare teams that commit to antiracism practices and refuse free drug samples by pharmaceutical companies, turning sales representatives away from their offices.

3. Nazi experimentation on Holocaust concentration camp prisoners, for example, is held up by historians and philosophers of science as an example of research that was epistemically sound in terms of methodology and morally unsound in terms of values and politics (Proctor 1999; Proctor 2000; Kourany 2010; Mills 2020). For example, Kourany (2010) discusses Nazi cancer research as an example where facts and values were troublingly separate. Yet Clough (2015) insists that facts and values cannot be separated as such. Instead, even by the criteria of the time, Nazi cancer research was empirically weak, and the weaknesses of the research stemmed from the moral failings of Nazi policies on coerced experimentation on vulnerable subjects.

4. As mentioned in chapter 5, membership in the Royal Society was exclusive to men of noble birth (with the exception of Queen Victoria). Women were first admitted as fellows in 1945 (Holmes 2010).

5. Boyle was said to have regarded aristocratic women as his equal in intellectually demanding religious discussions (Haraway 1997, 27).

6. In the legal context, eyewitness accounts of criminal activity have been shown to be inaccurate in many instances. Perception is an interpretive process, and even well-meaning eyewitnesses produce faulty recall due to unconscious cognitive biases. Physical evidence like DNA frequently undermines even the firmest eyewitness accounts (Chew 2018).

7. Scientists today know that peer review does not guard against fraud (Goodstein 2010, 17).

8. Historians of science can account for no more than four pneumatic engines (air pumps), in addition to the three owned by Boyle, in circulation in the decade following Boyle's first experiment. One pump was owned by Christian Huygens in The Hague, a second pump was located at Montmor Academy in Paris, and there may have been a pump in Cambridge and another owned by Henry Power in Halifax, England (Shapin and Schaffer 1984).

9. Boyle's pump was complicated, temperamental, and problematic to operate. Many demonstrations could only be performed with his technician, Robert Hooke, on hand (Jardine 2004).

10. The 2016 book and film adaptation *Hidden Figures* told the little-known true story of three Black American female mathmaticians, Dorothy Vaughan, Mary Jackson, and Katherine Johnson, who served a vital role in NASA during the early years of the US space program. Fighting gender and racial prejudice in the workplace, their heroic contributions were underacknowledged. There are many female "hidden figures" in the history of science whose stories need to be uncovered and/ or amplified. The stories of Black, Hispanic, Asian, Indigenous, and many other racialized people also deserve to be recognized, both for the contributions they made and for the lost opportunities that kept them from contributing to science.

11. This application of Merton's norms to individual behavioral expectations on scientists is inconsistent with Merton's thinking about scientific governance (personal communication with Heather Douglas).

12. Hwang Woo-Suk is a South Korean scientist whose revolutionary claims of having cloned human embryos and extracting stem cells from them were discredited as fabrications in 2005.

13. German physicist Jan Hendrik Schön rose to prominence after a series of apparent break-

throughs with semiconductors that were later determined to be fradulent. Before he was exposed, Schön had received numerous prizes and investigator awards for his research, all of which were later rescinded. Schon had roughly thirty papers withdrawn after a 2002 investigation revealed anomalies in his data sets that could not be attributed to honest errors. In June 2004, the University of Konstanz issued a press release stating that Schön's doctoral degree had been revoked due to "dishonorable conduct."

14. Marc Hauser is an American evolutionary biologist who researches primate behavior, animal cognition, and human behavior. He was found guilty of fabricating and falsifying data and subsequently resigned from his faculty position at Harvard University in 2011. He was also investigated by the US Office of Research Integrity and Health and Human Services because his research had been funded in part by government grants. Hauser was found to have fabricated data, manipulated experimental results, and published falsified findings.

15. See Douglas (2009, chapter 2) and Jasanoff (1990) on scientific advising to government in the United States.

16. Training and professionalization can also limit diversity of the expert pool by structural barriers like high tuition and restrictive student loan programs (Canadian Federation of Medical Students 2010), lack of representation among faculty (Prescod-Weinstein 2018), lack of family-friendly policies (Vogel 2019), and discriminatory and/or hostile work environments (Settles 2014).

17. Collins and Evans (2007) characterized this tension as a "problem of legitimation" for the employment of expert-driven decision-making in democratic societies. Specifically, decisions have low political legitimacy when an elite group decides for the public.

18. The lead author, Donald Braben, had just published a book on the topic, titled *Promoting the Planck Club: How Defiant Youth, Irreverent Researchers and Liberated Universities Can Foster Prosperity Indefinitely* (Braben 2014).

19. Hempel was unique among his cohort of the most influential twentieth-century philosophers of science for lengthy discussion of a case from medicine. Natural sciences were the preferred investigative domains for Carnap, Duhem, Feyerabend, Kuhn, Lakatos, Neurath, Poincare, Popper, and Quine (Gillies 2005). Hempel characterized Semmelweiss's investigation into the cause of puerperal fever as exemplary hypothetico-deductive reasoning. Gillies (2005) notes that Hempel did not offer an account for why Semmelweiss's findings were ignored by his colleagues and seeks to explain the resistance by an appeal to Kuhnian paradigms. Semmelweiss radically offered a causal theory that contradicted the paradigmatic framework of miasma and contagion theories of 1840 Viennese medicine.

20. The Conspira-Sea Cruise is a weeklong gathering of close to one hundred conspiracy theorists and curious followers on an ocean liner. Headliners offer musings and philosophies on a range of topics that include ancient intergalactic warfare, crop circles, magical vibrations, chemtrails, and the government's control of the weather (Greenberg 2016). The organization of these cruises is secretive—all web links to any official websites are broken—so my understanding of these cruises comes exclusively from freelance writers who have "infiltrated" and attended them and then written first-hand accounts of their cruise experiences (see Merlan [2016], Dickey [2016], Greenberg [2016]; see also Sturgess [2016] and Glaser [2016] for interviews with an undercover skeptic who attended the cruise gathering).

21. See "The Vaccine Autism Myth Started 20 Years Ago; Here's Why It Endures" in the February 28, 2018, issue of *Time* (Quick and Larson 2018). Medical blogger Skeptical Raptor frequently invokes the zombie reference regarding vaccine-skeptical communications (see, for example Skeptical Raptor [2013; 2018]).

22. Another maverick, Dr. Bob Sears, is also praised by his patients for engaging their questions about childhood vaccines. The *LA Times* reports: "During checkups, moms say, he makes small talk

with children in a high-pitched voice to soothe them, and he lets parents rattle off questions until they run out of things to ask" (Gutierrez 2019).

23. For considerations of testimonial injustice experienced by patients with disabilities, see Peña-Guzmán and Reynolds (2019).

24. Epistemic injustice lends itself to intersectional analyses of social identity groups and nonbinary gender categories. See Luvell Anderson (2017) on epistemic injustice and philosophy of race, and Miranda Fricker and Katharine Jenkins (2017) on epistemic injustice experienced by trans people.

25. Gaslighting means manipulating someone by psychological means into questioning their own sanity. Through denial, misdirection, and contradiction the victim is destabilized and their beliefs are delegitimized (Sweet 2019). The term originates in the 1938 stage play *Gas Light* (Hamilton 1938) and its British and American film adaptations, which chronicle systematic psychological manipulation of a victim by her husband. In the story, the husband attempts to convince the wife and others that she is insane by manipulating small elements of their home environment and insisting that she is mistaken or delusional when she points out these changes. The play's title refers to how the abusive husband slowly dims the gas lights in their home, while pretending nothing has changed, in an effort to make his wife doubt her own perceptions. He intends to have her assessed and institutionally committed. *Gaslighting* became a colloquial term to describe psychological manipulation of a victim to doubt their own judgment, and its usage entered the psychology literature in the 1970s to describe a form of manipulation of victims by their domestic partners as well as of children by their caregivers (Barton and Whitehead 1969; Smith and Sinanan 1972; Shengold 1979; Calef and Weinshel 1981). Gaslighting has been examined by sociologists in the context of social inequalities and power-laden domestic and intimate relationships (see Sweet 2019 for a review of sociology of gaslighting). Feminist philosopher Kate Abramson (2014) points to the gendering of victims of gaslighting due to women's social conditioning to be less confident about their views, beliefs, reactions, and perceptions than men. Gaslighting and epistemic injustice have been tied together by philosophers Nora Berenstain (2016), Rachel McKinnon (2017), and Kate Manne (2017).

26. Where does the troubling resistance of today's vaccine-refusing "mother warriors" diverge from the commendable epistemic resistance of women's health activists to patriarchal medicine? One difference is in the terms of inquiry. Where the latter engaged in open-minded and challenging engagement with expert knowledge in order to create critical dissent and fill gaps in knowledge about women's health, vaccine skepticism tends to take the form of "bad faith dissent" (De Melo-Martín and Intemann 2018). The arguments work to shut out, rather than critically engage, the scientific orthodoxy on vaccines.

27. Risk society was first described in Beck's *Risikogesellschaft* (1986), and then in the 1992 English translation, *Risk Society*.

### Conclusion. Rebuilding Trust

1. That language is also folded into a compelling vision of the Good Parent.

2. The language of "upstream" and "downstream" is familiar to researchers working on social determinants of health. In the classic public health parable credited to medical sociologist Irving Zola, a witness sees a man caught in a river current. The witness saves the man and is then quickly drawn to the rescue of more drowning people. After many have been rescued, the witness walks upstream to investigate why so many people have fallen into the river. The story illustrates the tension between public health's protection mandates to respond to emergencies (help people caught in the current) and its prevention and promotion mandates (stop people from falling into the river). Evidence is mounting that an upstream approach to health—one that addresses people's access to the determinants of health—will benefit everyone (Commission on Social Determinants of Health 2008). In 1986, the Ottawa Charter for

Health Promotion (World Health Organization 1986) captured the shift in public health's focus from individual risk factors and behaviors to the societal conditions that keep people healthy, such as adequate income, meaningful work, education, community connection, freedom from discrimination, adequate housing, and healthy food (Kickbusch 2003). Community groups and grassroots and nongovernmental organizations have been calling for collective, upstream action to reduce health disparities (Scutchfield and Howard 2011; Phelan, Link, and Tehranifar 2010). These actions bring multiple sectors and publics together to advance healthy public policies and programs. This upstream-focused public health has been called the "new public health" (Kickbusch 2003), as well as "population health," while others call it a return to public health's roots (Frank 1995). See Valles (2018) for the philosophy of population health.

3. For me, the biggest surprise of Nyhan et al.'s (2014) vaccine communications study (discussed in chapter 2) was not that none of them worked, but that these long-used communications methods had never been tested.

4. A collaboration between Wellcome Trust and Gallup World Poll, the 2018 Wellcome Global Monitor study surveyed over 140,000 individuals living in over 140 countries. Wellcome studied the publics' understanding of science, whether they trusted scientific individuals and institutions, what they believed was the impact of science on society, and their confidence in vaccinations. The study revealed a high overall global trust (72 percent) in scientists and healthcare professionals, as well as vaccines (79 percent); however, it also noted troubling trends, such as a loss in confidence regarding vaccine safety in higher income countries. Overall, the publics' engagement with science is influenced by a combination of culture, context, and background, suggesting that scientists and science communicators need to keep this diversity of attitudes to science and health in mind when engaging with the publics.

5. Note that the Wellcome Global Measure does not capture variations within populations, like the known lower levels of trust in healthcare providers among racialized people. See chapter 5.

6. "Billing codes" are used by healthcare professionals to receive payment for healthcare services in both private and public healthcare systems. Billing codes are also called "ICD codes" and "ICD-10 codes," which map the International Classification of Diseases onto billing in fee-per-diagnosis medical reimbursement systems for healthcare services.

7. The pressure placed on women to breastfeed and the shame many mothers feel when they do not succeed in doing so have been strongly criticized by feminist writers and scholars. See for example, Gordon (1989), Rosin (2009), Kukla (2006), and Hausman (2014). More recently, healthcare professionals have acknowledged the harms of "breast is best" messaging to mothers (Pearson 2019; Diez-Sampedro 2019; Chaput et al. 2016).

8. For a review of the term "mother blaming," see Hatfield (2019).

9. Reich similarly concludes that we must eradicate the culture of mother blaming (Reich 2016, 248–49).

10. Canada should take notice. Only three of its thirteen provinces and territories have school-entry requirements. Some provinces have jurisdiction to exclude children from school during an outbreak—see for example the Alberta Public Health Act—although such quarantine measures have been criticized for being too slow in practice to curb the spread of highly infectious diseases (see Born, Yiu, and Sullivan 2014).

11. There are libertarian arguments favoring mandatory vaccination. Briefly, one's freedom to choose is limited by others' right not to be harmed by your choices (J. Brennan 2018; Novak 2015). Bernstein (2017) disputes this position, claiming that the libertarian argument for compulsory vaccination ultimately fails (on libertarian grounds).

12. Vaccine compulsion without consent from the legal guardian is not justified.

13. While diversity and context are recognized in the development and enactment of vaccine

mandates, the ethics of vaccine mandates tend to be argued by reference to singular overarching values—whether utility, children's interests, or harm reduction. Navin and Attwell (2019) have explored this curious disconnect between the practice and the ethical analysis of the practice and defend value pluralism for the ethics of vaccine mandates.

14. California's Senate Bill 277 was passed in the midst of the notorious Disneyland measles outbreak of 2014 that resulted in 150 cases of measles throughout the United States, Mexico, and Canada. The California legislature capitalized on extreme public frustration over the outbreak and successfully passed the sweeping bill, which was unprecedented in its dramatic removal of all nonmedical (personal belief and religious) exemptions for school-entry vaccines for all public and private schools and daycare centers in California.

15. The State of New York enacted law repealing religious and personal belief exemptions in response to a major measles outbreak in New York City in 2018–2019. The political situation around the outbreak was politically volatile because the most affected areas were Orthodox Jewish communities, raising both the spectre of anti-Semitism in the public health response and concern about the safety of a marginalized religious group. Indeed, there was a rise of anti-Semitism being expressed in New York during that time (Green 2019). The legislation to remove all religious and personal belief exemptions to vaccines in New York State was passed while public emergency efforts were being enacted in New York City and neighboring Rockland County to curb the outbreak. The legislation was thereby introduced at a highly galvanized political moment. In addition to barring unvaccinated children from schools and daycares in both jurisdictions, New York City's public health emergency enabled New York City to introduce mandatory vaccinations for the most heavily hit neighborhoods, with a penalty of one thousand dollars to those who refused. One preschool was forced to close because it would not cooperate with requests for vaccination information. In Rockland County, unvaccinated children were barred from public places for thirty days, and noncomplying parents faced up to six months in jail or a five-hundred dollar fine. A judge later lifted the public spaces ban, saying that the outbreak did not qualify for an emergency order. There were roughly 150 confirmed cases at the time.

16. Personal belief exemptions are also called philosophical exemptions in some jurisdictions, but "philosophical" is surely a misnomer. Philosophy is the systematic investigation of ideas, not an expression of personal preferences.

17. See chapter 2, note 7.

18. For an analysis of the population impact of different mandatory vaccination policies in Europe, see Vaz et al. (2020).

19. See chapter 5, note 11.

20. The Public Health Agency of Canada organizes its public health competencies into seven categories: (1) Public Health Science; (2) Assessment and Analysis; (3) Policy & Program Planning, Implementation & Evaluation; (4) Partnerships, Collaboration & Advocacy; (5) Diversity & Inclusiveness; (6) Communication; (7) Leadership. The Public Health Agency of Canada's list of core competencies was developed in consultation with more than three thousand practitioners from across Canada.

21. Anti-oppressive practice is a progressive approach to social work that counters socioeconomic oppression and exclusion. These practices target individual, group, and institutional/structural oppression. See, for example, Dominelli (2002; 2009).

22. Physical distancing, also called "social distancing," is a nonpharmaceutical public health measure for preventing the spread of contagious disease by maintaining a physical distance between people and limiting close contact.

# REFERENCES

3M State of Science Index. 2019. *3M State of Science Report*. Survey, Saint Paul, MN: 3M. https://www.3m.com/3M/en_US/state-of-science-index-survey/.

Abatte, Janet. 2012. *Recoding Gender: Women's Changing Participation in Computing*. Cambridge, MA: MIT Press.

Abrams, Lindsay. 2014. "Study: Trying to Convince Parents to Vaccinate Their Kids Just Makes the Problem Worse." *Salon*, March 3, 2014. http://www.salon.com/2014/03/03/study_trying_to_convince_parents_to_vaccinate_their_kids_just_makes_the_problem_worse/.

Abramson, Kate. 2014. "Turning Up the Lights on Gaslighting." *Philosophical Perspectives* 28 (1): 1–30.

Achenbach, Joel. 2015. "Why Do Many Reasonable People Doubt Science?" *National Geographic*, March 2015. https://www.nationalgeographic.com/magazine/2015/03/science-doubters-climate-change-vaccinations-gmos/.

Agence Science-Presse. 2016. "Guerre à la science: Le temps de la contre-attaque." *Le Devoir*, September 6, 2016. https://www.ledevoir.com/societe/science/479314/la-guerre-a-la-science-le-temps-de-la-contre-attaque.

Almassi, Ben. 2012. "Climate Change, Climate Change, Epistemic Trust, and Expert Trustworthiness." *Ethics and the Environment* 17, no. 2 (Fall): 29–49.

Alsan, Marcella, and Marianne Wanamaker. 2017. "Tuskegee and the Health of Black Men." NBER Working Paper No. 22323. Cambridge, MA: National Bureau of Economic Research.

Alter, Charlotte. 2014. "Nothing, Not Even Hard Facts, Can Make Anti-Vaxxers Change Their Minds." *Time*, March 4, 2014.

Altman, Ian. 2017. "5 Reasons Why Workplace Diversity Is Good for Business." *Inc.*, March 17, 2017. https://www.inc.com/ian-altman/5-reasons-why-workplace-diversity-is-good-for-business.html.

American Academy of Arts and Sciences. 2014a. "American Academy Report Calls for More Research on Parental Decision-Making on Childhood Vaccines." *Summer 2014 Bulletin*. https://www.amacad.org/news/academy-report-calls-more-research-parental-decision-making-childhood-vaccines.

American Academy of Arts and Sciences. 2014b. *Public Trust in Vaccines*. Washington, DC: AAAS.

Anderson, Elizabeth. 2004. "Uses of Value Judgments in Science: A General Argument, with Lessons from a Case Study of Feminist Research on Divorce." *Hypatia* 19, no. 1 (February): 1–24.

Anderson, Elizabeth. 2006. "The Epistemology of Democracy." *Episteme* 3, nos. 1–2 (June): 8–22.

Anderson, Elizabeth. 2010. *The Imperative of Integration*. Princeton, NJ: Princeton University Press.

Anderson, Elizabeth. 2011. "Democracy, Public Policy, and Lay Assessments of Scientific Testimony." *Episteme* 8, no. 2 (June): 144–64.

Anderson, Luvell. 2017. "Epistemic Injustice and the Philosophy of Race." In *The Routledge Handbook of Epistemic Injustice*, edited by Ian James Kidd, José Medina, and Gaile Pohlhaus Jr., chapter 12. London: Routledge.

Angell, Marcia. 2005. *The Truth about Drug Companies: How They Deceive Us and What to Do About It*. New York: Penguin Random House.

Anonymous. 2014. "Entitled Rich Hollywood Assholes Are to Blame for Recent Whooping Cough Epidemic." *Data Lounge*, September 14, 2014. https://www.datalounge.com/thread/14385395 -entitled-rich-hollywood-assholes-are-to-blame-for-recent-whooping-cough-epidemic.

Antony, Louise. 1993. "Quine as Feminist: The Radical Import of Naturalized Epistemology." In *A Mind of One's Own: Feminist Essays on Reason and Objectivity*, edited by Louise Antony and Charlotte Witt, 185–226. Boulder, CO: Westview.

Armstrong, David. 2019. "Inside Purdue Pharma's Media Playbook: How It Planted the Opioid 'Anti-Story.'" *ProPublica*, November 19, 2019. https://www.propublica.org/article/ inside-purdue-pharma-media-playbook-how-it-planted-the-opioid-anti-story.

Atkinson, Sharyl. 2008. "How Independent Are Vaccine Defenders?" *CBS News*, July 25, 2008. https://www.cbsnews.com/news/how-independent-are-vaccine-defenders/.

Attwell, Katie, and Melanie Freeman. 2015. "I Immunise: An Evaluation of a Values-Based Campaign to Change Attitudes and Beliefs." *Vaccine* 33, no. 46 (November 17): 6235–40.

Attwell, Katie, and Mark C. Navin. 2019. "Childhood Vaccination Mandates: Scope, Sanctions, Severity, Selectivity, and Salience." *Millbank Quarterly* 97, no. 4 (December): 978–1014.

Attwell, Katie, Mark C. Navin, Pier L. Lopalco, Christine Jestin, S. Reiter, and Saad B. Omer. 2018. "Recent Vaccine Mandates in the United States, Europe and Australia: A Comparative Study." *Vaccine* 36, no. 48 (November 19): 7377–84.

Bacher, John C. 1993. *Keeping to the Marketplace: The Evolution of Canadian Housing Policy*. Montreal: McGill-Queen's University Press.

Baggini, Julian, and Simon Jenkins. 2019. "Is Reason the Slave of the Passions?" *Prospect Magazine*, May 4, 2019. https://www.prospectmagazine.co.uk/magazine/is-reason-the-slave-of-the-pass ions-philosophy-hume.

Bahm, Archie. 1971. "Science Is Not Value-Free?" *Policy Sciences* 2, no. 4 (December): 391–96.

Baier, Annette. 1986. "Trust and Antitrust." *Ethics* 96, no. 2 (January): 231–60.

Baier, Annette. 1991. "Trust and Its Vulnerabilities." In *Tanner Lectures on Human Values*, 13:109–36. Salt Lake City: University of Utah Press.

Baker, Sherry. 1999. "Five Baselines for Justification in Persuasion." *Journal of Mass Media Ethics* 14 (2): 69–94.

Baker, Sherry, and David L. Martinson. 2001. "The TARES Test: Five Principles for Ethical Persuasion." *Journal of Mass Media Ethics* 16 (2/3): 148–75.

Barad, Karen. 2007. *Meeting the Universe Halfway: Quantum Physics and the Entanglement of Matter and Meaning*. Durham, NC: Duke University Press.

Barton, Russell, and J. A. Whitehead. 1969. "The Gaslight Phenomenon." *Lancet* 293, no. 7608 (June 21): 1258–60.

Baum, Gary, and Eric Gall. 2014. "Hollywood's Vaccine Wars: L.A.'s 'Entitled' Westsiders Behind City's Epidemic." *Hollywood Reporter*, September 10, 2014. https://www.hollywoodreporter. com/features/los-angeles-vaccination-rates/?src=longreads.

Beatty, William. 2002. "Ridiculed Discoverers, Vindicated Mavericks." Amasci (website). http:// amasci.com/weird/vindac.html.

Beck, Ulrich. 1986. *Risikogesellshaft. Auf dem Weg in Eine Andere Moderne*. Frankfurt: Suhrkamp.

Beck, Ulrich. 1992. *Risk Society: Towards a New Modernity*. London: Sage.

Beck-Gernsheim, Elisabeth. 2000. "Health and Responsibility: From Social Change to Technological Change and Vice Versa." In *The Risk Society and Beyond: Critical Issues for Social*

*Theory*, edited by Barbara Adam, Ulrich Beck, and Joost van Loon, 122–35. London: Sage Publications.

Bekelman, Justin E., Yan Li, and Cary P. Gross. 2003. "Scope and Impact of Financial Conflicts of Interests in Biomedical Research: A Systematic Review." *Journal of the American Medical Association* 289 (4): 454–65.

Bell, Stephen, Andrew Hindmoor, and Frank Mols. 2010. "Persuasion as Governance: A State-Centric Relational Perspective." *Public Administration* 88, no. 3 (September): 851–70.

Berenstain, Nora. 2016. "Epistemic Exploitation." *Ergo: An Open Access Journal of Philosophy* 3:569–90.

Bergkamp, Lucas. 2016. "Post-Modernism's Troubled Relationship with Science." *Areo*, November 30, 2016. https://areomagazine.com/2016/11/30/post-modernisms-troubled-relationship-with -science/.

Bernstein, Justin. 2017. "The Case against Libertarian Arguments for Compulsory Vaccination." *Journal of Medical Ethics* 43 (11): 792–96.

Betsch, Cornelia, Frank Renkewitz, Tilmann Betsch, and Corina Ulshofer. 2010. "The Influence of Vaccine-Critical Websites on Perceiving Vaccination Risks." *Journal of Health Psychology* 15, no. 3 (April): 446–55.

Bhat-Schelbert Kavitha, Chyongchiou Jeng Lin, Annamore Matambanadzo, Kristin Hannibal, Mary Patricia Nowalk, and Richard K. Zimmerman. 2012. "Barriers to and Facilitators of Child Influenza Vaccine—Perspectives from Parents, Teens, Marketing and Healthcare Professionals." *Vaccine* 30, no. 14 (January 17): 2448–52.

Bjørnskov, Christian. 2006. "The Multiple Facets of Social Capital." *European Journal of Political Economy* 22, no. 1 (March): 22–40.

Blakemore, Erin. 2018. "Until 1975, 'Sexual Harassment' Was the Menace with No Name." History .com, January 8. https://www.history.com/news/until-1975-sexual-harassment-was-the-men ace-with-no-name.

Blank, Nina, Arthur L. Caplan, and Catherine Constable. 2013. "Exempting Schoolchildren from Immunizations: States with Few Barriers Had Highest Rates of Nonmedical Exemptions." *Health Affairs* 32, no. 7 (July): 1282–90.

Bloom, Barry R., Edgar Marcuse, and Seth Mnookin. 2014. "Addressing Vaccine Hesitancy." *Science* 334 (6182): 339.

Bloor, David. 2007. "Epistemic Grace, Anti-Relativism as Theology in Disguise." *Common Knowledge* 13, nos. 2–3 (Spring): 250–80.

Blume, Stuart. 2006. "Anti-Vaccination Movements and Their Interpretations." *Social Science and Medicine* 62, no. 3 (February): 628–42.

Bomey, Nathan. 2018. *After the Fact*. Amherst, MA: Prometheus Books.

Bonfield, John. 2015. "California's Rich, White Unvaccinated Kindergartners." *CNN*, December 30, 2015. https://www.cnn.com/2015/12/30/health/california-vaccine-refusers-white-and -wealthy/index.html.

Born, Karen, Verna Yiu, and Terrence Sullivan. 2014. "Provinces Divided Over Mandatory Vaccination for Children." *Healthy Debate*, May 22, 2014. https://healthydebate.ca/2014/05/topic/ health-promotion-disease-prevention/mandatory-school-entry-vaccinations.

Börzel, Tanja A., and Diana Panke. 2007. "Network Governance: Effective and Legitimate?" In *Theories of Democratic Network Governance*, edited by Eva Sorenson and Jacob Torfing, 153–66. London: Palgrave Macmillan.

Boseley, Sarah. 2018. "How Disgraced Anti-Vaxxer Andrew Wakefield Was Embraced by Trump's

America." *Guardian*, July 18, 2018. https://www.theguardian.com/society/2018/jul/18/how-disgraced-anti-vaxxer-andrew-wakefield-was-embraced-by-trumps-america.

Boseley, Sarah. 2019. "Survey Shows Crisis of Confidence in Vaccines in Parts of Europe." *Guardian*, June 19, 2019. https://www.theguardian.com/society/2019/jun/19/survey-shows-crisis-of-confidence-in-vaccines-in-parts-of-europe.

Boston Women's Health Collective. 1973. *Our Bodies, Ourselves.* New York: Simon and Schuster.

Bouie, Jamelle. 2015. "How to Deal with Anti-Vaxxers." *Slate*, February 2, 2015. http://www.slate.com/articles/news_and_politics/politics/2015/02/anti_vaxxers_resist_persuasion_if_they_refuse_we_have_to_force_them_to_vaccinate.html.

Bowers, Simon. 2018. "How Lobbying Blocked European Safety Checks for Dangerous Medical Implants." *BMJ* 363 (November 26): k4999.

Braben, Donald W. 2014. *Promoting the Planck Club: How Defiant Youth, Irreverent Researchers and Liberated Universities Can Foster Prosperity Indefinitely.* Hoboken, NJ: Wiley and Sons.

Braben, Donald W., John F. Allen, William Amos, et al. 2014. "We Need More Scientific Mavericks." *Guardian*, March 18, 2014. https://www.theguardian.com/science/2014/mar/18/we-need-more-scientific-mavericks.

Brandt, Allan M. 1978. "Racism and Research: The Case of the Tuskegee Syphilis Study." *Hastings Center Report* 8, no. 6 (December): 21–29.

Brandt, Allan M. 2007. *The Cigarette Century: The Rise, Fall, and Deadly Persistence of the Product That Defined America.* New York: Basic Books.

Brennan, Jason. 2018. "A Libertarian Case for Mandatory Vaccination." *Journal of Medical Ethics* 44, no. 1 (January): 37–43.

Brennan, Zachary. 2018. "FDA Director Moves to AstraZeneca." *Regulatory Focus*, April 18, 2018. https://www.raps.org/news-and-articles/news-articles/2018/4/fda-director-moves-to-astrazeneca.

Brewer, Noel T., Gretchen B. Chapman, Alexander J. Rothman, Julie Leask, and Allison Kempe. 2017. "Increasing Vaccination: Putting Psychological Science into Action." *Psychological Science in the Public Interest* 18, no. 3 (December): 149–207.

Britneff, Beatrice. 2020. "No Return to 'Normality' until Coronavirus Vaccine Is Available, Trudeau Says." *Global News*, April 9, 2020. https://globalnews.ca/news/6799110/coronavirus-covid-19-vaccine-return-to-normality-trudeau/.

Bronson, Kelly. 2013. "Framing the Debate: How Scientistism in the Language of the Law Binds Public-Biotechnology Engagement." PhD diss., York University.

Bronson, Kelly. 2014. "Reflecting on the Science of Science Communication." *Canadian Journal of Communication* 39 (4): 523–37.

Brossard, Dominique, and Bruce V. Lewenstein. 2009. "A Critical Appraisal of Models of Public Understanding of Science: Using Practice to Inform Theory." In *New Agendas in Science Communication*, edited by L. Kahlor, 11–39. Mahwah, NJ: Laurence Erlbaum.

Brown, Katrina F., Simon Kroll, Michael J. Hudson, Mary Ramsay, John Green, Susannah J. Long, Charles A. Vincent, Graham Fraser, and Nick Sevdalis. 2010. "Factors Underlying Parental Decisions about Combination Childhood Vaccinations Including MMR: A Systematic Review." *Vaccine* 28, no. 26 (June 11): 4235–48.

Brown, Matthew J. 2020. *Science and Moral Imagination: A New Ideal for Values in Science.* Pittsburgh: University of Pittsburgh Press.

Brownlee, Shannon. 2010. *Overtreated: Why Too Much Medicine Is Making Us Sicker and Poorer.* New York: Bloomsbury.

Brownlie, Julie, and Alexandra Howson. 2005. "Leaps of Faith and MMR: An Empirical Test of Trust." *Sociology* 39, no. 2 (April): 221–39.

Bruinius, Harry. 2018. "Who Made You an Expert? Is America's Distrust of 'Elites' Becoming More Toxic?" *Christian Science Monitor*, August 27, 2018. https://www.csmonitor.com/USA/Politics /2018/0827/Who-made-you-an-expert-Is-America-s-distrust-of-elites-becoming-more-toxic.

Brumback, Roger A. 2011. Review of *Deadly Choices: How the Anti-Vaccine Movement Threatens Us All*, by P. A. Offit. *Journal of Child Neurology* 26, no. 10 (October): 1329.

Brunk, Conrad G. 2006. "Public Knowledge, Public Trust: Understanding the 'Knowledge Deficit.'" *Community Genetics* 9:178–83.

Buck, Genna. 2017. "No One Listens to the Experts Anymore." *Metro Life* (Ottawa), March 23, 2017. https://www.readmetro.com/en/canada/ottawa/20170323/15/#book/15.

Calef, Victor, and Edward M. Weinshel. 1981. "Some Clinical Consequences of Introjection: Gaslighting." *Psychoanalytic Quarterly* 50 (1): 44–66.

Calligeros, Melissa. 2015. "Melbourne's Anti-Vaccination Hot Spots: Rich Suburbs Have Low Immunisation Rates." *Age*, December 15, 2015. https://www.theage.com.au/national/victoria /melbournes-antivaccination-hot-spots-rich-suburbs-have-low-immunisation-rates-2015 1214-glmuvo.html.

Canadian Biotechnology Secretariat. 2006. *Research Report: Public Engagement on the Future Government of Canada Role in Biotechnology*. Ottawa: Industry Canada, Decima Research. http:// www.ic.gc.ca/eic/site/icgc.nsf/vwapj/ResearchReport-Biotechnology.pdf/$file/ Research Report-Biotechnology.pdf.

Canadian Federation of Medical Students. 2010. "Diversity in Medicine in Canada: Building a Representative and Responsive Medical Community." Position paper. https://www.cfms.org/ files/position-papers/diversity_in_medicine_-_updated_2010__cait_c_.pdf.

Caplan, Arthur. 2015. "There Is No Other Side to the Vaccine Debate." *Chicago Tribune*, February 12, 2015. https://www.chicagotribune.com/opinion/commentary/ct-measles-vaccine-jenny-mccarthy -autism-ebola-perspec-0213-jm-20150212-story.html.

Carel, Havi H. 2016. *Phenomenology of Illness*. Oxford: Oxford University Press.

Carel, Havi H., and Ian J. Kidd. 2014. "Epistemic Injustice in Healthcare: A Philosophical Analysis." *Medicine, Healthcare, and Philosophy* 17, no. 4 (November): 529–40.

Carli, Linda L., Laila Alawa, YoonAh Lee, Bei Zhao, and Elaine Kim. 2016. "Stereotypes about Gender and Science: Women ≠ Scientists." *Psychology of Women Quarterly* 40, no. 2 (June): 244–60.

Carolan, Michael S. 2008. "The Bright-and Blind-Spots of Science: Why Objective Knowledge Is Not Enough to Resolve Environmental Controversies." *Critical Sociology* 34, no. 5 (September): 725–40.

Carrington, Damian. 2000. "Fatal Flaws." *New Scientist*, October 25, 2000. https://newscientist .com/article/dn94-fatal-flaws/.

Cartwright, Samuel A. 1851. "Report on the Diseases and Physical Peculiarities of the Negro Race." *New Orleans Medical and Surgical Journal* 7 (1851): 691–715.

Cassuto, Leonard. 2002. "Big Trouble in the World of 'Big Physics.'" *Guardian*, September 18, 2002. https://www.theguardian.com/education/2002/sep/18/science.highereducation.

Castelvecchi, Davide. 2015. "Physics Paper Sets Record with More than 5,000 Authors." *Nature*, May 15, 2015. https://www.nature.com/news/physics-paper-sets-record-with-more-than-5-000 -authors-1.17567.

CBC Radio. 2017. "CBC Radio, Just Five Minutes on the Internet Can Sow Seeds of Doubt about Vaccines." *CBC Radio*, October 27, 2017. https://www.cbc.ca/radio/whitecoat/an-outbreak

-of-doubt-1.4373395/just-five-minutes-on-the-internet-can-sow-seeds-of-doubt-about
-vaccines-1.4374871.

Center for Disease Control and Prevention. n.d. *Vaccines: VDP-VAC/combo/MMRV/FAQs for Pro-viders*. CDC. Accessed April 12, 2014. http://www.cdc.gov/vaccines/vpd-vac/combo-vaccines
/mmrv/vacopt-faqs-hcp.htm.

Chaput, Kathleen H., Alberto Nettel-Aguirre, Richard Musto, Carol E. Adair, and Susan C. Tough.
2016. "Breastfeeding Difficulties and Supports and Risk of Postpartum Depression in a Cohort
of Women Who Have Given Birth in Calgary: A Prospective Cohort Study." *Canadian Medical
Association Journal Open* 4, no. 1 (March 21): E103–E109.

Chen, Robert T., and Frank DeStefano. 1998. "Vaccine Adverse Events: Causal or Coincidental?"
*Lancet* 351, no. 9103 (February 28): 611–12.

Chen, Robert T., Suresh C. Rastogi, John R. Mullen, Scott W. Hayes, Stephen L. Cochi, Jerome
A. Donlon, and Steven G. Wassilak. 1994. "The Vaccine Adverse Events Reporting System
(VAERS)." *Vaccine* 12, no. 6 (May): 542–50.

Cheng, Maria. 2013. "Measles Surge in U.K. Years after Flawed Research." *USA Today*, May 20, 2013.
http://www.usatoday.com/story/news/world/2013/05/20/measles-uk-research/2327135/.

Chew, Stephen L. 2018. "Myth: Eyewitness Testimony Is the Best Kind of Evidence." *Association for
Psychological Science*, August 8, 2018. https://www.psychologicalscience.org/teaching/myth
-eyewitness-testimony-is-the-best-kind-of-evidence.html.

Chiou, Catherine, and Catherine Tucker. 2018. *Fake News and Advertising on Social Media: A Study
of the Anti-Vaccination Movement*. Cambridge, MA: National Bureau of Economic Research.

Clark, Anna. 2019. *The Poisoned City: Flint's Water and the American Urban Tragedy*. New York:
Macmillan Books.

Clarke, Christopher E. 2008. "A Question of Balance: The Autism-Vaccine Controversy in the Brit-ish and American Elite Press." *Science Communication* 30, no. 1 (September): 77–107.

Clements, C. John, and Scott Ratzan. 2003. "Misled and Confused? Telling the Public about Vac-cine Safety." *Journal of Medical Ethics* 29 (1): 22–26.

Clifton, Jim. 2019. "Do You Trust Science?" *Gallup*. June 19, 2019. https://news.gallup.com/opinion
/chairman/258329/trust-science.aspx.

Clough, Sharyn. 2003a. "A Hasty Retreat from Evidence: The Recalcitrance of Relativism in Fem-inist Epistemology." In *Siblings under the Skin: Feminism, Social Justice and Analytic Philosophy*,
edited by Sharyn Clough, 85–115. Aurora, CO: Davies Group.

Clough, Sharyn. 2003b. *Beyond Epistemology: A Pragmatic Approach to Feminist Science Studies*.
Lantham, MD: Rowman & Littlefield.

Clough, Sharyn. 2013. "Feminist Theories of Evidence and Biomedical Research Communities: A
Reply to Goldenberg." *Social Epistemology Review and Reply Collective* 2 (12): 72–76.

Clough, Sharyn. 2015. "Fact/Value Holism, Feminist Philosophy, and Nazi Cancer Research." *Fem-inist Philosophy Quarterly* 1 (1): Article 7. https://doi.org/10.5206/fpq/2015.1.7.

Code, Lorraine. 1991. *What Can She Know? Feminist Theory and the Construction of Knowledge*. Itha-ca, NY: Cornell University Press.

CNN Transcripts. 2011. "AMERICAN MORNING Autism Vaccine Study Fraud; Republicans
Rule the House; Bubbling Crude: Near $100 Per Barrel; Wild Horse Roundup; 'Golden' Gift.
Aired January 6, 2011–06:00 ET." *CNN*, January 6, 2018. http://transcripts.cnn.com/TRAN
SCRIPTS/1101/06/ltm.01.html.

Cohen, Roger. 2016. "The Age of Distrust." *New York Times*, September 19, 2016. https://www.ny
times.com/2016/09/20/opinion/the-age-of-distrust.html.

Cohn, Melvin, and Rodney E. Langman. 1990. "The Protecton: The Unit of Humoral Immunity Selected by Evolution." *Immunological Reviews* 115, no. 1 (June): 7–147.

Coleman, Patrick A. 2019. "Reminder Jenny McCarthy Helped Cause the Anti-Vaxxer Measles Outbreak." *Fatherly,* February 7, 2019. https://www.fatherly.com/health-science/jenny-mccarthy-masked-singer-measles-outbreak-anti-vaxxer/.

Colgrove, James. 2006. *State of Immunity: The Politics of Vaccination in 20th Century America.* Berkeley: University of California Press.

Collins, Harry. 2014. *Are We All Experts Now?* Amherst, NY: Prometheus Books.

Collins, Harry, and Robert Evans. 2002. "The Third Wave of Science Studies: Studies of Expertise and Experience." *Social Studies of Science* 32, no. 2 (April): 235–96.

Collins, Harry, and Robert Evans. 2007. *Rethinking Expertise.* Chicago: University of Chicago Press.

Collins, Harry, Robert Evans, and Martin Weinel. 2017. "STS as Science or Politics?" *Social Studies of Science* 47, no. 4 (August): 580–86.

Collins, Harry, and Martin Weinel. 2011. "Transmuted Expertise: How Technical Non-Experts Can Assess Experts and Expertise." *Argumentation* 25, no. 3 (August): 401–13.

Commission on Social Determinants of Health. 2008. *Closing the Gap in a Generation: Health Equity through Action on the Social Determinants of Health. Final Report.* Geneva: World Health Organization.

Committee on Public Understanding of Science. 1987. *COPUS Looks Forward—The Next Five Years.* London: Royal Society.

Conis, Elena. 2015a. "Vaccination Resistance in Historical Perspective." *American Historian,* August 2015. https://tah.oah.org/issue-5/vaccination-resistance/.

Conis, Elena. 2015b. *Vaccine Nation: America's Changing Relationship with Immunization.* Chicago: University of Chicago Press.

Connor, Clifford D. 2005. *A People's History of Science: Miners, Midwives, and "Low Mechanicks."* New York: PublicAffairs.

Cook, Bryan G., Garnett J. Smith, and Melody Tankersley. 2012. "Evidence-Based Practices in Education." In *APA Educational Psychology Handbook,* vol. 1, *Theories, Constructs, and Critical Issues,* edited by Karen R. Harris, Steve Graham, Tim Urdan, et al., 495–527. Washington, DC: American Psychological Association.

Cook, John. 2016. "Countering Climate Science Denial and Communicating Scientific Consensus." In *Oxford Encyclopedia of Climate Change Communication.* London: Oxford University Press. https://doi.org/10.1093/acrefore/9780190228620.013.314.

Cook, John, Dana Nuccitelli, Sarah A. Green, Mark Richardson, Barbel Winkler, Rob Painting, Robert Way, Peter Jacobs, and Andrew Skuce, 2013. "Quantifying the Consensus on Anthropogenic Global Warming in the Scientific Literature." *Environmental Research Letters* 8, no. 2 (April–June): 024024. https://doi.org/10.1088/1748-9326/8/2/024024.

Cook, John, Sander van der Linden, Edward Maibach, and Stefan Lewandowsky. 2018. *The Consensus Handbook.* George Mason University Center for Climate Change Communication. https://doi.org/10.13021/G8MM6P.

Corben, Paul, and Julie Leask. 2018. "Vaccination Hesitancy in the Antenatal Period: A Cross-Sectional Survey." *BMC Public Health* 18, article no. 566. https://doi.org/10.1186/s12889-018-5389-6.

Corbie-Smith, Giselle, Stephen B. Thomas, and Diane Marie M. St. George. 2002. "Distrust, Race and Research." *Archives of Internal Medicine* 162, no. 21 (November 25): 2458–63.

Corbie-Smith, Giselle, Stephen B. Thomas, Mark V. Williams, and Sandra Moody-Ayers. 1999. "Attitudes and Beliefs of African Americans toward Participation in Medical Research." *Journal of General Internal Medicine* 14, no. 9 (September): 537–46.

Cournoyer, Barry R. 2007. *The Evidence-Based Social Work Skills Book.* Boston: Cengage Learning.

Cramer, Katherine J. 2016. *The Politics of Resentment: Rural Consciousness and the Rise of Scott Walker.* Chicago: University of Chicago Press.

Crease, Robert P. 2000. "Why Science Thrives on Criticism." *Physics World*, May 1, 2000. http://physicsworld.com/cws/article/print/2000/may/01/why-science-thrives-on-criticism.

Crease, Robert P. 2004. "The Paradox of Trust in Science." *Physics World* 17 (3): 18.

Crowe, Kelly. 2020. "Prominent Scientist Dares to Ask: Has the COVID-19 Response Gone Too Far? *CBC*, March 19, 2020. https://www.cbc.ca/news/health/coronavirus-covid-pandemic-response-scientists-1.5502423.

Dalton, Russell J. 2004. *Democratic Challenges, Democratic Choices: The Erosion of Political Support in Advanced Industrial Democracies.* Oxford: Oxford University Press.

Daly, Jeanne. 2005. *Evidence Based Medicine and the Search for a Science of Clinical Care.* Berkeley: University of California Press.

Daston, Lorraine, and Peter Galison. 2010. *Objectivity.* Cambridge, MA: Zone Books.

Davies, William. 2016. "The Age of Post-Truth Politics." *New York Times*, August 24, 2016. https://www.nytimes.com/2016/08/24/opinion/campaign-stops/the-age-of-post-truth-politics.html.

De Bakker, Dinny H., Dayline S. V. Coffie, Eibert R. Heerdink, Liset van Dijk, and Peter P. Groenewegen. 2007. "Determinants of the Range of Drugs Prescribed in General Practice: A Cross-Sectional Analysis." *BMC Health Services Research* 7 (August 22): 132.

Deer, Brian. 2004. "Revealed: MMR Research Scandal." *Sunday Times*, February 22, 2004. http://www.thetimes.co.uk/tto/health/article1879347.ece.

Deer, Brian. 2011a. "Secrets of the MMR Scare: How the Case against the MMR Vaccine Was Fixed." *British Medical Journal* 342:c5347.

Deer, Brian. 2011b. "Secrets of the MMR Scare: How the Vaccine Crisis Was Meant to Make Money." *British Medical Journal* 342:c5258.

Deer, Brian. 2011c. "Secrets of the MMR Scare: The *Lancet*'s Two Days to Bury Bad News." *British Medical Journal* 342:c7001.

De Graff, John. 2014. "Co-Author of *Affluenza:* 'I'm Appalled by the Ethan Couch Decision.'" *Time*, December 14, 2014. https://web.archive.org/web/20171231034624/http://ideas.time.com/2013/12/14/co-author-of-affluenza-im-appalled-by-the-ethan-couch-decision/.

De Graff, John, David Wann, and Thomas H. Naylor. 2001. *Affluenza: The All-Consuming Epidemic.* San Francisco: Berrett-Koehler.

De Melo-Martín, Inmaculeda, and Kristen Intemann. 2018. *The Fight against Doubt: How to Bridge the Gap between Scientists and the Public.* Oxford University Press.

Dempsey, Amanda F., Sarah Schaffer, Dianne Singer, Amy Butchart, Matthew Davis, and Gary L. Freed. 2011. "Alternative Vaccination Schedule Preferences among Parents of Young Children." *Pediatrics* 128, no. 5 (November): 848–56.

Department of Health. 1998. "MMR Vaccine Is Not Linked to Crohn's Disease or Autism." Press release, March 24, 1998. http://www.doh.gov.uk/pub/docs/doh/plcmo2.pdf.

Descartes, Rene. (1637) 1998. *Discourse on Method*, 3rd ed. Translated by Donald A. Cross. Indianapolis: Hackett.

Descartes, Rene. (1641) 1993. *Meditations on First Philosophy*, 3rd ed. Translated by Donald A. Cross. Indianapolis: Hackett.

De Vrieze, Jop. 2017. "Bruno Latour, a Veteran of the 'Science Wars,' Has a New Mission." *Science Magazine*, October 10, 2017. https://www.sciencemag.org/news/2017/10/bruno-latour-veteran-science-wars-has-new-mission.

Dewey, John. (1922) 1982. "Review of Public Opinion by Walter Lippmann." In *John Dewey: The Middle Works 1899–1924*, vol. 13, *1921–1922*, edited by Jo Ann Boydston, 337–44. Carbondale: Southern Illinois University Press.

Dewey, John. (1925) 1982. "Practical Democracy. Review of Walter Lippmann's book The Phantom Public." In *John Dewey, Philosophy and Democracy: The Later Works 1925–1953*, vol. 2, *1925–1927*, edited by Jo Ann Boydston, 213–20. Carbondale: Southern Illinois University Press.

Dewey, John. 1927. *The Public and Its Problems*. New York: Holt.

Dickey, Bronwen. 2016. "Climb Aboard, Ye Who Seek the Truth!" *Popular Mechanics*, August 17, 2016. https://www.popularmechanics.com/culture/a21919/conspiracy-theory-cruise/.

Diez-Sampedro, Ana, Monica Flowers, Maria Olenick, Tatayana Maltseva, and Guillermo Valdes. 2019. "Women's Choice Regarding Breastfeeding and its Effect on Well-Being." *Nursing for Women's Health* 23, no. 5 (October 1): 383–89.

Doc Bastard. 2019. "Busting Vaccine Myths." *Stories from the Trauma Bay* (blog), March 29, 2019. http://www.docbastard.net/2019/03/busting-vaccine-myths.html.

Dominelli, Lena. 2002. *Anti-Oppressive Social Work Theory and Practice*. New York: Palgrave Macmillan.

Dominelli, Lena. 2009. "Anti-Oppressive Practice: The Challenges of the Twenty-First Century." In *Social Work: Themes, Issues and Critical Debates*, 3rd ed., edited by Robert Adams, Lena Dominelli, and Malcolm Payne, 49–60. London: Red Globe.

Dominus, Susan. 2011. "The Crash and Burn of an Autism Guru." *New York Times Magazine*, April 20, 2011. https://www.nytimes.com/2011/04/24/magazine/mag-24Autism-t.html.

Douglas, Heather. 2000. "Inductive Risk and Values in Science." *Philosophy of Science* 67, no. 4 (December): 559–79.

Douglas, Heather. 2004. "The Irreducible Complexity of Objectivity." *Synthese* 138, no. 3 (February): 453–73.

Douglas, Heather. 2009. *Science, Policy, and the Value-Free Ideal*. Pittsburgh: University of Pittsburgh Press.

Douglas, Heather. 2016. "Values in Science." In *Oxford Handbook of Philosophy of Science*, edited by Paul Humphreys, 609–30. Oxford: Oxford University Press.

Douglas, Heather. 2017. "Science, Values, and Citizens." In *Eppur si muove: Doing History and Philosophy of Science with Peter Machamer*, edited by Marcus P. Adams, Zvi Beiner, Uljana Feest, and Jacqueline A. Sullivan, 83–96. New York: Springer Berlin Heidelberg.

Douglas, Mary. 1970. *Natural Symbols: Explorations in Cosmology*. New York: Pantheon Books.

Douglas, Mary, and Aaron Wildavsky. 1982. *Risk and Culture: An Essay on the Selection of Technological and Environmental Dangers*. Berkley: University of California Press.

Drummond, Caitlin, and Baruch Fischhoff. 2017. "Science Knowledge and Polarization." *Proceedings of the National Academy of Sciences* 114 (36): 9587–92.

Dubé, Eve, Caroline Laberge, Marise Guay, Paul Bramadat, Réal Roy, and Julie Bettinger. 2013. "Vaccine Hesitancy: An Overview." *Human Vaccines & Immunotherapeutics* 9, no. 8 (August): 1763–73.

Dubé, Eve, Maryline Vivion, Chantal Sauvageau, Arnaud Gagner, Raymond Gagnon, and Maryse Guay. 2015. "'Nature Does Things Well, Why Should We Interfere?' Vaccine Hesitancy among Mothers." *Qualitative Health Research* 26, no. 3 (February): 411–25.

Duff, Michelle. 2019. "In an Affluent Corner of Auckland, a GP Struggles against Vaccine Disinformation." *Stuff*, September 4, 2019. https://www.stuff.co.nz/national/health/114994080/in-an-affluent-corner-of-auckland-a-gp-struggles-against-vaccination-disinformation.

Duhem, Pierre. (1906) 1962. *The Aim and Structure of Physical Theory*. Translated by Philip P. Wiener. Princeton, NJ: Princeton University Press.

Duncan, David Ewing. 2007. "The Anti-Science President." *MIT Technology Review*, July 12, 2007. https://www.technologyreview.com/s/408236/the-anti-science-president/.

Dupré, John. 1993. *The Disorder of Things, Metaphysical Foundations of the Disunity of Science*. Cambridge, MA: Harvard University Press.

Dupuis, John. 2013. "The Canadian War on Science: A Long Unexaggerated Devastating Chronological Indictment." *ScienceBlogs* (blog), May 20, 2013. https://scienceblogs.com/confessions/2013/05/20/the-canadian-war-on-science-a-long-unexaggerated-devastating-chronological-indictment.

Durbach, Nadja. 2000. "They Might as Well Brand Us: Working Class Resistance to Compulsory Vaccination in Victorian England." *Social History of Medicine* 13, no. 1 (April): 45–63.

Durbach, Nadja. 2002. "Class, Gender, and the Conscientious Objector to Vaccination, 1898–1907." *Journal of British Studies* 41, no. 1 (January): 58–83.

Durbach, Nadja. 2004. *Bodily Matters: The Anti-Vaccination Movement in England, 1853–1907*. Durham, NC: Duke University Press.

Editorial Board. 2017. "President Trump's War on Science." *New York Times*, September 19, 2017. https://www.nytimes.com/2017/09/09/opinion/sunday/trump-epa-pruitt-science.html.

Editors. 2015. "The Science is Clear: Anti-Vaxxers Are Immune to the Truth." *Globe and Mail*, February 13, 2015. http://www.theglobeandmail.com/opinion/editorials/the-science-is-clear-anti-vaxxers-are-immune-to-the-truth/article22987563/.

Editors of the *Lancet*. 2010. "Retraction—Ileal-Lymphoid-Nodular Hyperplasia, Non-Specific Colitis, and Pervasive Developmental Disorder in Children." *Lancet* 375, no. 9713 (February 6): 445.

Edward Jenner Society. 2019. "About Edward Jenner." Jenner Institute. https://www.jenner.ac.uk/edward-jenner.

Edwards, Kari, and Edward E. Smith. 1996. "A Disconfirmation Bias in the Evaluation of Arguments." *Journal of Personality and Social Psychology* 71 (1): 5–24.

Elliott, Carl. 2004. "Pharma Goes to the Laundry: Public Relations and the Business of Medical Education." *Hastings Center Report* 24, no. 5 (September–October): 18–23.

Engs, Ruth Clifford. 2000. *Clean Living Movements: American Cycles of Health Reform*. Westport, CT: Praeger.

Engs, Ruth Clifford. 2003. *The Progressive Era's Health Reform Movement: A Historical Dictionary*. Westport, CT: Praeger.

Epstein, Deborah, and Lisa A. Goodman. 2019. "Discounting Women: Doubting Domestic Violence Survivors' Credibility and Dismissing Their Experiences." *University of Pennsylvania Law Review* 167 (2): 399–461.

European Commission 2008. *Public Engagement in Science*. Brussels: Directorate-General for Research.

Evans, Geoff, and John Durant. 1995. "The Relationship between Knowledge and Attitudes in the Public Understanding of Science in Britain." *Public Understanding of Science* 4, no. 1 (January): 57–74.

Evans, M., H. Stoddart, L. Condon, E. Freeman, M. Grizzell, and R. Mullen. 2001. "Parents' Perspectives on the MMR Immunisation: A Focus Group Study." *British Journal of General Practice* 51, no. 472 (November): 904–10.

Evans, Robert G., Morris L. Barer, and Theodore R. Marmor, eds. 1994. *Why Are Some People Healthy and Others Not?* New York: Aldine de Gruyter.

Evidence-Based Medicine Working Group. 1992. "Evidence-Based Medicine: A New Approach to Teaching the Practice of Medicine." *Journal of the American Medical Association* 268, no. 17 (November 4): 2420–25.

Eyb, Lyn. 2014. "Australia Wages Relentless War on Science." *Salon*, April 24, 2014. https://www.salon.com/2014/04/24/australia_wages_relentless_war_on_science_partner/.

Ezrahi, Yaron. 1990. *The Descent of Icarus: Science and the Transformation of Contemporary Democracy*. Cambridge, MA: Harvard University Press.

Fausto-Sterling, Anne. 1985. *Myths of Gender: Biological Theories about Women and Men*. New York: Basic Books.

Favilli, Elena, and Francesca Cavallo. *Good Night Stories for Rebel Girls: 100 Tales of Extraordinary Women*. Vol. 1. New York: Rebel Girls.

Fawkes, Johanna. 2007. "Public Relations Models and Persuasion Ethics: A New Approach." *Journal of Communication Management* 11 (4): 313–31.

Fein, Steven, and Steven J. Spencer. 1997. "Prejudice as Self-Image Maintenance: Affirming the Self through Derogating Others." *Journal of Personality and Social Psychology* 73 (1): 31–44.

Fenton, Siobhan. 2016a. "Doctors Ignore Women's Pain." *Independent*, July 27, 2016. https://www.independent.co.uk/life-style/health-and-families/health-news/how-sexist-stereotypes-mean-doctors-ignore-womens-pain-a7157931.html.

Fenton, Siobhan. 2016b. "Period Pain Is Officially as Bad as a Heart Attack—So Why Have Doctors Ignored It? The Answer Is Simple." *Independent*, February 16, 2016. https://www.independent.co.uk/voices/period-pain-is-officially-as-bad-as-a-heart-attack-so-why-have-doctors-ignored-it-the-answer-is-a6883831.html.

Festinger, Leon, Henry Riecken, and Stanley Schachter. 1956. *When Prophecy Fails: A Social and Psychological Study of a Modern Group That Predicted the Destruction of the Word*. New York: Harper-Touchstone.

Fetters, Ashley, 2018. "The Doctor Doesn't Listen to Her. But the Media Is Starting to." *Atlantic*, August 10, 2018. https://www.theatlantic.com/family/archive/2018/08/womens-health-care-gaslighting/567149/.

Fischer, Bill. 2015. "The End of Expertise." *Harvard Business Review*, October 19, 2015. https://hbr.org/2015/10/the-end-of-expertise.

Fischer, Kari. 2019. "Opinion: What You Believe about 'Science Denial' May Be All Wrong." *Scientist*, February 11, 2019. https://www.the-scientist.com/news-opinion/opinion--what-you-believe-about-science-denial-may-be-all-wrong-65448.

Fisher, Colleen, Katie Attwell, and Michael J. Wise. 2014. "Vaccinations Are a Vital Part of Ethical 'Alternative' Lifestyles." *Conversation*, January 29, 2014. https://theconversation.com/vaccinations-are-a-vital-part-of-ethical-alternative-lifestyles-22385.

Fitzpatrick, Michael. 2004a. *MMR and Autism: What Parents Need to Know*. London: Routledge.

Fitzpatrick, Michael. 2004b. "MMR: Investigating the Interests." *Spiked*, February 23, 2004. https://www.spiked-online.com/2004/02/23/mmr-investigating-the-interests-2/.

Fitzpatrick, Michael. 2004c. "MMR: Risk, Choice, Chance." *British Medical Bulletin* 69, no. 1 (June): 143–53.

Fitzpatrick, Michael. 2004d. "Jabs and Junk Science." *Guardian*, September 8, 2004.

Fitzpatrick, Michael. 2009. *Defeating Autism: A Damaging Delusion*. London: Routledge.

Fletcher, Jackie. n.d. "Re: Jabs and Junk Science by Michael Fitzpatrick." *Jabs. Justice Awareness and Basic Support* (blog). Accessed May 1, 2015. http://www.jabs.org.uk/pages/jabswrites.asp.

Foley, Jonathan. 2017. "The War for Science." *Scientific American Blog* (blog), February 20, 2017. https://blogs.scientificamerican.com/guest-blog/the-war-for-science/.

Foley, Jonathan, and Christine Arena. 2017. "How to Defeat Those Who Are Waging War on Science: Here Are Five Meaningful Steps You Can Take." *Scientific American Blog* (blog), February 27, 2017. https://blogs.scientificamerican.com/guest-blog/how-to-defeat-those-who-are-waging-war-on-science/.

Fowler, P. B. S. 1997. "Evidence Based Everything." *Journal of Evaluation in Clinical Practice* 3, no. 3 (August): 239–43.

Frakt, Austin. 2020. "Bad Medicine: The Harm That Comes from Racism." *New York Times*, January 13, 2020. https://nytimes.com/2020/01/13/upshot/bad-medicine-the-harm-that-comes-from-racism.html.

Frank, John W. 1995. "Why 'Population Health'?" *Canadian Journal of Public Health* 86, no. 3 (May–June): 162–64.

Frankl, Michelle M. 2013. "Don't Buy the Alternative Medicine in 'The Boy with a Thorn in His Joints.'" *Slate*, February 7, 2013. https://slate.com/technology/2013/02/curing-chemophobia-dont-buy-the-alternative-medicine-in-the-boy-with-a-thorn-in-his-joints.html.

Freed, Gary, Sarah T. Clark, Amy T. Butchart, Dianne C. Singer, and Matthew M. Davis. 2010. "Parental Vaccine Safety Concerns in 2009." *Pediatrics* 125, no. 4 (April): 654–59.

Freimuth Vicki S., Amelia Jamison, Gregory Hancock, Donald Musa, Karen Hilyard, and Sandra Crouse Quinn. 2017. "The Role of Risk Perception in Flu Vaccine Behavior among African American and White Adults in the United States." *Risk Analysis* 37, no. 11 (November): 2150–63.

Freimuth Vicki S., Amelia Jamison, Gregory Hancock, and Sandra Crouse Quinn. 2017. "Determinants of Trust in Flu Vaccine for African Americans and Whites." *Social Science & Medicine* 193 (November): 70–79.

Freimuth, Vicki S., Sandra Crouse Quinn, Stephen B. Thomas, Cole Galen, Eric Zook, and Ted Duncan. 2001. "African Americans' Views on Research and the Tuskegee Syphilis Study." *Social Science & Medicine* 52, no. 5 (March): 797–808.

Fricker, Miranda. 2007. *Epistemic Injustice: Power & the Ethics of Knowing*. London: Oxford University Press.

Fricker, Miranda, and Katharine Jenkins. 2017. "Epistemic Injustice, Ignorance, and Trans Experience." In *Routledge Companion to Feminist Philosophy*, edited by Ann Gary, Serene J. Khader, and Alison Stone. Abingdon: Routledge.

Fuller, Steve. 1987. "On Regulating What Is Known: A Way to Social Epistemology." *Synthese* 73, no. 1 (October): 145–84.

Fuller, Steve. 1988. *Social Epistemology*. Bloomington: Indiana University Press.

Fuller, Steve. 1992. "Social Epistemology and the Research Agenda of Science Studies." In *Science as Practice and Culture*, edited by Andrew Pickering, 390–428. Chicago: University of Chicago Press.

Fukayama, Francis. 2017. "The Emergence of a Post-Fact World." *Pacific Standard*, January 12, 2017. https://www.project-syndicate.org/onpoint/the-emergence-of-a-post-fact-world-by-francis-fukayama-2017-01.

Galiston, Peter. 2016. "Practice All the Way Down." In *Kuhn's "Structure of Scientific Revolutions" at Fifty: Reflections on a Science Classic*, edited by Robert J. Richards and Lorraine Daston, 42–69. Chicago: University of Chicago Press.

Gass, Nick. 2016. "Trump: 'The Experts Are Terrible.'" *Politico*, April 4, 2016. https://www.politico.com/blogs/2016-gop-primary-live-updates-and-results/2016/04/donald-trump-foreign-policy-experts-221528.

Gatenby, Alex. 2019. "Debunking Vaccination Myths for Parents." *BBC News*, April 3, 2019. https://www.bbc.com/news/health-47787908.

Gellin, Bruce G., Edward W. Maibach, and Edward K. Marcus. 2000. "Do Parents Understand Immunization? A National Telephone Survey." *Pediatrics* 106 (5): 1097–102.

General Medical Council. 2010. *Andrew Wakefield: Determination of Serious Professional Misconduct.* www.gmc-uk.org/Wakefield_SPM_and_SANCTION.pdf_32595267.pdf.

George, John. 2011. "CHOP Doctor Who Developed Rotavirus Vaccine Honored." *Philadelphia Business Journal*, June 29, 2011. https://www.bizjournals.com/philadelphia/blog/john-george/2011/06/bio-award-goes-to-doctor-who-developed.html.

Georgiou, Aristos. 2019. "Anti-Vaxxers Are Targeting Doctors in Online Hate Campaigns." *Newsweek*, February 28, 2019. https://www.newsweek.com/anti-vaxxers-are-targeting-doctors-online-hate-campaigns-1347045.

Gerber, Jeffery S., and Paul A. Offit. 2009. "Vaccines and Autism: A Tale of Shifting Hypotheses." *Clinical Infectious Diseases* 48, no. 4 (February 15): 456–61.

Giddens, Anthony. 1990. *The Consequences of Modernity.* Stanford, CA: Stanford University Press.

Giddens, Anthony. 1999. "Risk and Responsibility." *Modern Law Review* 62, no. 1 (January): 1–10.

Giddens, Anthony, and Christopher Pierson. 1998. *Conversations with Anthony Giddens: Making Sense of Modernity.* Stanford, CA: Stanford University Press.

Gillies, Donald A. 2005. "Hempelian and Kuhnian Approaches in the Philosophy of Medicine: The Semmelweis Case." *Studies in History and Philosophy of Science Part C: Studies in History and Philosophy of Biological and Biomedical Science* 36, no. 1 (March): 159–81.

Gilson, Lucy. 2003. "Trust and the Development of Healthcare as a Social Institution." *Social Science and Medicine* 56, no. 7 (April): 1453–68.

Ginty, Molly M. 2004. "Our Bodies, Ourselves Turns 35 Today." *Women's eNews*, May 4, 2004. https://web.archive.org/web/20090903164405/http://www.womensenews.org/article.cfm/dyn/aid/1820/context/archive.

Glaser, April. 2016. "A Skeptic Infiltrates a Cruise for Conspiracy Theorists." *Wired*, April 9, 2016. https://www.wired.com/2016/02/conspira-sea-cruise-know-truth/.

Glenza, Jessica. 2018. "Disgraced Anti-Vaxxer Andrew Wakefield Aims to Advance His Agenda in Texas Election." *Guardian*, February 26, 2018. https://www.theguardian.com/us-news/2018/feb/26/texas-vaccinations-safety-andrew-wakefield-fear-elections.

Godlee, Fiona. 2006. "Can We Tame the Monster?" *British Medical Journal* 333 (July 6). https://doi.org/10.1136/bmj.333.7558.0-f.

Goetzsche, Peter. 2013. *Deadly Medicines and Organised Crime: How Big Pharma Has Corrupted Healthcare.* New York: Radcliffe.

Goldacre, Ben. 2012. *Bad Pharma: How Drug Companies Mislead Doctors and Harm Patients.* New York: Farrar, Straus and Giroux.

Goldenberg, Maya J. 2005. "Evidence-Based Ethics? On Evidence-Based Practice and the 'Empirical Turn' from Normative Bioethics." *BMC Medical Ethics* 6 (1): 11.

Goldenberg, Maya J. 2008. "Health." In *Oxford Encyclopedia of Women in World History*, edited by Bonnie G. Smith, 440–42. Oxford: Oxford University Press.

Goldenberg, Maya J. 2014. "Diversity in Epistemic Communities: A Response to Clough." *Social Epistemology Review and Reply Collective* 3 (5): 25–30.

Goldenberg, Maya J. 2015. "How Can Feminist Theories of Evidence Assist Clinical Reasoning and Decision-Making?" *Social Epistemology* 29 (1): 3–30.

Goldenberg, Maya J. 2017. "A Lack of Trust, Not of Science, behind Vaccine Resistance." *Toronto Star*, November 9, 2017. https://www.thestar.com/opinion/commentary/2017/11/09/a-lack-of-trust-not-of-science-behind-vaccine-resistance.html.

Goldenberg, Maya J., and Christopher McCron. 2017. "'The Science is Clear!' Media Uptake of Health Research into Vaccine Hesitancy." In *Knowing and Acting in Medicine*, edited by Robyn Bluhm, 113–32. Lanham, MD: Rowman & Littlefield.

Goldman, Alvin. 1987. "Foundations of Social Epistemics." *Synthese* 73, no. 1 (October): 109–44.

Goldman, Alvin. 1997. *Knowledge in a Social World*. Oxford: Oxford University Press.

Goldman, Alvin. 2001. "Experts: Which Ones Should You Trust?" *Philosophy and Phenomenological Research* 63, no. 1 (July): 85–110.

Goodman, Ashley, Kim Fleming, Nicole Markwick, Tracey Morrison, Louise Lagimodiere, Thomas Kerr, and the Western Aboriginal Harm Reduction Society. 2017. "'They Treated Me Like Crap and I Know It Was Because I Was Native': The Healthcare Experiences of Aboriginal Peoples Living in Vancouver's Inner City." *Social Science and Medicine* 178, no. 4 (April): 87–94.

Goodnough, Abby, and Margot Sanger-Katz. 2019. "As Tens of Thousands Died, F.D.A. Failed to Police Opioids." *New York Times*, December 30, 2019. https://www.nytimes.com/2019/12/30/health/FDA-opioids.html.

Goodstein, David. 2010. *On Fact and Fraud: Tales from the Front Lines of Science*. Princeton, NJ: Princeton University Press.

Gordon, Jane. 1989. "Choosing to Breastfeed: Some Feminist Questions." *Resources for Feminist Research/Documentation sur la recherche féministe* 18 (2): 10–12.

Gore, Al. 2007. *The Assault on Reason*. New York: Penguin.

Gould, Stephen Jay. 1996. *The Mismeasure of Man*. New York: W. W. Norton.

Goyal, Monika K., Nathan Kupperman, Sean D. Cleary, Stephen J. Teach, and James M. Chamberlain. 2015. "Racial Disparities in Pain Management of Children with Appendicitis in Emergency Departments." *JAMA Pediatrics* 169, no. 11 (November): 996–1002.

Grasswick, Heidi. 2010. "Scientific and Lay Communities: Earning Epistemic Trust through Knowledge Sharing." *Synthese* 177, no. 3 (December): 387–409.

Gray, Andy, Jerome Hoffman, and Peter R. Mansfield. 2010. "Pharmaceutical Sales Representatives." In *Understanding and Responding to Pharmaceutical Promotion: A Practical Guide*, edited by Barbara Mitzes, Dee Mangin, and Lisa Hayes, 61–80. Amsterdam: Health Action International.

Green, Emma. 2019. "Measles Can Be Contained. Anti-Semitism Cannot." *Atlantic*, May 25, 2019. https://www.theatlantic.com/politics/archive/2019/05/orthodox-jews-face-anti-semitism-after-measles-outbreak/590311/.

Greenberg, Annie Georgia. 2016. "These Are the Most Out-There Conspiracy Theories We've Ever Heard." *Refinery 29*, July 6, 2016. https://www.refinery29.com/en-us/2016/07/102450/conspiracy-theorist-theories.

Greenberg, Josh, Eve Dubé, and Michelle Driedger. 2017. "Vaccine Hesitancy: In Search of the Risk Communication Comfort Zone." *PLoS Currents*, March 3. ecurrents.outbreaks.0561a011117a1d1f9596e24949e8690b.

Greenhalgh, Trisha. 2004. "A Critical Appraisal of the Wakefield et al Paper." Brian Deer (website). http://briandeer.com/mmr/lancet-greenhalgh.htm.

Griffiths, Andrew, and Raymond F. Zammuto. 2005. "Institutional Governance Systems and Variations in National Competitive Advantage: An Integrative Framework." *Academy of Management Review* 30, no. 4 (October): 823–42.

Grinnell, Richard M., and Yvonne A. Unrau. 2010. *Social Work Research and Evaluation: Foundations of Evidence-Based Practice*, 9th ed. New York: Oxford University Press.

Gross, Charles. 2011. "Disgrace: On Marc Hauser." *Nation*, December 21, 2011. https://www.thenation.com/article/archive/disgrace-marc-hauser/.

Gross, Paul R., and Norman Levitt. 1994. *Higher Superstition: The Academic Left and Its Quarrels with Science*. Baltimore: Johns Hopkins University Press.

Grundy, Quinn. 2018. *Infiltrating Healthcare: How Marketing Works Underground to Influence Nurses*. Baltimore: Johns Hopkins University Press.

Gutierrez, Melody. 2019. "Dr. Bob Sears' Views on Vaccines Have Inspired Loyal Followers—And a Crush of Criticism." *Los Angeles Times*, September 3, 2019. https://www.latimes.com/california/story/2019-09-02/bob-sears-controversial-views-on-vaccines-inspire-critics-and-fans.

Habakus, Louise Kuo, and Mary Holland, 2012. "Introduction." In *Vaccine Epidemic: How Corporate Greed, Biased Science, and Coercive Government Threaten Our Human Rights, Our Health, and Our Children*, edited by Louise Kuo Habakus and Mary Holland, 1–10. New York: Skyhorse.

Hacking, Ian. 1999. *The Social Construction of What?* Cambridge, MA: Harvard University Press.

Haelle, Tara. 2015a. "15 Myths about Anti-Vaxxers, Debunked—Part 1." *Forbes*, February 17, 2015. https://www.forbes.com/sites/tarahaelle/2015/02/17/15-myths-about-anti-vaxxers-debunked-part-1/#3fef5de82474.

Haelle, Tara. 2015b. "15 Myths about Anti-Vaxxers, Debunked—Part 2." *Forbes*, February 18, 2015. https://www.forbes.com/sites/tarahaelle/2015/02/18/15-myths-about-anti-vaxxers-debunked-part-2/#6720ado265de.

Haelle, Tara. 2015c. "15 Myths about Anti-Vaxxers, Debunked—Part 3." *Forbes*, February 19, 2015. https://www.forbes.com/sites/tarahaelle/2015/02/19/15-myths-about-anti-vaxxers-debunked-part-3/#6d90eb722748.

Hahn, Robert A., and Benedict I. Truman. 2015. "Education Improves Public Health and Promotes Health Equity." *International Journal of Health Services* 45 (4): 657–78.

Haller, John S., Jr. 1972. "The Negro and the Southern Physician: A Study of Medical and Racial Attitudes." *Medical History* 16, no. 3 (July): 238–53.

Hamilton, Clive, and Richard Denniss. 2001. *Affluenza: The All-Consuming Epidemic*. Crows Nest, New South Wales: Allen & Unwin.

Hamilton, Patrick. 1938. *Gaslight*. London: Samuel French.

Hannaford, Alex. 2013. "Autism Inc.: The Discredited Science, Shady Treatments and Rising Profits behind Alternative Autism Treatments." *Texas Observer*, January 30, 2013. http://www.texasobserver.org/autism-inc-the-discredited-science-shady-treatments-and-rising-profits-behind-alternative-autism-treatments/.

Haraway, Donna. 1996. "Modest Witness: Feminist Diffractions in Science Studies." In *The Disunity of Science: Boundaries, Contexts, and Power*, by Peter Galison and David J. Stump, 428–42. Palo Alto, CA: Stanford University Press.

Haraway, Donna. 1997. *Modest_Witness@Second_Millennium. FemaleMan_Meets_OncoMouse: Feminism and Technoscience*. New York: Routledge.

Harding, S. 1991. *Whose Science? Whose Knowledge? Thinking from Women's Lives*. Ithaca, NY: Cornell University Press.

Harding, Sandra. 1993. "Rethinking Standpoint Epistemology: What Is Strong Objectivity?"

In *Feminist Epistemologies*, edited by Linda Alcoff and Elizabeth Potter, 49–82. New York: Routledge.

Hardwig, John. 1985. "Epistemic Dependence." *Journal of Philosophy* 82, no. 7 (July): 335–49.

Hardwig, John. 1991. "The Role of Trust in Knowledge." *Journal of Philosophy* 88, no. 12 (December): 693–708.

Hardwig, John. 1994. "Toward an Ethics of Expertise." In *Professional Ethics and Social Responsibility*, edited by Daniel Wueste, 83–101. Lanham, MD: Rowman & Littlefield, 1994.

Harel, Amos. 2020. "The Expert Who Says Israel Is Overreacting to Coronavirus." *Haaretz*, March 19, 2020. https://www.haaretz.com/israel-news/.premium-the-expert-who-says-israel-is-overreacting-to-coronavirus-1.8689010.

Hargreaves, Ian, Justin Lewis, and Tammy Speers. 2003. *Towards a Better Map: Science, the Public, and the Media*. London: Economic and Social Research Council.

Harris, Gardiner. 2008. "Measles Cases Grow in Number, and Officials Blame Parents' Fear of Autism." *New York Times*, August 21, 2008. http://www.nytimes.com/2008/08/22/health/research/22measles.html?_r=0.

Harris, Sam. 2011. *The Moral Landscape: How Science Can Determine Human Values*. New York: Free Press.

Hatfield, Tammy. 2017. "Mother-Blaming." In *SAGE Encyclopedia of Marriage, Family, and Couples Counseling*, vol. 3, edited by Jon Carlson and Shannon B. Dermer, 1105–7. Thousand Oaks, CA: SAGE.

Hausman, Bernice L. 2014. *Mother's Milk: Breastfeeding Controversies in American Culture*. New York: Routledge.

Hausman, Bernice L. 2019. *Anti/Vax: Reframing the Vaccination Controversy*. Ithaca, NY: Cornell University Press.

Hausman, Daniel M., and Brynn Welch. 2010. "Debate: To Nudge or Not to Nudge." *Journal of Political Philosophy* 18 (1): 123–36.

Hawkins, Kirk. 2010. *Venezuela's Chavismo and Populism in Comparative Perspective*. Cambridge, UK: Cambridge University Press.

Health 2.0. 2018. "One Size Fits All Is Out, Precision Health Is In." http://health2con.com/news-iteam/8992-2-2/.

Health Canada. 2011. *Misconceptions about Vaccine Safety*. Ottawa: Government of Canada. http://healthycanadians.gc.ca/health-sante/medicine-medicament/misconception-eng.php.

Hegde, Sonia T., Abram L. Wagner, Philippa J. Clarke, R. C. Potter, R. G. Swanson, and M. L. Boulton. 2019. "Neighborhood Influence on the Fourth Dose of Diphtheria-Tetanus-Pertussis Vaccination." *Public Health* 167 (February): 41–49.

Helft, Laura, and Emily Willingham. 2014. "What Is Herd Immunity?" *PBS*, September 5, 2014. https://www.pbs.org/wgbh/nova/article/herd-immunity/.

Hempel, Carl. 1965. "Science and Human Values." In *Aspects of Scientific Explanation and Other Essays in Philosophy of Science*, by Carl Hempel, 81–96. New York: Free Press.

Hempel, Carl. 1966. *The Philosophy of Natural Science*. Upper Saddle River, NJ: Prentice Hall.

Hendricks, Scott. 2018. "Is Postmodernism Really Anti-Science?" *Big Think*, October 15, 2018. https://bigthink.com/culture-religion/is-postmodernism-really-anti-science.

Herrick, Charles N. 2004. "Objectivity versus Narrative Coherence: Science, Environmental Policy, and the U.S. Data Quality Act." *Environmental Science & Policy* 7, no. 5 (October) 419–33.

Herrick, Charles, and Dale Jamieson. 1995. "The Social Construction of Acid Rain: Some Implications for Science/Policy Assessment." *Global Environmental Change* 5, no. 2 (May): 105–12.

Hicks, Daniel J. 2017. "Scientific Controversies as Proxy Politics." *Issues in Science and Technology* 33, no. 2 (Winter). Online at https://issues.org/scientific-controversies-as-proxy-politics/.

Hicks, Mar. 2017. *Programmed Inequality: How Britain Discarded Women Technologists and Lost Its Edge in Computing.* Cambridge, MA: MIT Press.

Hobson-West, Pru. 2003. "Understanding Vaccination Resistance: Moving beyond Risk." *Health, Risk & Society* 5 (3): 273–83.

Hobson-West, Pru. 2007. "'Trusting Blindly Can Be the Biggest Risk of All': Organised Resistance to Childhood Vaccination in the UK." *Sociology of Health & Illness* 29, no. 2 (March): 198–215.

Hoffman, Kelly M., Sophie Trawalter, Jordan R. Axt, and M. Norman Oliver. 2016. "Racial Bias in Pain Assessment and Treatment Recommendations, and False Beliefs about Biological Differences between Blacks and Whites." *PNAS Proceedings of the National Academies of Science* 113, no. 16 (April 19): 4296–301.

Hofstader, Richard. 1963. "Anti-Intellectualism in American Life." New York: Albert A. Knopf.

Holland, Mary. 2012. "Who Is Dr. Andrew Wakefield?" In *Vaccine Epidemic: How Corporate Greed, Biased Science, and Coercive Government Threaten Our Human Rights, Our Health, and Our Children,* edited by Louise Kuo Habakus and Mary Holland, 223–29. New York: Skyhorse.

Holmes, Richard. 2010. "The Royal Society's Lost Women Scientists." *Guardian*, November 21, 2010. https://www.theguardian.com/science/2010/nov/21/royal-society-lost-women-scientists.

Holton, Richard. 1994. "Deciding to Trust, Coming to Believe." *Australasian Journal of Philosophy* 72 (1): 63–76.

Horgan, John. 2015. "Everyone, Even Jenny McCarthy, Has the Right to Challenge 'Scientific Experts.'" *Scientific American Blog* (blog), March 19, 2015. https://blogs.scientificamerican.com/cross-check/everyone-even-jenny-mccarthy-has-the-right-to-challenge-8220-scientific-experts-8221/.

Horner, Robert H., Edward G. Carr, James Halle, Gail McGee, Samuel Odom, and Mark Wolery. 2005. "The Use of Single-Subject Research to Identify Evidence-Based Practice in Special Education." *Exceptional Children* 71 (2): 165–79.

Horton, Richard. 2004. *MMR: Science and Fiction: Exploring the Vaccine Crisis.* London: Granta.

House of Lords. 2000. *Science and Society.* London: House of Lords.

House of Lords. 2004. *Science in Society Report 2004.* London: House of Lords.

Howard, Beth. 2005. "10 Vaccine Myths—Busted." *Baby Talk* 70, no. 7 (September): 52–56.

Howard, Matthew O., Curtis J. McMillen, and David E. Pollio. 2003. "Teaching Evidence-Based Practice: Toward a New Paradigm for Social Work Education." *Research on Social Work Practice* 13, no. 2 (March): 234–59.

Huff, Ethan. 2012. "Neurosurgeon Issues Public Challenge to Vaccine Zealots: Inject Yourselves with All Shots You Say Children Should Get!" *Natural News*, March 23, 2012. http://www.naturalnews.com/035335_vaccines_Dr_Blaylock_children.html.

Hughes, Robert. 1993. *Culture of Complaint: The Fraying of America.* New York: Oxford University Press.

Hume, David. (1739) 1975. *A Treatise of Human Nature.* Edited by L. A. Selby-Bigge. Oxford: Clarendon Press.

Hviid, Anders, Jørgen Vinsløv, and Morten Frisch. 2019. "Measles, Mumps, Rubella Vaccination and Autism: A National Cohort Study." *Annals of Internal Medicine* 170 (8): 513–20.

Ignatofsky, Rachel. 2016. *Women in Science: 50 Fearless Pioneers Who Changed the World.* Emeryville, CA: Ten Speed Press.

Inquiring Minds. 2014. "Harry Collins: Why Googling Doesn't Make You a Scientific Expert."

*Inquiring Minds* (podcast), May 29, 2014. https://www.mixcloud.com/InquiringMinds
/36-harry-collins-why-googling-doesnt-make-you-a-scientific-expert/.

Institute of Medicine. 2003. *Unequal Treatment: Confronting Racial and Ethnic Disparities in Health-care*. Washington, DC: The National Academies Press. https://doi.org/10.17226/10260.

Intemann, Kirstin. 2009. "Why Diversity Matters: Understanding and Applying the Diversity Component of the National Science Foundation's Broader Impacts Criterion." *Social Epistemology* 23 (3–4): 249–66.

Irwin, Alan. 1995. *Citizen Science: A Study of People, Expertise and Sustainable Development*. London: Routledge.

Irwin, Alan, and Brian Wynne. 1996. *Misunderstanding Science? The Public Reconstruction of Science and Technology*. Cambridge, UK: Cambridge University Press.

Irzik, Gürol, and Faik Kurtulumus. 2019. "What Is Epistemic Public Trust in Science?" *British Journal of Philosophy of Science* 70, no. 4 (December): 1145–66.

Jackson, Jeffry T., Kirsten Dellinger, Kathryn McKee, and Annette Trefzer. 2016. "Interdisciplinary Perspectives on the Global South and Global North." In *The Sociology of Development Handbook*, edited by Gregory Hooks, 129–52. Oakland: University of California Press.

Jacoby, Susan. 2008. *The Age of American Unreason*. New York: Vintage Books.

Jamison, Amelia M., Sandra Crouse Quinn, and Vicki S. Freimuth. 2019. "'You Don't Trust a Government Vaccine': Narratives of Institutional Trust and Influenza Vaccination among African American and White Adults." *Social Science & Medicine* 221 (January): 87–94.

Janko, Matthew. 2012. "Vaccination: A Victim of Its Own Success." *Virtual Mentor* 14 (1): 3–4.

Jardine, Lisa. 2004. *The Curious Life of Robert Hooke: The Man Who Measured London*. New York: HarperCollins.

Jasanoff, Sheila. 1987. "Contested Boundaries in Policy-Relevant Science." *Social Studies of Science* 17 (2): 195–230.

Jasanoff, Sheila. 1990. *The Fifth Branch*. Cambridge, MA: Harvard University Press.

Jasanoff, Sheila. 1995. *Science at the Bar: Law, Science, and Technology in America*. Cambridge, MA: Harvard University Press.

Jasanoff, Sheila. 2003. "Technologies of Humility: Citizen Participation in Governing Science." *Minerva* 41, no. 3 (September): 223–44.

Jasanoff, Sheila, ed. 2004. *States of Knowledge: The Co-Production of Science and Social Order*. London: Routledge.

Jasanoff, Sheila. 2005. *Design by Nature: Science and Democracy in Europe and the United States*. Princeton, NJ: Princeton University Press.

Jasanoff, Sheila, and Hilton R. Simmet. 2017. "No Funeral Bells: Public Reason in a 'Post-Truth' Age." *Social Studies of Science* 47 (5): 751–70.

Johnson, Jenna. 2017. "The Tale of a Trump Falsehood: How His Voter Fraud Claim Spread Like a Virus." *Washington Post*, January 31, 2017. https://www.courant.com/politics/hc-ap-trump
-voter-falsehood-spreads-20170131-story.html.

Johnston, Josephine. 2010. "Financial Conflicts of Interest in Biomedical Research." In *Trust and Integrity in Biomedical Research: The Case of Financial Conflicts of Interest*, edited by Thomas H. Murray and Josephine Jonston, 3–32. Baltimore: Johns Hopkins University Press.

Joint Task Group on Public Health Human Resources. 2005. "Building the Public Health Workforce for the 21st Century: A Pan-Canadian Framework for Public Health Human Resources Planning." http:// www.phac-aspc.gc.ca/php-psp/pdf/building_the_public_health_workforce
_fo_%20the21stc_e.pdf.

Jones, Abbey M., Saad B. Omer, Robert A. Bednarczyk, Neal A. Halsey, Lawrence H. Moulton, and Daniel A. Salmon. 2012. "Parents' Source of Vaccine Information and Impact on Vaccine Attitudes, Beliefs, and Nonmedical Exemptions." *Advances in Preventive Medicine.* Open access, Article ID 932741. https://doi.org/10.1155/2012/932741.

Jones, James H. 1993. *Bad Blood: The Tuskegee Syphilis Experiment.* New York: Free Press.

Jones, Karen. 1996. "Trust as an Affective Attitude." *Ethics* 107, no. 1 (October): 4–25.

Jost, John T., Jack Glaser, Arie W. Kruglanski, and Frank J. Sulloway. 2003. "Political Conservatism as Motivated Social Cognition." *Psychological Bulletin* 129 (3): 339–75.

Kahan, Dan. 2010. "Fixing the Communications Failure." *Nature* 463, 296–97.

Kahan, Dan. 2011. "What Is Motivated Reasoning? How Does It Work? Dan Kahan Answers." *Discovery Magazine Blog* (blog), May 5, 2011. http://blogs.discovermagazine.com/intersection/2011/05/05/what-is-motivated-reasoning-how-does-it-work-dan-kahan-answers/#.XXOhVChKhPY.

Kahan, Dan. 2012. "Cultural Cognition as a Conception of the Cultural Theory of Risk." In *Handbook of Risk Theory: Epistemology, Decision Theory, Ethics and Social Implications of Risk,* edited by Sabine Roeser, Hillerbrand Sabine, Rafaela, Per Sandin, and Martin Peterson, 725–60. Amsterdam: Springer Netherlands.

Kahan, Dan. 2015. "You Can Change the Minds of Climate Change Skeptics. Here's How." *Washington Post,* February 23, 2015. https://www.washingtonpost.com/news/monkey-cage/wp/2015/02/23/you-can-change-the-minds-of-climate-change-skeptics-heres-how/.

Kahan, Dan M., and Donald Braman. 2003. "More Statistics, Less Persuasion: A Cultural Theory of Gun-Risk Perceptions." *University of Pennsylvania Law Review* 151, no. 4 (April): 1291–327.

Kahan, Dan M., Donald Braman, G. L. Cohen, J. Gastil, and Paul Slovic. 2010. "Who Fears the HPV Vaccine, Who Doesn't, and Why? An Experimental Study of the Mechanisms of Cultural Cognition." *Law & Human Behavior* 34:501–16.

Kahan, Dan M., Donald Braman, John Gastil, Paul Slovic, and C. K. Mertz. 2007. "Culture and Identity-Protective Cognition: Explaining the White Male Effect in Risk Perception." *Journal of Empirical Legal Studies* 4 (3): 465–505.

Kahan, Dan M., Donald Braman, Paul Slovic, John Gastil, and Geoff Cohen. 2009. "Cultural Cognition of the Risks and Benefits of Nanotechnology." *Nature Nanotechnology* 4:87–90.

Kahan, Dan M., Hank Jenkins-Smith, and Donald Braman. 2011. "Cultural Cognition of Scientific Consensus." *Journal of Risk Research* 14 (2): 147–74.

Kahan, Dan M., Hank Jenkins-Smith, Tor Tarantola, and Carol L. Silva, 2015. "Geoengineering and Climate Change Polarization: Testing a Two-Channel Model of Science Communication." *Annals of the American Academy of Political & Social Science* 658 (March): 192–222.

Kahan, Dan M., Ellen Peters, Maggie Wittlin, Paul Slovic, Lisa Larrimore Ouellette, Donald Braman, and Gregory Mandel. 2012. "The Polarizing Impact of Science Literacy and Numeracy on Perceived Climate Change Risks." *Nature Climate Change* 2:732–35.

Kakutani, Michiko. 2017. "'The Death of Expertise' Explores How Ignorance Became a Virtue." *New York Times,* March 21, 2017. https://www.nytimes.com/2017/03/21/books/the-death-of-expertise-explores-how-ignorance-became-a-virtue.html.

Kant, Immanuel. (1790) 2016. *Critique of Judgment.* Translated by Werner S. Pluhar. Indianapolis: Hackett.

Kappel, Klemens. 2014. " The Proper Role of Science in Liberal Democracy." Unpublished conference paper. https://www.academia.edu/7017103/The_Proper_Role_of_Science_in_Liberal_Democracy.

Karlamanglasta, Soumya. 2019. "Anti-Vaccine Activists Have Doctors 'Terrorized into Silence' with Online Harassment." *Los Angeles Times*, March 17, 2019. https://www.latimes.com/local/california/la-me-ln-vaccine-attacks-20190317-story.html.

Kaufman, Martin. 1967. "The American Anti-Vaccinationists and Their Arguments." *Bulletin of the History of Medicine* 41, no. 5 (September–October): 463–78.

Kaufman, Sharon R. 2010. "Regarding the Rise in Autism: Vaccine Safety Doubt, Conditions of Inquiry, and the Shape of Freedom." *Ethos* 38 (1): 8–32.

Kayyem, Juliette. 2019. "Anti-Vaxxers are Dangerous. Make Them Face Isolation, Fines, Arrests." *Washington Post*, April 30, 2019. https://www.washingtonpost.com/opinions/2019/04/30/time-get-much-tougher-anti-vaccine-crowd/.

Keller, Evelyn Fox. 1983. *A Feeling for the Organism: The Life and Work of Barbara McClintock*. San Francisco: W. H. Freeman.

Kickbusch, Ilona. 2003. "The Contribution of the World Health Organization to a New Public Health and Health Promotion." *American Journal of Public Health* 9, no. 3 (March): 383–88.

Kidder, F. Key. 2010. "Science and Public Trust." *Lab Manager*, September 9, 2010. http://www.labmanager.com/business-management/2010/09/science-the-public-trust?fw1pk=2#.V3KNObgrKhc.

Kierkegaard, Søren. 1985. *Fear and Trembling*. Translated by Alastair Hannay. New York: Penguin.

Kierkegaard, Søren. 1992. *Concluding Unscientific Postscript to Philosophical Fragments*. Translated by Howard V. Hong and Edna Hong. Princeton, NJ: Princeton University Press.

Kirby, David. 2006. *Evidence of Harm: Mercury in Vaccines and the Autism Epidemic*. New York: St. Martin's Griffin.

Kirkey, Sharon. 2019. "Ontario's Mandatory Class for Parents Seeking Vaccine Exemptions Has 'Zero Conversions.'" *National Post*, March 15, 2019. https://nationalpost.com/news/ontarios-mandatory-class-for-parents-seeking-vaccine-exemptions-has-zero-conversions.

Kitcher, Philip. 1990. "The Division of Cognitive Labor." *Journal of Philosophy* 87, no. 1 (January): 5–22.

Kitcher, Philip. 1993. *The Advancement of Science: Science without Legend, Objectivity without Illusions*. New York: Oxford University Press.

Kitcher, Philip. 2001. *Science, Truth, and Democracy*. New York: Oxford University Press.

Kitcher, Philip. 2011a. *Science in a Democratic Society*. Amherst, NY: Prometheus Books.

Kitcher, Philip. 2011b. *The Ethical Project*. Cambridge, MA: Harvard University Press.

Koch, Deborah. 2009. "Why Paul Offit Isn't Flexible on Vaccines." *U.S. News & World Report*, January 9, 2009. http://health.usnews.com/health-news/blogs/on-medicine/2009/01/05/why-paul-offit-isnt-flexible-on-vaccines.

Koertge, Noretta, ed. 2000. *A House Built on Sand: Exposing Postmodernist Myths about Science*. Oxford: Oxford University Press.

Kofman, Ava. 2018. "Bruno Latour, the Post-Truth Philosopher, Mounts a Defense of Science." *New York Times*, October 25, 2018. https://www.nytimes.com/2018/10/25/magazine/bruno-latour-post-truth-philosopher-science.html.

Kourany, Janet A. 2010. *Philosophy of Science after Feminism*. Oxford: Oxford University Press.

Kovner, Anthony R., Jeffery Elton, and John Billings. 2000. "Evidence-Based Management." *Frontiers of Health Services Management* 16, no. 4 (Summer): 3–26.

Kovner, Anthony R., and Thomas G. Rundall. 2006. "Evidence-Based Management Reconsidered." *Frontiers of Health Services Management* 22, no. 3 (Spring): 3–21.

Kruger, Justin, and David Dunning. 1999. "Unskilled and Unaware of It: How Difficulties in Recognizing One's Own Incompetence Leads to Inflated Self-Assessments." *Journal of Personality and Social Psychology* 77 (6): 1121–34.

Krystal, Arthur. 2014. "The Shrinking World of Ideas." *Chronicle of Higher Education*, November 21, 2014. https://www.chronicle.com/article/the-shrinking-world-of-ideas/.

Kuhl, Stefan. 1994. *The Nazi Connection: Eugenics, American Racism, and German Socialism*. New York: Oxford University Press.

Kuhn, Thomas. 1962. *The Structure of Scientific Revolutions*. Chicago: University of Chicago Press.

Kukla, Rebecca. 2006. "Ethics and Ideology in Breastfeeding Advocacy Campaigns." *Hypatia* 21, no. 1 (Winter): 157–80.

Kunda, Ziva. 1990. "The Case for Motivated Reasoning." *Psychological Bulletin* 108, no. 3 (November): 480–98.

Kuntz, Ted. 2017. "Letter: Toronto Star Influenza Vaccine Claims Not Supported by Evidence." *Vaccine Choice Canada*, November 13, 2017. https://vaccinechoicecanada.com/media/letter_toronto_star_flu_vaccine_claims_not_supported_by_evidence/.

Lam, Bourree. 2015. "Vaccines Are Profitable, So What?" *Atlantic*, February 10, 2015. https://www.theatlantic.com/business/archive/2015/02/vaccines-are-profitable-so-what/385214/.

Lareo, Inés, and Ana Montoya Reyes. 2007. "Scientific Writing: Following Robert Boyle's Principles in Experimental Essays–1704 and 1998." *Revista Alicantina de Estudios Ingleses* 20:119–37.

Largent, Mark A. 2012. *Vaccine: The Debate in Modern America*. Baltimore: Johns Hopkins University Press.

Largent, Mark A. 2013. "Prof. Largent Blog Post: 'Is Jenny McCarthy a Threat to Public Health?'" James Madison College, July 26, 2013. https://jmc.msu.edu/contact/faculty-news-article.php?id=46.

Larson, Heidi J., Richard M. Clarke, Caitlin Jarrett, Elisabeth Eckersberger, Zachary Levine, Will S. Schulz, and Pauline Peterson. 2018. "Measuring Trust in Vaccination: A Systematic Review." *Human Vaccines & Immunotherapeutics* 14 (7): 1599–609.

Larson, Heidi, Louis Z. Cooper, Juhani Eskola, Samuel L. Katz, and Scott Ratzan. 2011. "Addressing the Vaccine Confidence Gap." *Lancet* 378, no. 9790 (August 6): 536–35.

Larson, Heidi J., Alexandre de Figueiredo, Emilie Karafllakis, and Mahesh Rawal. 2018. *State of Vaccine Confidence in the EU. A Report to the European Commission*. Luxembourg: Luxembourg Publication Office of the European Union. https://ec.europa.eu/health/sites/health/files/vaccination/docs/2018_vaccine_confidence_en.pdf.

Larson, Heidi J., William S. Schulz, Joseph D. Tucker, and David M. Smith. 2015. "Measuring Vaccine Confidence: Introducing a Global Vaccine Confidence Index." *PLoS Currents Outbreaks*, February 25. https://doi.org/10.1371/currents.outbreaks.ce0f6177bc97332602a8e3fe7d7f7cc4.

Latour, Bruno. 1987. *Science in Action: How to Follow Scientists and Engineers through Society*. Cambridge, MA: Harvard University Press.

Latour, Bruno. 2004. "Why Has Critique Run Out of Steam? From Matters of Fact to Matters of Concern?" *Critical Inquiry* 30, no. 2 (Winter): 225–48.

Latour, Bruno. 2015. "Telling Friends from Foes at the Time of the Anthropocene." In *The Anthropocene and the Global Environment Crisis—Rethinking Modernity in a New Epoch*, edited by Clive Hamilton, Christophe Bonneuil, and François Gemenne, 145–55. London: Routledge.

Latour, Bruno, and Steve Woolgar. 1979. *Laboratory Life: The Construction of Scientific Facts*. Beverley Hills, CA: Sage.

Laudan, Larry. 1984. *Science and Values: The Aims of Science and Their Role in Scientific Debate*. Berkeley: University of California Press.

Layton, David, Edgar Jenkins, Sally Macgill, and Angela Davey. 1993. *Inarticulate Science? Perspectives on the Public Understanding of Science and Some Implications for Science Education.* Nafferton: Studies in Education Ltd.

Leach, Melissa. 2005. "MMR Mobilisation: Science and Citizens in a British Vaccine Controversy." IDS Working Paper No. 247. Brighton: Institute of Development Studies. http://www.drc-citizenship.org/system/assets/1052734466/original/1052734466-leach.2005-mmr.pdf?1289493597.

Leach, Melissa, and James Fairhead. 2007. *Vaccine Anxieties: Global Health, Child Health & Society.* London: Earthscan.

Leach, Melissa, and James Fairhead. 2008. "Understandings of Immunization: Some West African Perspectives." *Bulletin of the World Health Organization* 86, no. 6 (June): 418.

Leask, Julie. 2011. "Target the Fence-Sitters." *Nature* 473 (May 26): 443–45.

Leask, Julie, Kinnersley Paul, Jackson Cath, Cheater Francine, Bedford Helen, and Greg Rowles. 2012. "Communicating with Parents about Vaccination: A Framework for Health Professionals." *BMC Pediatrics* 12:154. https://doi.org/10.1186/1471-2431-12-154.

Lee, Thomas H., Elizabeth A. McGlynn, and Dana Gelb Safran. 2019. "A Framework for Increasing Trust between Patients and the Organizations That Care for Them." *JAMA* 321 (6): 539–40.

Lehrer, Keith. 1977. "Social Information." *Monist* 60, no. 4 (October): 473–87.

LeMieux, Juliana. 2016. "Why Won't This Andrew Wakefield Nightmare End?" *American Council on Science and Health Blog* (blog) May 17, 2016. http://acsh.org/news/2016/05/17/why-wont-the-andrew-wakefield-nightmare-end/.

Lenzer, Jeanne. 2004. "Scandals Have Eroded US Public's Confidence in Drug Industry." *British Medical Journal* 329, no. 7460 (July 31): 247.

Lenzer, Jeanne. 2017. *The Danger within Us: America's Untested, Unregulated Medical Device Industry and One Man's Battle to Survive It.* New York: Little, Brown.

Levitt, Norman. 1999. *Prometheus Bedeviled: Science and the Contradictions of Contemporary Culture.* New Brunswick, NJ: Rutgers University Press.

Lewandowsky, Stephan, Gilles E. Gignac, and Samuel Vaughan. 2012. "The Pivotal Role of Perceived Scientific Consensus in Acceptance of Science." *Nature Climate Change* 3: 399–404.

Lewandowsky, Stephan, Klaus Oberauer, and Gilles E. Gignac. 2013. "NASA Faked the Moon Landing—Therefore, (Climate) Science Is a Hoax: An Anatomy of the Motivated Rejection of Science." *Psychological Science* 24 (5): 622–33.

Lewenstein, Bruce T., ed. 1992. *When Science Meets the Public.* Washington, DC: American Association for the Advancement of Science.

Lewis, J. David, and Andrew Weigert. 1985. "Trust as a Social Reality." *Social Forces* 63, no. 4 (June): 967–85.

Lewis, Ricki. 2004. "Vaccines: Victims of Their Own Success?" *Scientist*, July 19, 2004. https://www.the-scientist.com/feature/vaccines-victims-of-their-own-success-49782.

Lexchin, Joel. 2013. "Health Canada and the Pharmaceutical Industry: A Preliminary Analysis of the Historical Relationship." *Healthcare Policy* 9, no. 2 (November): 22–29.

Lexchin, Joel. 2016. *Private Profits versus Public Policy: The Pharmaceutical Industry and the Canadian State.* Toronto: University of Toronto Press.

Lexchin, Joel. 2017. *Doctors in Denial: Why Big Pharma and Canadian Medical Profession Are Too Close for Comfort.* Toronto: Lorimer.

Lexchin, Joel. 2019. "Health Canada and Big Pharma: Too Close for Comfort." *Conversation*, August 12, 2019. https://theconversation.com/health-canada-and-big-pharma-too-close-for-comfort-120965.

Lexchin, Joel, Lisa Bero, Benjamin Djulbegovic, and Otavio Clark.2003. "Pharmaceutical Industry Sponsorship and Research Outcome and Quality: Systematic Review." *British Medical Journal* 326 (7400): 1167.

Light, Donald W. 2020. "Addressing Healthcare Disparities: A Radical Perspective and Proposal." *Frontiers in Sociology*, April 28. https://doi.org/10.3389/fsoc.2020.00029.

Lindley, Megan C., Pascale M. Wortley, and Barbara H. Bardenheier. 2006. "The Role of Attitude in Understanding Disparities in Adult Influenza Vaccination." *American Journal of Preventive Medicine* 31, no. 4 (October): 281–85.

Lindsay, Sally, and Hubertus Vrijhoef. 2009. "A Sociological Focus on Expert Patients." *Health Sociology Review* 18 (2): 139–44.

Link, Bruce G., and Jo Phelan. 1995. "Social Conditions as Fundamental Causes of Disease." *Journal of Social Behavior* 35:80–94.

Lippmann, Walter. 1922. *Public Opinion*. New York: Macmillan.

Lippmann, Walter. 1925. *The Phantom Public*. New York: Harcourt Brace.

Logel, Christine, and Gerry L. Cohen. 2012. "The Role of the Self in Physical Health: Testing the Effect of a Values-Affirmation Intervention on Weight Loss." *Psychological Science* 23, no. 1 (January 1): 53–55.

Logel, Christine, Gregory M. Walton, Jennifer M. Peach, Steven J. Spencer, and Mark P. Zanna. 2012. "Unleashing Latent Ability: Implications of Stereotype Threat for College Admissions." *Educational Psychologist* 47 (1): 42–50.

London Royal Society. 1985. *The Public Understanding of Science: Report of a Working Party*. London: London Royal Society.

Longino, Helen. 1990. *Science as Social Knowledge*. Bloomington: Indiana University Press.

Longino, Helen. 1993. "Subjects, Knowledge, and Power: Description and Prescription in Feminist Philosophies of Science." In *Feminist Epistemologies*, edited by Linda Alcoff and Elizabeth Potter, 101–20. New York: Routledge.

Longino, Helen. 2002. *The Fate of Knowledge*. Princeton, NJ: Princeton University Press.

Lord, Charles G., Lee Ross, and Mark R. Lepper. 1979. "Biased Assimilation and Attitude Polarization—Effects of Prior Theories on Subsequently Considered Evidence." *Journal of Personality and Social Psychology* 37 (11): 2098–109.

Luhmann, Niklas. 1979. *Trust and Power*. Translated by Howard H. Davis, John Raffan, and Kathryn Rooney. Chichester: Wiley and Sons.

Lupton, Deborah. 1995. *The Imperative of Health: Public Health and the Regulated Body*. London: Sage.

Luthy, Karlen E., Renea L. Beckstand, and Neil E. Peterson. 2009. "Parental Hesitation as a Factor in Delayed Childhood Immunization." *Journal of Pediatric Health Care* 23, no. 6 (November–December): 388–93.

MacDonald, Noni, and SAGE Working Group on Vaccine Hesitancy. 2015. "Vaccine Hesitancy: Definition, Scope, Determinants." *Vaccine* 33, no. (August 14): 4161–64.

MacDougall, Heather, and Laurence Monnais. 2017. "Not without Risk: The Complex History of Vaccine Resistance in Central Canada, 1885–1960." In *Public Health in the Age of Anxiety: Religious and Cultural Roots of Vaccine Hesitancy in Canada*, edited by Paul Bramadat et al., 129–63. Toronto: University of Toronto Press.

Malaysian Vaccines Exposed. n.d. *Malaysian Vaccines Exposed*. Accessed September 2, 2019. https://www.facebook.com/MalaysiaVaccine/.

Mammoser, Gigen. 2019. "Fact or Fiction: Debunking the Latest Anti-Vax Myths." *Healthline*, March

7, 2019. https://www.healthline.com/health-news/the-latest-anti-vax-conspiracies-could-be
-harmful-to-kids.

Mance, Henry. 2016 "Britain Has Had Enough of Experts, Says Gove." *Financial Times*, June 3, 2016.
https://www.ft.com/content/3be49734-29cb-11e6-83e4-abc22d5d108c.

Manne, Kate. 2017. *Down Girl: The Logic of Misogyny*. New York: Oxford University Press.

Marcum, James A. 2005. *Thomas Kuhn's Revolution*. London: Continuum.

Marston, Greg, and Rob Watts. 2003. "Tampering with the Evidence: A Critical Appraisal of Evidence-Based Policy-Making." *The Drawing Board: An Australian Review of Public Affairs* 3 (3):
143–63.

Martin, Emily. 1996. "The Egg and the Sperm: How Science Has Constructed a Romance Based on
Stereotypical Male-Female Roles." In *Feminism and Science*, edited by Evelyn Fox Keller and
Helen Longino, 103–20. Oxford: Oxford University Press.

Martinson, Brian C., Anderson, Melissa C., and Raymond de Vries. 2005. "Scientists Behaving
Badly." *Nature* 435:737–38.

Martucci, Jessica, and Anne Barnhill. 2016. "Unintended Consequences of Invoking 'Natural' in Breast
Feeding Promotion." *Pediatrics* 137, no. 4 (April): e20154154. https://doi.org/10.1542/peds.2015-4154.

Masters, Geoff N. 2018. "The Role of Evidence in Teaching and Learning." *2009–2019 ACER Research Conferences* 2. https://research.acer.edu.au/research_conference/RC2018/13august/2.

McCallum, Jan M., Dhananjaya M. Arekere, B. Lee Green, Ralph V. Katz, and Brian M. Rivers.
2006. "Awareness and Knowledge of the US Public Health Service Syphilis Study at Tuskegee:
Implications for Biomedical Research." *Journal of Healthcare for the Poor and Underserved* 17,
no. 4 (November): 716–33.

McCarthy, Jenny. 2009. *Mother Warriors: A Nation of Parents Healing Autism against the Odds*. Boston: Dutton Penguin.

McGarity, Thomas O., and Wendy E. Wagner. 2008. *Bending Science: How Special Interests Corrupt
Public Health Research*. Cambridge, MA: Harvard University Press.

McGregor, Russell. 1997. *Imagined Destinies: Aboriginal Australians and the Doomed Race Theory,
1900–1972*. Melbourne: Melbourne University Press.

McGuire, Wendy L. 2005. "Beyond EBM: New Directions for Evidence-Based Public Health." *Perspectives in Biology and Medicine* 48, no. 4 (Autumn): 557–69.

McLaren, Angus. 1990. *Our Own Master Race: Eugenics in Canada, 1885–1945*. Toronto: McClelland
and Stewart.

McLeod, Carolyn. 2002. *Self-Trust and Reproductive Autonomy*. Cambridge, MA: MIT Press.

McKinnon, Rachel. 2017. "Allies Behaving Badly." In *The Routledge Handbook of Epistemic Injustice*,
edited by Ian James Kidd, José Medina, and Gaile Pohlhaus Jr., 167–74. London: Routledge.

McNeil, Maureen. 2007. *Feminist Cultural Studies of Science and Technology*. New York: Routledge.

McNutt, Louise-Ann, Christina Desemone, erica DeNicola, et al. 2016. "Affluence as a Predictor of
Vaccine Refusal and Underimmunization in California Private Kindergartens." *Vaccine* 34, no.
14 (March 29): 1733–38.

McWilliam, James. 2015. "How the Term 'Anti-Science' Distorts America's Relationship with
Technology." *Pacific Standard*, December 30, 2015. https://psmag.com/environment/
how-the-term-anti-science-distorts-americas-relationship-with-technology.

Meier, Cecile. 2017. "Immunisation Rates Declining in Canterbury's Wealthiest Areas." *Stuff*,
March 13, 2013. https://www.stuff.co.nz/national/health/90334313/immunisation-rates-de
clining-in-canterburys-wealthiest-areas.

Mercer, David. 2008. "Science, Legitimacy, and 'Folk Epistemology' in Medicine and Law: Parallels between Legal Reforms to the Admissibility of Expert Evidence and Evidence-Based Medicine." *Social Epistemology* 22 (4): 405–23.

Mercola, Joseph. 2009. "Vaccine Doctor Given at Least $30 Million Dollars to Push Vaccines?" Mercola.com, June 25, 2009. http://articles.mercola.com/sites/articles/archive/2009/06/25/vaccine-doctor-given-at-least-30-million-dollars-to-push-vaccines.aspx.

Merlon, Anna. 2016. "Sail (Far) Away: At Sea with America's Largest Floating Gathering of Conspiracy Theorists." *Jezebel*, February 25, 2016. https://jezebel.com/sail-far-away-at-sea-with-americas-largest-floating-1760900554.

Merton, Robert. (1942) 1973. "The Normative Structure of Science." In *The Sociology of Science: Theoretical and Empirical Investigations*, edited by Robert K. Merton, 267–78. Chicago: University of Chicago Press.

Merry, Sally Engel. 2016. *The Seductions of Quantification: Measuring Human Rights, Gender Violence, and Sex Trafficking*. Chicago: University of Chicago Press.

Mesch, Gustavo S., and Kent P. Schwirian. 2015. "Confidence in Government and Vaccination Willingness in the USA." *Health Promotion International* 30, no. 2 (June): 213–21.

Messina, Alex. 2007. "Public Relations, the Public Interest and Persuasion." *Journal of Communications Management* 11 (1): 29–52.

Miller, Clark A. 2017. "It's Not a War on Science." *Issues in Science and Technology* 33, no. 3 (Spring). Available at https://issues.org/perspective-its-not-a-war-on-science/.

Miller, Gerald R. 1989. "Persuasion and Public Relations: 2 'Ps' in a Pod?" In *Public Relations Theory*, edited by Carl H. Botan and Vincent Hazleton Jr., 45–81. New York: Routledge.

Miller, Steve. 2001. "Public Understanding of Science at the Crossroads." *Public Understanding of Science* 10:115–20.

Mills, James. 2020. "Pandora's Box Closed: The Royal Air Force Institute of Aviation Medicine and Nazi Medical Experiments on Human Beings during World War II." *Studies in History and Philosophy of Science Part C: Studies in History and Philosophy of Biological and Biomedical Sciences* 79 (February): 101190.

Mimiko, N. Oluwafemi. 2012. *Globalization: The Politics of Global Economic Relations and International Business*. Durham, NC: Carolina Academic.

Misztal, Barbara A. 1996. *Trust in Modern Societies: Search for Bases of Social Order*. Cambridge, UK: Polity.

Mnookin, Seth. 2011. *The Panic Virus: The True Story behind the Vaccine-Autism Controversy*. New York: Simon and Schuster.

Mooney, Chris. 2005. *The Republican War on Science*. New York: Basic Books.

Mooney, Chris. 2011. "The Science of Why We Don't Believe Science." *Mother Jones*, May/June. https://www.motherjones.com/politics/2011/04/denial-science-chris-mooney/.

Mooney, Chris. 2014a. "This Is Why You Have No Business Challenging Scientific Experts." *Mother Jones*, May 30, 2014. https://www.motherjones.com/environment/2014/05/harry-collins-inquiring-minds-science-studies-saves-scientific-expertise/.

Mooney, Chris. 2014b. "Study: You Can't Change an Anti-Vaxxer's Mind." *Mother Jones*, March 3, 2014. http://www.motherjones.com/environment/2014/02/vaccine-denial-psychology-back-fire-effect.

Mooney, Chris, and Sheril Kirshenbaum. 2009. *Unscientific America: How Scientific Illiteracy Threatens Our Future*. New York: Basic Books.

Mollering, Guido. 2001. "The Nature of Trust: From Georg Simmel to a Theory of Expectation, Interpretation and Suspension." *Sociology* 35 (2): 403–20.

Mollering, Guido. 2006. "Trust, Institutions, Agency: Towards a Neoinstitutional Theory of Trust." In *Handbook of Trust Research*, edited by Reinhard Bachmann and Akbar Zaheer, 355–76. Cheltenham, UK: Edward Elgar.

Mols, Frank, S. Alexander Haslam, Joanda Jetten, and Niklas K. Steffens. 2015. "Why a Nudge Is Not Enough: A Social Identity Critique of Governance." *European Journal of Political Research* 54:81–98.

Morgan, Andrew J., and Gregory A. Poland. 2011. "The Jenner Society and the Edward Jenner Museum: Tributes to a Physician-Scientist." *Vaccine* 295 (December 30): D152–D154.

Mosby, Ian. 2013. "Administering Colonial Science: Nutrition Research and Human Biomedical Experimentation in Aboriginal Communities and Residential Schools, 1942–1952." *Histoire sociale/Social History* 46 (91): 145–72.

Moynihan, Ray, and Allan Cassels. 2005. *Selling Sickness*. Sydney: Greystone Books.

Moynihan, Ray, and David Henry. 2006. "The Fight against Disease Mongering: Generating Knowledge for Action." *PloS* 3, no. 4 (April): e91. https://doi.org10.1371/journal.pmed.0030191.

Moynihan, Ray, Alexandra Lai, Huw Jarvis, Geraint Duggan, Stephanie Goodrick, Elaine Beller, and Lisa Bero. 2018. "Moynihan: Undisclosed Financial Ties between Guideline Writers and Pharmaceutical Companies: A Cross-Sectional Study across 10 Disease Categories." *BMJ Open* 9 (2): e025864.

Mueller, Benjamin. 2020. "As Europe Shuts Down, Britain Takes a Different, and Contentious, Approach." *New York Times*, March 13, 2020. https://www.nytimes.com/2020/03/13/world/europe/coronavirus-britain-boris-johnson.html.

Munro, Geoffrey, and Peter H. Ditto. 1997. "Biased Assimilation, Attitude Polarization, and Affect in Reactions to Stereotype-Relevant Scientific Information." *Personality and Social Psychology Bulletin* 23 (6): 636–53.

Murch, Simon H., Andrew Anthony, David H. Cassen, Moshin Malik, Mark Berelowitz, Amar P. Dhillon, Michael A. Thompson, Alan Valentine, Susan E. Davies, and John A. Walker-Smith. "Retraction of an Interpretation." *Lancet* 363, no. 9411 (March 6): 750.

Murdoch, Lydia. 2014. *The Daily Life of Victorian Women*. Santa Barbara, CA: Greenwood.

Mykhalovskiy, Eric, and Lorna Weir. 2004. "The Problem of Evidence-Based Medicine: Directions for Social Medicine." *Social Science & Medicine* 59, no. 5 (September): 1059–69.

Narine, Shari. 2013. "Racism, Mistrust Keep Aboriginal People from Healthcare." Ammsa.com. https://ammsa.com/publications/windspeaker/racism-mistrust-keep-aboriginal-people-health-care.

Narruhn, Robin, and Terri Clark. 2020. "Epistemic Injustice: A Philosophical Analysis of Women's Reproductive Healthcare in a Somali-American Community." *Advances in Nursing Science* 43, no. 1 (January–March): 86–100.

Nass, Meryl. 2011. "Wakefield Witch Hunt: What's Up?" *Anthrax Vaccine Blogspot* (blog), January 9, 2011. http://anthraxvaccine.blogspot.ca/2011/01/wakefield-witch-hunt-whats-up.html.

National Academy of Sciences, National Academy of Engineering, and Institute of Medicine. 2007. *Beyond Bias and Barriers: Fulfilling the Potential of Women in Academic Science and Engineering*. Washington, DC: National Academies Press.

National Research Council. 2010. *Advancing the Science of Climate Change*. Washington, DC: National Academies Press.

National Science Board. 1981. *Science Indicators—1980*. Washington, DC: Government Printing Office.

National Science Board. 1983. *Science Indicators—1982*. Washington, DC: Government Printing Office.

National Science Board. 1986. *Science Indicators—1985*. Washington, DC: Government Printing Office.

National Science Foundation. 1995. *NSF in a Changing World: The National Science Foundation's Strategic Plan* (NSF 95–24). Washington, DC: National Science Foundation.

Navin, Mark C. 2015. *Values and Vaccine Refusal.* New York: Routledge.

Navin, Mark, and Katie Attwell. 2019. "Vaccine Mandates, Value Pluralism, and Policy Diversity." *Bioethics* 33 (9): 1042–49.

Navin, Mark, and Mark Largent. 2017. "Improving Nonmedical Vaccine Exemption Policies: Three Case Studies." *Public Health Ethics* 10, no. 3 (November): 225–34.

Nelson, Hilde Lindemann. 2001. *Damaged Identities, Narrative Repair.* Ithaca, NY: Cornell University Press.

Nelson, Lynn Hankinson. 1990. *Who Knows: From Quine to Feminist Empiricism.* Philadelphia: Temple University Press.

Neuman, Jennifer, Deborah Korenstein, Joseph S. Ross, and Salomeh Kayhani. 2011. "Prevalence of Financial Conflicts of Interest among Panel Members Producing Clinical Practice Guidelines in Canada and United States: Cross Sectional Study." *British Medical Journal* 343:d5621.

Nichols, Tom. 2014. "The Death of Expertise." *Federalist*, January 17, 2014. https://thefederalist.com/2014/01/17/the-death-of-expertise/.

Nichols, Tom. 2017a. *The Death of Expertise.* New York: Oxford University Press.

Nichols, Tom. 2017b. "How America Lost Faith in Expertise." *Foreign Affairs*, March/April. https://www.foreignaffairs.com/articles/united-states/2017-02-13/how-america-lost-faith-expertise.

Nickerson, Raymond S. 1998. "Confirmation Bias: A Ubiquitous Phenomenon in Many Guises." *Review of General Psychology* 2 (2): 175–220.

Nisbet, Matthew C., and Dietram A. Scheufele. 2009. "What's Next for Science Communication? Promising Directions and Lingering Distractions." *American Journal of Botany* 96, no. 10 (October): 1767–78.

Norris, Pippa. 2007. "Skeptical Patients: Performance, Social Capital, and Culture." In *The Trust Crisis in Healthcare: Causes, Consequences and Cures*, edited by D. A. Shore, 32–48. New York: Oxford University Press.

Novak, Jake. 2015. "A Libertarian Argument FOR Vaccine Laws." *CNBC*, February 10, 2015. https://www.cnbc.com/2015/02/10/a-libertarian-argument-for-vaccine-laws-commentary.html.

Nwaubani, Adaobi Tricia. 2016. "Nigeria Fights Myths, Fear in Polio Vaccine Drive." *Thomas Reuters Foundation News*, November 18, 2016. http://news.trust.org/item/20161118151643-vg74z.

Nyhan, Brendan, and Jason Riefler. 2018. "The Roles of Information Deficits and Identity Threat in the Prevalence of Misperception." *Journal of Elections, Political Opinion and Parties* 29 (2): 222–44.

Nyhan, Brendan, Jason Riefler, Sean Richey, and Gary L. Freed. 2014. "Effective Messages in Vaccine Promotion: A Randomized Trial." *Pediatrics* 133, no. 4 (April): e835–e842.

Oakley, Ann. 2002. "Social Science and Evidence-Based Everything: The Case of Education." *Educational Review* 54 (3): 277–86.

Office of Disease Prevention and Health Promotion. 2020. *Healthy People 2020.* https://www.healthypeople.gov/?_ga=2.260604237.1367656718.1588094069-066450360.1588094069.

Offit, Paul A. 2007a. "The Risk of Being Risk Averse." *Philadelphia Inquirer*, June 12, 2007.

Offit, Paul A. 2007b. "Thimerosal and Vaccines—A Cautionary Tale." *New England Journal of Medicine* 357:1278–79.

Offit, Paul A. 2008a. *Autism's False Prophets: Bad Science, Risky Medicine, and the Search for the Cure.* New York: Columbia University Press.

Offit, Paul A. 2008b. "Inoculated against Facts." *New York Times*, March 31, 2008. http://www.nytimes.com/2008/03/31/opinion/31offit.html.

Offit, Paul A. 2008c. "Vaccines and Autism Revisited—The Hannah Poling Case." *New England Journal of Medicine* 358:2089–91.

Offit, Paul A. 2011a. *Deadly Choices: How the Anti-Vaccine Movement Threatens Us All.* New York: Basic Books.

Offit, Paul A. 2011b. "Junk Science Isn't a Victimless Crime." *Wall Street Journal,* January 11, 2011. https://www.wsj.com/articles/SB10001424052748703779704576073744290909186.

Offit, Paul A. 2014. "The Anti-Vaccination Epidemic." *Wall Street Journal,* September 25, 2014.

Offit, Paul A., and Louis M. Bell. 1999. *Vaccines: What Every Parent Should Know.* New York: Wiley.

Offit, Paul A., and Susan E. Coffin. 2003. "Communicating Science to the Public: MMR Vaccine and Autism." *Vaccine* 22, no. 1 (December 8): 1–6.

Offit, Paul A., and Charles J. Hackett. 2003. "Addressing Parents' Concerns: Do Vaccines Cause Allergic or Autoimmune Diseases?" *Pediatrics* 111, no. 3 (March): 653–59.

Offit, Paul A., and Rita K. Jew. 2003. "Addressing Parents' Concerns: Do Vaccines Contain Harmful Preservatives, Adjuvants, Additives, or Residuals?" *Pediatrics* 112, no. 6 (December): 1394–97.

Offit, Paul A., and Charlotte Moser. 2011. *Vaccines and Your Child: Separating Fact from Fiction.* New York: Columbia University Press.

Offit, Paul A., Jessica Quarles, Michael A. Gerber, Charles J. Hackett, Edgar K. Marcuse, Tobias R. Kollman, Bruce G. Gellin, and Sarah Landry. 2002. "Addressing Parents' Concerns: Do Multiple Vaccines Overwhelm or Weaken the Infant's Immune System?" *Pediatrics* 109, no. 1 (January): 124–29.

Omer, Saad B., Cornelia Betsch, and Julie Leask. 2019. "Mandate Vaccination with Care." *Nature* 571 (July 25): 469–74.

Omer, Saad, William K. Y. Pan, Neal A. Halsey, Shannon Stokley, Lawrence H. Moulton, Ann Marie Navar, Mathew Pierce, and Daniel A. Salmon. 2006. "Nonmedical Exemptions to School Immunization Requirements: Secular Trends and Association of State Policies with Pertussis Incidence." *Journal of the American Medical Association* 296 (14): 1757–63.

O'Neill O. 2002. *A Question of Trust: BBC Reith Lectures 2002.* Cambridge, UK: Cambridge University Press.

Opel, Douglas J., Rita Mangione-Smith, James A. Taylor, Carolyn Korfiatis, Cheryl Wiese, Sheryl Catz, and Diane P. Martin. . 2011. "Development of a Survey to Identify Vaccine-Hesitant Parents." *Human Vaccines and Immunotherapeutics* 7, no. 4 (April): 419–25.

Oreskes, Naomi. 2004a. "The Scientific Consensus on Climate Change." *Science* 306 (5702): 1686.

Oreskes, Naomi. 2004b. "Undeniable Global Warming." *Washington Post,* December 26, 2004. http://www.washingtonpost.com/wp-dyn/articles/A26065-2004Dec25.html.

Oreskes, Naomi, and Erik M. Conway. 2010. *Merchants of Doubt: How a Handful of Scientists Obscured the Truth on Issues from Tobacco Smoke to Global Warming.* New York: Bloomsbury.

Orr, Colin, and Andrew F. Beck. 2017. "Measuring Vaccine Hesitancy in a Minority Community." *Clinical Pediatrics* 56, no. 8 (July): 784–88.

Ortutay, Barbara. 2019. "Vaccine Wars: Social Media Battle Outbreak of Bogus Claims." *Seattle Gazette,* April 5, 2019. https://www.post-gazette.com/news/health/2019/04/05/Vaccines-social-media-battle-outbreak-bogus-claims-effects/stories/201904050113.

Otto, Shawn Lawrence. 2012. "Antiscience Beliefs Jeopardize U.S. Democracy." *Scientific American,* November 1, 2012. https://www.scientificamerican.com/article/antiscience-beliefs-jeopardize-us-democracy/.

Otto, Shawn Lawrence. 2016. *The War on Science: Who's Waging It, Why It Matters, What We Can Do about It.* Minneapolis, MN: Milkweed Editions.

Pagan, Camille Noe. 2018. "When Doctors Downplay Women's Health Concerns." *New York Times*, May 3, 2018. https://www.nytimes.com/2018/05/03/well/live/when-doctors-downplay-womens-health-concerns.html.

Parker, Laura. 2017. "Why a 'War on Science' Puts Us All at Risk." *National Geographic*, April. https://news.nationalgeographic.com/2017/04/david-titley-science-climate-change-sea-level-rise/.

Parmar, Tarnjit. 2019. "Low Vaccination Rates in Wealthier Vancouver-Area Neighbourhoods." *City News*, February 16, 2019. https://www.citynews1130.com/2019/02/16/measles-affluence/.

Patient.co.uk. n.d. *MMR Immunisation—What Is the MMR Vaccine?* Accessed April 12, 2014. http://www.patient.co.uk/health/mmr-immunisation.

Payer, Lynn. 1992. *Disease-Mongers: How Doctors, Drug Companies, and Insurers Are Making You Sick*. Hoboken, NJ: John Wiley and Sons.

PBS NewsHour. 2017. "The Problem with Thinking You Know More than Experts." *PBS*, April 14, 2017. https://www.pbs.org/newshour/show/problem-thinking-know-experts.

Pead, P. J. 2003. "Benjamin Jesty: New Light in the Dawn of Vaccination." *Lancet* 362, no. 9401 (December 20): 2104–9.

Pearson, Catherine. 2019. "The Pressure to Breastfeed Can Hurt Moms. And Doctors Are Finally Realizing It." *Huffington Post*, September 19, 2019. https://www.huffingtonpost.ca/entry/breastfeeding-pressure-women-mental-health-doctor_l_5d811672e4b00d69059fc2d0.

Pelletier, Roxanne, Karin H. Humpries, Avi Shimony, Simon L Bacon, Kim L Lavoie, Doreen Rabi, Igor Karp, Meytal Avgil Tsadok, and Louise Pilote. 2014. "Sex-Related Differences in Access to Care for Patients with Premature Acute Coronary Syndrome." *Canadian Medical Association Journal* 186 (7): 497–504.

Pellum, Kimberly Brown. 2019. *Black Women in Science: A Black History Book for Kids*. Emeryville, CA: Rockridge.

Peña-Guzmán, David M., and Joel Michael Reynolds. 2019. "The Harm of Ableism: Medical Error and Epistemic Injustice." *Kennedy Institute of Ethics Journal* 29 (3): 205–42.

Penneta, Enzo. 2015. "Guerra Alla Scienza." *Critica Scientifica*, March 15, 2015. https://www.enzopennetta.it/2015/03/21612/.

Persaud, Nav. 2014. "Questionable Content of an Industry-Supported Medical School Lecture Series: A Case Study." *Journal of Medical Ethics* 40 (2014): 414–18.

Peters, Richard G., Vincent T. Covello, and David B. McCallum. 1997. "The Determinants of Trust and Credibility in Environmental Risk Communication: An Empirical Study." *Risk Analysis* 17, no. 1 (February): 43–54.

Petersen, Alan, and Deborah Lupton. 1996. *The New Public Health: Health and Self in the Age of Risk*. London: Sage.

Pharr, Susan J., and Robert D. Putnam. 2000. *Disaffected Democracies: What's Troubling Trilateral Countries?* Princeton, NJ: Princeton University Press.

Phelan, Jo C., Bruce H. Link, and Parisa Tehranifar. 2009. "Social Conditions as Fundamental Causes of Health Inequalities: Theory, Evidence, and Policy Implications." *Journal of Health and Social Behavior* 51 (Suppl): S28–40.

Pielke, Robert A., Jr. 2004a. "The Cherry Pick." *Ogmius Newsletter* 8 (May 2004): 1–2. https://sciencepolicy.colorado.edu/ogmius/archives/issue_8/ogmius.pdf.

Pielke, Robert A., Jr. 2004b. "When Scientists Politicize Science: Making Sense of Controversy over *The Skeptical Environmentalist*." *Environmental Science & Policy* 7, no. 5 (October): 405–17.

Pielke, Robert A., Jr. 2007. *The Honest Broker: Making Sense of Science in Policy and Politics*. Cambridge, UK: Cambridge University Press.

Piller, Charles. 2018. "FDA's Revolving Door: Companies Often Hire Agency Staffers Who Managed Their Successful Drug Reviews." *Science*, July 5, 2018. https://www.sciencemag.org/news/2018/07/fda-s-revolving-door-companies-often-hire-agency-staffers-who-managed-their-successful.

Pinch, Trevor J., and Wiebe E. Bijker. 1984. "The Social Construction of Facts and Artefacts: Or How the Sociology of Science and the Sociology of Technology Might Benefit Each Other." *Social Studies of Science* 14 (3): 399–441.

Pluckrose, Helen. 2017. "How French Intellectuals Ruined the West: Postmodernism and Its Impact, Explained." *Areo*, March 27, 2017. https://areomagazine.com/2017/03/27/how-french-intellectuals-ruined-the-west-postmodernism-and-its-impact-explained/#_ftn11.

Poltorak, Mike, Melissa Leach, James Fairhead, and Jackie Cassell. 2005. "MMR Talk and Vaccination Choices: An Ethnographic Study in Brighton." *Social Science & Medicine* 61, no. 3 (August): 709–19.

Popper, Karl. (1963) 2002. *Conjectures and Refutations: The Growth of Scientific Knowledge*. London: Routledge.

Prescod-Weinstein, Chandra. 2018. "Defying the Odds." *Inside Higher Education*, March 9, 2018. https://www.insidehighered.com/advice/2018/03/09/mentors-and-role-models-can-attract-minority-students-fields-where-they-may-not.

Prislin, Radmila, James A. Dyer, Craig H. Blakely, and Charles D. Johnson. 1998. "Immunization Status and Sociodemographic Characteristics: The Mediating Role of Beliefs, Attitudes, and Perceived Control." *American Journal of Public Health* 88, no. 12 (December): 1821–26.

Proctor, Robert N. 1999. *The Nazi War on Cancer*. Princeton, NJ: Princeton University Press.

Proctor, Robert N. 2000. "Nazi Science and Nazi Medical Ethics: Some Myths and Misconceptions." *Perspectives in Biology and Medicine* 43, no. 3 (Spring): 335–46.

Prothero, Donald. 2013. *Reality Check: How Science Deniers Threaten Our Future*. Bloomington: Indiana University Press.

Public Health. 2019. "Vaccine Myths Debunked." *Public Health*. https://www.publichealth.org/public-awareness/understanding-vaccines/vaccine-myths-debunked/.

Public Health Agency of Canada. 2007. *Core Competencies for Public Health in Canada: Release 1.0*. Ottawa: PHAC. https://www.phac-aspc.gc.ca/php-psp/ccph-cesp/pdfs/zcard-eng.pdf.

Public Health Agency of Canada. 2011. *Your Immunization Schedule–Immunize Your Child–Public Health Agency of Canada*. http://www.phac-aspc.gc.ca/im/iyc-vve/is-cv-eng.php.

Public Health Agency of Canada. 2018. *A Parent's Guide to Vaccination*. Ottawa: Public Health Agency of Canada. https://www.canada.ca/content/dam/phac-aspc/documents/services/publications/healthy-living/parent-guide-vaccination/pgi-gpv-eng.pdf.

Putnam, Hillary. 2002. *The Collapse of the Fact/Value Dichotomy and Other Essays*. Cambridge, MA: Harvard University Press.

Qaisar, Farah. 2019. "People Trust Science, Says Landmark Study, but There Are Troubling Trends." *Massive Science*, June 21, 2019. https://massivesci.com/articles/trust-in-science-vaccination-climate-change-pseudoscience/.

Quart, Alissa. 2013. "Adventures in Neurohumanities." *Nation*, May 12, 2013. https://www.thenation.com/article/adventures-neurohumanities/.

Quick, Jonathan, and Heidi Larson. 2018. "The Vaccine-Autism Myth Started 20 Years Ago. Here's Why It Still Endures Today." *Time*, February 28, 2018. http://time.com/5175704/andrew-wakefield-vaccine-autism.

Quinn, Sandra Crouse. 1997. "Belief in AIDS as a Form of Genocide: Implications for HIV Prevention Programs for African Americans." *Journal of Health Education* 28 (Supp): S6–12.

Quinn, Sandra Crouse, Amelia M. Jamison, Vicki S. Freimuth, An Ji, and Gregory R. Hancock. 2017. "Determinants of Influenza Vaccination among High-Risk Black and White Adults." *Vaccine* 35, no. 51 (December 18): 7154–59.

Quinn, Sandra Crouse, Amelia Jamison, Vicki S. Freimuth, Ji An, Gregory R. Hancock, and Donald Musa. 2017. "Exploring Racial Influences on Flu Vaccine Attitudes and Behavior: Results of a National Survey of White and African American Adults." *Vaccine* 35, no. 8 (February 22): 1167–74.

Quinn, Sandra Crouse, Amelia Jamison, Donald Musa, Karen Hilyard, and Vicki S. Freimuth. 2016. "Exploring the Continuum of Vaccine Hesitancy between African American and White Adults: Results of a Qualitative Study." *PLoS Currents* 8 (December 29): ecurrents. outbreaks.3e4a5ea39d8620494e2a2c874a3c4201.

Rainford, John, and Josh Greenberg. 2015. "Taking Off the Gloves." *Policy Options*, July 6, 2015. http://policyoptions.irpp.org/magazines/clearing-the-air/rainford-greenberg/.

Ranalli, Brent. 2012. "Climate Science, Character, and the "Hard-Won" Consensus." *Kennedy Institute of Ethics Journal* 22 (2): 183–210.

Ranji, Usha, Caroline Rosenzweig, Ivette Gomez, and Alina Salganicoff. 2018. *2017 Kaiser Women's Health Survey*. Kaiser Family Foundation, March 18.

Ray, Wayne A., and C. Michael Stein. 2006. "Reform of Drug Regulation: Beyond an Independent Drug Safety Board." *New England Journal of Medicine* 354:194–201.

Reich, Jennifer. 2016. *A Calling the Shots: Why Parents Reject Vaccines*. New York: New York University Press.

Reay, Diane. 2018. "Race and Elite Universities in the UK." In *Dismantling Race in Higher Education: Racism, Whiteness, and Decolonizing the Academy*, edited by Jason Arday and Heidi Safia-Mirza, 46–66. London: Palgrave Macmillan.

Resnick, David, Adi Shamoo, and Sheldon Krimsky. 2006. "Fraudulent Human Embryonic Stem Cell Research in South Korea: Lessons Learned." *Accountability Research* 13 (1): 101–9.

Ridley, Matt. 2011a. "Scientific Heresy." Angus Millar Lecture of the Royal Society of the Arts, Edinburgh. http://www.bishop-hill.net/storage/ScientificHeresy.pdf.

Ridley, Matt. 2011b. "Is That Scientific Heretic a Genius—Or a Loon?" *Wall Street Journal*, November 12, 2011. https://www.wsj.com/articles/SB10001424052970204554204577702389308832871.

Ritzer, George. 2013. *Introduction to Sociology*. Thousand Oaks, CA: Sage.

Robbins, Bruce, and Andrew Ross. 1996. "Mystery Science Theater." *Lingua Franca*, July– August. http://linguafranca.mirror.theinfo.org/9607/mst.html.

Roberts, Laura Weiss. 2000. "Evidence-Based Ethics and Informed Consent in Mental Illness Research." *Archives of General Psychiatry* 57, no. 6 (June): 540–42.

Roger, Charles Barclay. 2010. "The Truth about Public Trust in Government." *Open Democracy*, August 13. https://www.opendemocracy.net/en/truth-about-public-trust-in-government/.

Rolin, Kristina. 2002. "Gender and Trust in Science." *Hypatia* 17, no. 4 (Autumn): 95–118.

Rosenberg, Andrew A., and Kathleen Rest. 2018. "The Trump Administration's War on Science Agencies Threatens the Nation's Health and Safety." *Scientific American*, January 1, 2018. https://www.scientificamerican.com/article/the-trump-administration-rsquo-s-war-on-science-agencies-threatens-the-nation-rsquo-s-health-and-safety/.

Rosenbaum, Lisa. 2015a. "Reconnecting the Dots—Reinterpreting Industry-Physician Relation." *New England Journal of Medicine* 372 (19): 1860–64.

Rosenbaum, Lisa. 2015b. "Understanding Bias—The Case for Careful Study." *New England Journal of Medicine* 372 (20): 1959–63.

Rosenbaum, Lisa. 2015c. "Beyond Moral Outrage: Weighing the Trade-Offs of COI Regulations." *New England Journal of Medicine* 372 (21): 2064–68.

Rosin, Hannah. 2009. "The Case against Breastfeeding." *Atlantic*, April. https://www.theatlantic.com/magazine/archive/2009/04/the-case-against-breast-feeding/307311/.

Rothman, David, and Sheila Rothman. 2009. "The Willowbrook Hepatitis Studies." In *Ethical Issues in Modern Medicine: Contemporary Readings in Bioethics*, 7th ed, edited by Bonnie Steinbock, John Arras, and Alex John London, 749–53. Boston: McGraw-Hill.

Rothstein, Bo, and Dietlind Stolle. 2008. "The State and Social Capital: An Institutional Theory of Generalized Trust." *Comparative Politics* 40, no. 4 (July): 441–59.

Royal Society of Public Health. 2018. *Moving the Needle: Promoting Vaccination Uptake through the Life Course*. London: Royal Society of Public Health. https://www.rsph.org.uk/static/uploaded/3b82db00-a7ef-494c-85451e78ce18a779.pdf.

Rudner, Richard. 1953. "The Scientist Qua Scientist Makes Value Judgments." *Philosophy of Science* 20, no. 1 (January): 1–6.

SAGE Working Group on Vaccine Hesitancy. 2014. *Report of the SAGE Working Group on Vaccine Hesitancy*. November 12, 2014. Geneva: World Health Organization.

Saini, Angela. 2019. *Superior: On the Return of Race Science*. Boston: Beacon.

Salmon, Daniel A., Lawrence H. Moulton, Saad B. Omer, M. Patricia DeHart, Shannon Stokley, and Neal A. Halsey. 2005. "Factors Associated with Refusal of Childhood Vaccines among Parents of School-Aged Children: A Case-Control Study." *Archives of Pediatrics and Adolescent Medicine* 159, no. 5 (May): 470–76.

Sarewitz, Daniel. 2004. "How Science Makes Environmental Controversies Worse." *Environmental Science & Policy* 7, no. 4 (October): 385–403.

Sarewitz, Daniel. 2010. "The Trouble with Climate Science." *Slate*, March 21, 2010. https://slate.com/technology/2010/03/science-won-t-tell-us-what-to-do-about-climate-change-but-it-can-make-the-controversy-worse.html.

Sarewitz, Daniel, and Robert A. Pielke Jr. 2000. "Breaking the Global-Warming Gridlock." *Atlantic Monthly* 286 (1): 55–64.

Satti, Wiriya. 2018. "No Jab, No Play: Health Researchers Register Rise in Vaccinations Following Welfare Cuts." *ABC News*, September 12, 2018. https://www.abc.net.au/news/2018-09-13/vaccinations-no-jab-no-pay-takes-effect/10169684.

Saurette, Paul, and Shane Gunster. 2011. "Ears Wide Shut: Epistemological Populism." *Canadian Journal of Political Science* 44, no. 1 (March): 195–218.

Sayre, Anne. 1975. *Rosalind Franklin and DNA*. New York: Norton.

Schafer, Arthur M. 2004. "Biomedical Conflicts of Interest: A Defence of the Sequestration Thesis." *Journal of Medical Ethics* 30, no. 1 (February): 8–24.

Schechter, Alan N., James B. Wyngaarden, John T. Edsaal, John Maddox, Arnold S. Relman, Angel Marcia, and Walter W. Stewart. 1989. "Colloquium on Scientific Authorship: Rights and Responsibilities." *FASEB Journal* 3, no. 2 (February): 209–17.

Scheman, Naomi. 2001. "Epistemology Resuscitated: Objectivity as Trustworthiness." In *Engendering Rationalities*, edited by Nancy Tuana and Sandra Morgen, 23–52. Albany: State University of New York Press.

Schroeder, Doris, Julie Cook, François Hirsch, Solveig Fenet, and Vasantha Muthuswamy. 2018. *Ethics Dumping: Case Studies from North-South Research Collaboration*. Springer Open. https://link.springer.com/book/10.1007%2F978-3-319-64731-9.

Schulz-Hardt, Stefan, Dieter Frey, Carsten Lüthgens, and Serge Moscovici. 2000. "Biased Information Search in Group Decision Making." *Journal of Personality and Social Psychology* 78, no. 4 (April): 655–69.

Schuster, Melanie, Jehani Eskola, Phillipe Duclos, and SAGE Working Group on Vaccine Hesitancy 2015. "Review of Vaccine Hesitancy: Rationale, Remit and Methods." *Vaccine* 33, no. 34 (August 14): 4157–60.

Scott-Mumby, Keith. n.d. "Witch Hunt!" *Alternative Doctor.com*. Accessed January 14, 2019. http://www.alternative-doctor.com/vaccination/witchhunt.html.

Scruton, Roger. 2013. "Scientism in the Arts and Humanities." *New Atlantis* (Fall): 33–46.

Scutchfield, F. Douglas, and Alex F. Howard A. 2010. "Moving on Upstream: The Role of Health Departments in Addressing Socioecologic Determinants of Disease." *American Journal of Preventive Medicine* 40 (Suppl 1): S80–S83.

Sears, Robert W. 2007. *The Vaccine Book: Making the Right Decision for Your Child*. New York: Little, Brown.

Selinger, Evan. 2011. *Expertise: Philosophical Reflections*. Chicago: Automatic/VIP Press.

Selinger, Evan, and Robert Crease, eds. 2007. *The Philosophy of Expertise*. New York: Columbia University Press.

Settles, Isis H. 2014. "Women in STEM: Challenges and Determinants of Success and Well-Being." *American Psychological Association*. https://www.apa.org/science/about/psa/2014/10/women-stem.

Shahi, Ankur, Fareen Karachiwalla, and Nagma Grewal, 2019. "Walking the Walk: The Case for Internal Equity, Diversity, and Inclusion Work within the Canadian Public Health Sector." *Health Equity* 3 (1): 183–85.

Shahzad, Asif, and Jibran Ahmad. 2019. "Monstrous Rumors Stoke Hostility to Pakistan's Anti-Polio Drive." *Financial Times*, May 2, 2019. https://www.reuters.com/article/us-pakistan-polio/monstrous-rumors-stoke-hostility-to-pakistans-anti-polio-drive-idUSKCN1S9051.

Shapin, Steven. 1984. "Pump and Circumstance." *Social Studies of Science* 14 (4): 481–520.

Shapin, Steven. 1995. "Trust, Honesty, and the Authority of Science." In *Society's Choices: Social and Ethical Decision Making in Biomedicine*, edited by Ruth Ellen Bulgar, Elizabeth Meyer Bobby, and Harvey V. Fineberg, 388–408. Washington, DC: National Academies Press.

Shapin, Steven, and Simon Schaffer. 1984. *Leviathan and the Air-Pump: Hobbes, Boyle, and the Experimental Life*. Princeton, NJ: Princeton University Press.

Shaywitz, David A., and Thomas P. Stossel. 2009. "It's Time to Fight the 'PharmaScolds.'" *Wall Street Journal*, April 8, 2009. https://www.wsj.com/articles/SB123914780537299005.

Shengold, Leonard L. 1979. "Childhood Abuse and Deprivation: Soul Murder." *Journal of the American Psychological Association* 27 (3): 533–59.

Sherman, David K., and Geoffrey L. Cohen. 2006. "The Psychology of Self-Defense: Self-Affirmation Theory." In *Advances in Experimental Social Psychology*, vol. 38, edited by M. P. Zanna, 183–242. New York: Academic Press.

Sherman, David K., Kimberly A. Hartson, Kevin R. Binning, Valerie Purdie-Vaughns, Julio Garcia, Suzanne Taborsky-Barba, Sarah Tomassetti, A. David Nussbaum, and Geoffrey L. Cohen. 2013. "Deflecting the Trajectory and Changing the Narrative: How Self-Affirmation Affects Academic Performance and Motivation under Identity Threat." *Journal of Personality and Social Psychology* 104, no. 4 (April): 591–618.

Shetterly, Margot Lee. 2016. *Hidden Figures: The American Dream and the Untold Story of the Black Women Mathematicians Who Helped Win the Space Race*. New York: HarperCollins.

Shiu, Irene, Allison Kennedy, Karen Wooten, Benjamin Schwartz, and Deborah Gust. 2005.

"Factors Influencing African-American Mothers' Concerns about Immunization Safety: A Summary of Focus Group Findings." *Journal of the National Medical Association* 97, no. 5 (May): 657–66.

Shiu, Irene M., Eric S. Weintraub, and Deborah A. Gust. 2006. "Parents Concerned about Vaccine Safety: Differences in Race/Ethnicity and Attitudes." *American Journal of Preventative Medicine* 31, no. 3 (September): 244–51.

Shore, David A., ed. 2007. *The Trust Crisis in Healthcare: Causes, Consequences, and Cures.* New York: Oxford University Press.

Siddiqui, Mariam, Daniel A. Salmon, and Saad B. Omer. 2013. "Epidemiology of Vaccine Hesitancy in the United States." *Human Vaccines and Immunotherapies* 9, no. 12 (December): 2643–48.

Simmel, Georg. (1900) 1978. *The Philosophy of Money.* London: Routledge.

Sismondo, Sergio. 2018. *Ghost Managed Medicine: Big Pharma's Invisible Hands.* Manchester: Mattering.

Skeptical Raptor. 2013. "The Zombie Apocalypse of Antivaccine Lies–They Just Won't Die." *Skeptical Raptor* (blog), September 21, 2013. https://www.skepticalraptor.com/skepticalraptorblog.php/zombie-apocalypse-antivaccine-lies-they-die/.

Skeptical Raptor. 2017. "Anti-Vaccine Doctors—Naming Names and Listing Lists." *Skeptical Raptor* (blog), July 6, 2017. https://www.skepticalraptor.com/skepticalraptorblog.php/anti-vaccine-doctors-naming-names/.

Skeptical Raptor. 2018. "Zombie Anti-Vaccine Research Returns from the Dead—Real Science Laughs." *Skeptical Raptor* (blog), December 10, 2018. https://www.skepticalraptor.com/skepticalraptorblog.php/zombie-anti-vaccine-research-real-science-laughs/.

Skloot, Rebecca. 2011. *The Immortal Life of Henrietta Lax.* New York: Crown.

Slater, Matthew H., and Andrea Borghini. 2011. "Introduction: Lessons from the Scientific Butchery." In *Carving Nature at Its Joints: Natural Kinds in Metaphysics and Science*, edited by Joseph Keim Campbell, Michael O'Rourke, and Matthew H. Slater. Cambridge, MA: MIT Press.

Slavin, Robert E. 2002. "Evidence-Based Educational Policies: Transforming Educational Practice and Research." *Educational Researcher* 31 (7): 15–21.

Slovic, Paul. 2000. *The Perception of Risk.* New York: Earthscan.

Smith, Charles G., and Kenneth Sinanan. 1972. "The 'Gaslight Phenomenon' Reappears: A Modification of the Ganser Syndrome." *British Journal of Psychology* 120, no. 559 (June): 685–86.

Smith, Lena H. 2018. "Anti-Vaxxers Face Backlash as Measles Cases Surge." *Washington Post*, February 25, 2018. https://www.washingtonpost.com/national/health-science/anti-vaxxers-face-backlash-as-measles-cases-surge/2019/02/25/e2e986c6-391c-11e9-a06c-3ec8ed509d15_story.html.

Smith, Philip J., Susan Y. Chu, and Lawrence E. Barker. 2004. "Children Who Received No Vaccine. Who Are They and Where Do They Live." *Pediatrics* 114, no. 1 (July): 187–95.

Smith, Sandra Susan. 2010. "Race and Trust." *Annual Review of Sociology* 36:453–75.

Smolkin, Doran. 2008. "Puzzles about Trust." *Southern Journal of Philosophy* 46, no. 3 (Fall): 431–49.

Sobo, Elisa J. 2015. "Social Cultivation of Vaccine Refusal and Delay among Waldorf (Steiner) School Parents." *Medical Anthropology Quarterly* 29, no. 3 (September): 381–99.

Sobo, Elisa J., Arianna Huhn, Autumn Sannwald, and Lori Thurman. 2016. "Information Curation among Vaccine Cautious Parents: Web 2.0, Pinterest Thinking, and Pediatric Vaccination Choice." *Medical Anthropology* 35, no. 6 (November–December): 529–46.

Soekov, Kimberley. 2018. "Kids in Sydney's Richest Suburbs Less Likely to Be Vaccinated." *10 Daily*, October 24, 2018. https://10daily.com.ua/news/australia/a181024tqd/kids-in-sydneys-richest-suburbs-less-likely-to-be-vaccinated-20181024.

Sokal, Alan. 1996. "Transgressing the Boundaries: Towards a Transformative Hermeneutics of Quantum Gravity." *Social Text* 46/47 (Spring–Summer): 217–52.

Sokal, Alan, and Jean Bricmont. 1999. *Fashionable Nonsense: Postmodern Intellectuals' Abuse of Science.* New York: Picador.

Solomon, Miriam. 2001. *Social Epistemology.* Cambridge, MA: MIT Press.

Solomon, Miriam. 2006. "Norms of Epistemic Diversity." *Episteme* 3, no. 1 (June): 23–36.

Specter, Michael. 2010. *Denialism: How Irrational Thinking Harms the Planet and Threatens Our Lives.* London: Penguin.

Stafford, Tom. 2015. "Throwing Science at Anti-vaxxers Just Makes Them More Hardline." *Conversation*, February 19, 2015. http://theconversation.com/throwing-science-at-anti-vaxxers-just-makes-them-more-hardline-37721.

Stamp, Nikki. 2018. "Women with Heart Diseases Are Dismissed and Its Killing Them." *Guardian*, June 14, 2018. https://www.theguardian.com/commentisfree/2018/jun/14/women-with-heart-diseases-are-dismissed-and-its-killing-them.

Stanley, Dick. 2003. "What Do We Know about Social Cohesion: The Research Perspective of the Federal Government's Social Cohesion Research Network." *Canadian Journal of Sociology* 28, no. 1 (Winter): 5–17.

Steele, Claude M. 1988. "The Psychology of Self-Affirmation: Sustaining the Integrity of the Self." In *Advances in Experimental Social Psychology* 21, edited by L. Berkowitz, 261–302. San Diego, CA: Academic Press.

Steenhuysen, Julie, Peter Eisler, Allison Martell, and Stephanie Nebehay. 2020. "Race for Coronavirus Vaccine Draws Billions Worldwide, with Focus on Speed." *Global News*, April 25, 2020. https://globalnews.ca/news/6868824/research-coronavirus-vaccine/.

Steinman, Michael A., G. Michael Harper, Mary-Margaret Chren, C. Seth Landefeld, and Lisa A. Bero. 2007. "Characteristics and Impact of Drug Detailing for Gabapentin." *PLoS Medicine* 4, no. 4 (April): e134.

Stirling, Andrew. 1997. "Multi-Criteria Mapping: Mitigating the Problems of Environmental Valuation?" In *Valuing Nature? Economics, Ethics, and the Environment*, edited by John Foster, 186–210. London: Routledge.

Stirling, Andrew. 2010. "Keep it Complex." *Nature* 468:1029–31.

Stirling, Andy, and Sue Mayer. 1999. *Rethinking Risk: A Pilot Multi-Criteria Mapping of a Genetically Modified Crop in Agricultural Systems in the UK.* Sussex, UK: Science Policy Research Unit, University of Sussex.

Stone, Tanya Lee. 2018. *Who Says Women Can't Be Computer Programmers? The Story of Ada Lovelace.* New York: Henry Holt.

Stossell, Thomas P. 2015. *Pharmaphobia: How the Conflict of Interest Myth Undermines American Medical Innovation.* Lanham, MD: Rowman & Littlefield.

Stote, Karen. 2012. "The Coercive Sterilization of Aboriginal Women in Canada." *American Indian Culture and Research* 36 (3): 117–50.

Strauss, Matt. 2020. "Herd Immunity Might Still Be Key in the Fight against Coronavirus." *Spectator*, March 26, 2020. https://www.spectator.co.uk/article/herd-immunity-might-still-be-key-in-the-fight-against-coronavirus.

Street, Richard L., Kimberley J. O'Malley, Lisa A. Cooper, and Paul Haidet. 2008. "Understanding Concordance in Patient-Physician Relationships: Personal and Ethnic Dimensions of Shared Identity." *Annals of Family Medicine* 6, no. 3 (May–June): 198–205.

Sturgess, Kyle. 2016. "A Skeptic on the ConspiraSea Cruise—Interview With Colin McRoberts."

*Skeptical Inquirer*, Feb 15, 2016. https://skepticalinquirer.org/exclusive/a-skeptic-on-the-conspirasea-cruiseinterview-with-colin-mcroberts/.

Sullivan Commission. 2004. *Missing Persons: Minorities in the Health Professions, A Report of the Sullivan Commission on Diversity in the Healthcare Workforce.* Atlanta, GA: Morehouse School of Medicine.

Sunstein, Cass R., and Adrian Vermeule. 2009. "Conspiracy Theories: Causes and Cures." *Journal of Political Philosophy* 17 (2): 202–27.

Sweet, Paige L. 2019. "The Sociology of Gaslighting." *American Sociological Review* 84 (5): 851–75.

Swope, Carolyn. 2018. "The Problematic Role of Public Health in Urban Renewal in Washington, DC's Urban Renewal." *Public Health Reports* 133 (6): 707–14.

Taber, Charles S., and Milton Lodge. 2006. "Motivated Skepticism in the Evaluation of Political Beliefs." *American Journal of Political Science* 50, no. 3 (July): 755–76.

Taverne, Dick. 2005. *The March of Unreason: Science, Democracy and the New Fundamentalism.* London: Oxford University Press.

Taylor, Ginger. 2010. "Anatomy of a Witch Hunt." *Adventures in Autism* (blog), February 12, 2010. http://adventuresinautism.blogspot.ca/2010/02/anatomy-of-witch-hunt.html.

Thagard, Paul. 1999. *How Scientists Explain Disease.* Princeton, NJ: Princeton University Press.

Thaler, Richard H., and Cass R. Sunstein. 2008. *Nudge: Improving Decisions about Health, Wealth, and Happiness.* New Haven, CT: Yale University Press.

Tidyman, P. 1826. "A Sketch of the Most Remarkable Disease of the Negroes of the Southern States." *Philadelphia Journal of Medical and Physical Sciences* 3 (6): 306–38.

Timmermans, Stefan, and Marc Berg. 2003. *The Gold Standard: The Challenge of Evidence-Based Medicine and the Standardization of Healthcare.* Philadelphia: Temple University Press.

Thomas, Stephen B., and Sandra Crouse Quinn. 1991. "The Tuskegee Study, 1932 to 1972: Implications for HIV Education and AIDS Risk Education Programs in the Black Community." *American Journal of Public Health* 81 (11): 1491–504.

Thompson, Michael, Richard Ellis, and Aaron Wildavsky. 1990. *Cultural Theory.* Boulder, CO: Westview.

Togher, Leanne, Corina Yiannoukas, Michelle Lincoln, Emma Power, Natalie Munro, Patricia McCabe, Pratiti Ghosh, Linda Worrall, Elizabeth Ward, Alison Ferguson, Elisabeth Harrison, and Jacinta Douglas. 2011. "Evidence-Based Practice in Speech-Language Pathology Curricula: A Scoping Study." *International Journal of Speech-Language Pathology* 13, no. 6 (December): 459–68.

Tran, Lucky, Rachel Alter, and Tony Flattum-Reimers. 2019. "Anti-Vaxx Propaganda Is Flooding the Internet. Will Tech Companies Act?" *Guardian*, March 5, 2019. https://www.theguardian.com/commentisfree/2019/mar/05/anti-vaxx-propaganda-internet-tech.

Trauner, Joan B. 1978. "The Chinese as Medical Scapegoats in San Francisco, 1870–1905." *California History* 57, no. 1 (Spring): 70–87.

Trowther, David. 2003. *MMR and Acquired Autism (Autistic Enterocolitis): A Briefing Note.* http://www.whale.to/a/pdf/thrower.html.

Turner, Chris. 2013. *The War on Science: Muzzled Scientists and Willful Blindness in Stephen Harper's Canada.* Toronto: Greystone Books.

Turner, Stephen. 2001. "What is the Problem with Experts?" *Social Studies of Science* 31, no. 1 (February): 123–49.

Tweedy, Damon. 2015. *Black Man in a White Coat: A Doctor's Reflections on Race and Medicine.* New York: Picador.

Union of Concerned Scientists. 2004. *Restoring Science Integrity in Policy Making*. February 18. https://cdn.americanprogress.org/wp-content/uploads/kf/UCSSTATEMENT.PDF.

US National Commission on Excellence in Education. 1983. *A Nation at Risk: The Imperative for Educational Reform—A Report to the Nation and the Secretary of Education, United States Department of Education*. Washington, DC: National Commission on Excellence in Education.

Valente, Adriana, Tommaso Castellani, Maja Larsen, and Arja R. Aro. 2015. "Models and Visions of Science–Policy Interaction: Remarks from a Delphi Study in Italy." *Science and Public Policy* 42, no. 2 (April): 228–41.

Valles, Sean. 2018. *Philosophy of Population Health*. New York: Routledge.

vanden Heuvel, Katrina. 2004. "Bush's War on Science." *Nation*, July 20, 2004. https://www.thenation.com/article/bushs-war-science/.

vanden Heuvel, Katrina. 2013. "Jenny McCarthy's Vaccination Fear-Mongering and the Cult of False Equivalence." *Nation*, July 22, 2013. https://www.thenation.com/article/archive/jenny-mccarthys-vaccination-fear-mongering-and-cult-false-equivalence/.

Vaz, Olivia M., Mallory K. Ellingson, Paul Weiss, Samuel M. Jenness, Azucena Bardají, Robert A. Bedarczyk, and Saad B. Omer. 2020. "Mandatory Vaccination in Europe." *Pediatrics* 145, no. 2 (February): e20190620.

Vernon, Jamie L. 2011. "'Deathers' Offer a Unique Case Study for the Formulation of the Denialist Mentality." *Discover Magazine*, May 6, 2011. https://www.discovermagazine.com/the-sciences/deathers-offer-a-unique-case-study-for-the-formulation-of-the-denialist-mentality.

The Vienna Report. 2019. "Medical Professionals Speak Out." *The Vienna Report* (blog). http://theviennareport.us/medical-professionals-speak-out.

Vogel, Gretchen. 2011. "Jon Hendrick Shon Loses His PhD." *Science*, September 19, 2011. https://www.sciencemag.org/news/2011/09/jan-hendrik-sch-n-loses-his-phd.

Vogel, Lauren. 2015. "Broken Trust Drives Health Disparities." *Canadian Medical Association Journal* 187, no. 1 (January 6): E9–E10. https://doi.org/10.1503/cmaj.1094950.

Vogel, Lauren. 2019. "Starting a Family during Residency? Leave Policies Complicate the Choice." *Canadian Medical Association Journal* 191, no. 5 (February 4): E146–47. https://doi.org/10.1503/cmaj.109-5709.

von Zweck, Claudia. 1999. "The Promotion of Evidence-Based Occupational Therapy Practice in Canada." *Canadian Journal of Occupational Therapy* 66, no. 5 (December): 208–13.

Wagner, Abram L., Nina B. Masters, Gretchen J. Domek, Joseph L. Mathew, Xiaodong Sun, Edwin J. Asturias, Jia Ren, Zhuoying Huang, Ingrid L. Contreras-Roldan, Berhanu Gebremeskel, and Matthew L. Boulton. 2019. "Comparisons of Vaccine Hesitancy across Five Low-and Middle-Income Countries." *Vaccines* 7, no. 4 (October 18): 155.

Waismann, Friedrich. 1951. "Verifiability." In *Logic and Language, the First Series*, edited by Antony Flew. Hoboken, NJ: Blackwell.

Wakefield, Andrew. 2010. *Callous Disregard: Autism and Vaccines—The Truth behind a Tragedy*. New York: Skyhorse.

Wakefield, Andrew J., Simon H. Murch, Andrew Anthony, J. Linnell, D. M. Casson, M. Malik, M. Berelowitz, A. P. Dhillon, M. A. Thompson, P. Harvey, A. Valentine, S. E. Davies, and J. A. Walker-Smith. 1998. "Ileal-Lymphoid-Nodular Hyperplasia, Non-Specific Colitis, and Pervasive Developmental Disorder in Children." *Lancet* 351, no. 9103 (February 28): 637–41.

Wallerstein, Nina, and Bonnie Duran. 2010. "Community-Based Participatory Research Contributions to Intervention Research: The Intersection of Science and Practice to Improve Health Equity." *American Journal of Public Health* 100 (Supp 1): S40–S46.

Walters, Joanna. 2016."Texas Scientist and Evangelical Takes to the Web to Convert Climate Cynics." *Guardian*, November 6, 2016. https://www.theguardian.com/science/2016/nov/06/katharine-hayhoe-climate-scientist-evangelical-christian.

Ward, Paul R., Katie Attwell, Samantha B. Meyer, Philippa Rokkas, and Julie Leask. 2017. "Understanding the Perceived Logic of Care by Vaccine-Hesitant and Vaccine-Refusing Parents: A Qualitative Study in Australia." *PLoS ONE* 12, no. 10 (October 12): e0185955.

Weeks, Carly. 2017. "Billboards Posted by Anti-Vaccine Group in GTA Being Removed, Advertising Company Says." *Globe and Mail*, February 27, 2017. https://www.theglobeandmail.com/canada/article-billboards-posted-by-anti-vaccine-group-in-gta-being-removed/.

Welch, Gilbert. 2011. *Overdiagnosed: Making People Sick in the Pursuit of Health*. Boston: Beacon.

Wellcome Global Monitor. 2019. *Wellcome Global Monitor 2018*. Survey, London: Wellcome. https://wellcome.ac.uk/reports/wellcome-global-monitor/2018.

Whiting, Alex. 2019. "How France Is Persuading Its Citizens to Get Vaccinated." *Mosaic*, June 19, 2019. https://mosaicscience.com/storyhow-france-persuading-its-citizens-gt-vaccinated-measles-antivax-vaccines-vaccination/.

Whyte, Kyle Powys, and Robert R. Crease. 2010. "Trust, Expertise and the Philosophy of Science." *Synthese* 177:411–25.

Wilholt, Torsten. 2013. "Epistemic Trust in Science." *British Journal of Philosophy of Science* 64, no. 2 (June): 233–53.

Williams, Joseph P. 2018. "Why America Needs More Black Doctors." *U.S. News*, August 31, 2018. https://www.usnews.com/news/healthiest-communities/articles/2018-08-31/why-america-needs-more-black-doctors.

Wilson, Mark. 2016. "The New England Journal of Medicine: Commercial Conflict of Interest and Revisiting the Vioxx Scandal." *Indian Journal of Medical Ethics* 1, no. 3 (July–September): 1–5.

Wodak, Ruth. 2015a. "Argumentation, Political." In *The International Encyclopedia of Political Communication*, 1st ed., edited by Gianpietro Mazzoleni. Hoboken: Wiley. https://doi.org/10.1002/9781118541555.wbiepc080.

Wodak, Ruth. 2015b. *The Politics of Fear: What Right-Wing Populist Discourses Mean*. London: SAGE.

World Health Organization. 1986. *Ottawa Charter for Health Promotion: First International Conference on Health Promotion Ottawa, 21 November 1986*. https://www.healthpromotion.org.au/images/ottawa_charter_hp.pdf.

World Health Organization. 1993. *The ICD-10 Classification of Mental and Behavioural Disorders: Diagnostic Criteria for Research*. Geneva: World Health Organization.

World Health Organization. 2016. *International Statistical Classification of Diseases and Related Health Problems, 10th revision*. 5th edition. Vol 1: Tabular List. Geneva: World Health Organization.

World Health Organization. 2019. "Ten Threats to Global Health." https://www.who.int/emergencies/ten-threats-to-global-health-in-2019.

World Health Organization. 2020. *International Classification of Diseases (ICD) Information Sheet*. https://www.who.int/classifications/icd/factsheet/en/.

Wyatt, Ronald. 2013. "Pain and Ethnicity." *Virtual Mentor: American Medical Association Journal of Ethics* 15 (5): 449–54. https://journalofethics.ama-assn.org/article/pain-and-ethnicity/2013-05.

Wylie, Alison, and Lynne Hankinson Nelson. 2007. "Coming to Terms with the Values of Science: Insights from Feminist Science Studies Scholarship." In *Value-Free Science: Ideals and Illusions*, edited by Harold Kincaid, John Dupré, and Alison Wylie, 58–86. Oxford: Oxford University Press.

Wynne, Brian. 1991. "Knowledges in Context." *Science, Technology, & Human Values* 16 (1): 111–21.

Wynne, Brian. 1992. "Misunderstood Misunderstanding: Social Identities and the Public Uptake of Science." *Public Understanding of Science* 1 (3): 281–304.

Wynne, Brian. 1995. "The Public Understanding of Science." In *Handbook of Science and Technology Studies*, edited by Sheila Jasanoff, Gerald Markle, James C. Petersen, and Trevor Pinch, 380–92. E. Thousand Oaks, CA: Sage.

Wynne, Brian. 1996. "May the Sheep Safely Graze? A Reflexive View of the Expert-Lay Knowledge Divide." In *Risk, Environment, Modernity: Towards a New Ecology*, edited by Scott Lash, Scott, Bronislaw Szerszynski, and Brian Wynne, 44–83. London: Sage.

Wynne, Brian. 2006. "Public Engagement as a Means of Restoring Public Trust in Science—Hitting the Notes, but Missing the Music?" *Community Genetics* 9, no. 3 (February): 178–83.

Yaqub, Ohid, Sophie Castle-Clarke, Nick Sevdalis, and Joanna Chataway. 2014. "Attitudes to Vaccination: A Critical Review." *Social Science & Medicine* 112 (July): 1–11.

Ylä-Anttila, Tuuka. 2018. "Populist Knowledge: 'Post-Truth' Repertoires of Contesting Epistemic Authorities." *European Journal of Cultural and Political Sociology* 5 (4): 356–88.

Yong, Ed. 2020. "The U.K.'s Coronavirus 'Herd Immunity' Debacle." *Atlantic*, March 16, 2020. https://www.theatlantic.com/health/archive/2020/03/coronavirus-pandemic-herd-immunity-uk-boris-johnson/608065/.

# INDEX

Related Health Problems (ICD), 35, 190n22, 201n6; medical schools, 139, 140; Michigan Care Improvement Registry, 10; National Vaccine Information Center (NVIC), 26; Sullivan Commission on Diversity in the Healthcare Workforce (USA), 180; United States Public Health Service, 190n24; US Office of Research Integrity and Health and Human Services, 199n14; Vaccinate Your Family: The Next Generation of Every Child by Two, 173

medicine: academic, 30, 134, 135, 166; evidence-based, 94, 95; industry-influenced, 133–35, 182; modern, 165; and science, 17; Viennese, 199n19

Merton, Robert, 147–48, 149, 198n11

misinformation, 129–30, 139, 165, 170; debunking, 16, 139. See also vaccine: myths

MMR-autism debate, 22, 23, 27, 31, 190n14. See also under vaccines

Monsanto, 105, 106. See also genetically modified organisms (GMOs)

Mooney, Chris, 41, 42

mother blaming, 174. See also parents

morality, relational aspects of, 114; and integrity, 196n5; and psychology, 191n2

motivated reasoning, 45–49, 191n1

multi-criteria mapping (MCM), 103, 104

natural lifestyle, 14, 59, 173

Nazis, 132, 198n3

Nichols, Tom, 71, 72, 74–75, 86, 163, 164, 192n2

Nigeria, 8, 185n2

Nobel Prize, the, 146, 154

nonmedical exemptions, 7, 34, 104–5, 112, 130, 202nn14–16; and administrative obstacles, 67, 177–78

Nyhan, Brendan, 41–46, 51, 54, 69, 201n3

Offit, Dr. Paul, 7, 25–27, 28, 30, 189n10, 190n15

organizations: American scientific, 190n18; Commission of Conservation's public health committee, 197n21; ESRC commissioned report, 190n14; Informed Consent Action Network (iCAN), 35; Race Betterment Foundation, 197n20. See also medical organizations; scientific institutions

outreach, 12, 21, 23, 25, 38, 192n9; efforts, 22, 25, 30, 37, 40, 42, 57, 169; public, 26, 55, 69

pain tolerance, 139–40, 156

pandemic response, 169, 202n22

parents, 31–32, 33, 35, 36, 38–39, 117, 135; mothers, 157–58, 173–74, 201n9; Parent Attitudes about Childhood Vaccines (PACV), 8, 186n13. See also good parenting

patients, 6, 172, 180, 200n23

pediatricians, 33, 34

peer review, 64, 97, 121, 129, 130, 144, 161, 198n7; blind, 148; and publication, 123, 126, 162